D1070428

Drug Hypersensitivity

Guest Editor

WERNER J. PICHLER, MD

MEDICAL CLINICS
OF NORTH AMERICA

www.medical.theclinics.com

July 2010 • Volume 94 • Number 4

SAUNDERS an imprint of ELSEVIER, Inc.

W.B. SAUNDERS COMPANY
A Division of Elsevier Inc.

1600 John F. Kennedy Boulevard • Suite 1800 • Philadelphia, Pennsylvania 19103-2899

http://www.theclinics.com

MEDICAL CLINICS OF NORTH AMERICA Volume 94, Number 4
July 2010 ISSN 0025-7125, ISBN-13: 978-1-4377-2464-6

Editor: Rachel Glover
Developmental Editors: Theresa Collier and Donald Mumford

Medical Clinics of North America (ISSN 0025-7125) is published bimonthly by Elsevier Inc., 360 Park Avenue South, New York, NY 10010-1710. Months of issue are January, March, May, July, September, and November. Periodicals postage paid at New York, NY, and additional mailing offices. Subscription prices are USD 204 per year for US individuals, USD 361 per year for US institutions, USD 105 per year for US students, USD 259 per year for Canadian individuals, USD 469 per year for Canadian institutions, USD 165 per year for Canadian students, USD 314 per year for international individuals, USD 469 per year for international institutions and USD 165 per year for international students. To receive student/resident rate, orders must be accompanied by name of affiliated institution, date of term, and the *signature* of program/residency coordinator on institution letterhead. Orders will be billed at individual rate until proof of status is received. Foreign air speed delivery is included in all *Clinics* subscription prices. All prices are subject to change without notice. **POSTMASTER:** Send address changes to *Medical Clinics of North America*, Elsevier Health Sciences Division, Subscription Customer Service, 3251 Riverport Lane, Maryland Heights, MO 63043. **Customer Service: Telephone: 1-800-654-2452** (U.S. and Canada); **1-314-447-8871** (outside U.S. and Canada). **Fax: 1-314-447-8029.** **E-mail: journalscustomerservice-usa@elsevier.com** (for print support); **journalsonlinesupport-usa@ elsevier.com** (for online support).

Reprints. For copies of 100 or more of articles in this publication, please contact the Commercial Reprints Department, Elsevier Inc., 360 Park Avenue South, New York, NY 10010-1710. Tel.: 212-633-3812; Fax: 212-462-1935; E-mail: reprints@elsevier.com.

Medical Clinics of North America is also published in Spanish by McGraw-Hill Interamericana Editores S. A., P.O. Box 5-237, 06500 Mexico, D.F., Mexico.

Medical Clinics of North America is covered in *MEDLINE/PubMed (Index Medicus), Current Contents, ASCA, Excerpta Medica, Science Citation Index, and ISI/BIOMED.*

Printed in the United States of America.

GOAL STATEMENT
The goal of *Medical Clinics of North America* is to keep practicing physicians up to date with current clinical practice by providing timely articles reviewing the state of the art in patient care.

ACCREDITATION
The *Medical Clinics of North America* is planned and implemented in accordance with the Essential Areas and Policies of the Accreditation Council for Continuing Medical Education (ACCME) through the joint sponsorship of the University of Virginia School of Medicine and Elsevier. The University of Virginia School of Medicine is accredited by the ACCME to provide continuing medical education for physicians.

The University of Virginia School of Medicine designates this educational activity for a maximum of 15 *AMA PRA Category 1 Credits*™ for each issue, 90 credits per year. Physicians should only claim credit commensurate with the extent of their participation in the activity.

The American Medical Association has determined that physicians not licensed in the US who participate in this CME activity are eligible for a maximum of 15 *AMA PRA Category 1 Credits*™ for each issue, 90 credits per year.

Credit can be earned by reading the text material, taking the CME examination online at http://www.theclinics.com/home/cme, and completing the evaluation. After taking the test, you will be required to review any and all incorrect answers. Following completion of the test and evaluation, your credit will be awarded and you may print your certificate.

FACULTY DISCLOSURE/CONFLICT OF INTEREST
The University of Virginia School of Medicine, as an ACCME accredited provider, endorses and strives to comply with the Accreditation Council for Continuing Medical Education (ACCME) Standards of Commercial Support, Commonwealth of Virginia statutes, University of Virginia policies and procedures, and associated federal and private regulations and guidelines on the need for disclosure and monitoring of proprietary and financial interests that may affect the scientific integrity and balance of content delivered in continuing medical education activities under our auspices.

The University of Virginia School of Medicine requires that all CME activities accredited through this institution be developed independently and be scientifically rigorous, balanced and objective in the presentation/discussion of its content, theories and practices.

All authors/editors participating in an accredited CME activity are expected to disclose to the readers relevant financial relationships with commercial entities occurring within the past 12 months (such as grants or research support, employee, consultant, stock holder, member of speakers bureau, etc.). The University of Virginia School of Medicine will employ appropriate mechanisms to resolve potential conflicts of interest to maintain the standards of fair and balanced education to the reader. Questions about specific strategies can be directed to the Office of Continuing Medical Education, University of Virginia School of Medicine, Charlottesville, Virginia.

The faculty and staff of the University of Virginia Office of Continuing Medical Education have no financial affiliations to disclose.

The authors/editors listed below have identified no professional or financial affiliations for themselves or their spouse/partner:
Jaqueline Adam, MSc; Andreas J. Bircher, MD; Miguel Blanca, MD, PhD; Barbara Daubner, MSc; Pascal Demoly, MD, PhD; Lars E. French, MD; Thomas Gentinetta, MSc; Rachel Glover (Acquisitions Editor); R.M. Guéant-Rodriguez, MD, PhD; Thomas Harr, MD; Oliver V. Hausmann, MD; Kazuhisa Hirahara, MD; G. Iohom, MD, PhD; Tadashi Ishida, MD; Yoko Kano, MD, PhD; Monika Keller, PhD; M. Lambert, MD; Ticha Limsuwan, MD; J.M. Malinovsky, MD, PhD; P.M. Mertes, MD, PhD; Mauro Pagani, MD; M.A. Regnier-Kimmoun, MD; Mario Sánchez-Borges, MD; Kathrin Scherer, MD; Benno Schnyder, MD; Cornelia S. Seitz, MD; Tetsuo Shiohara, MD, PhD; K. Tajima, MD; Maria J. Torres, MD, PhD; Axel Trautmann, MD; Andrew Wolf, MD (Test Author); and Daniel Yerly, PhD.

The authors/editors listed below identified the following professional or financial affiliations for themselves or their spouse/partner:
Werner J. Pichler, MD (Guest Editor) is an industry funded research/investigator, consultant, and stockholder for ADR-AC GmbH, Holligenstr. 91, 3008 Bern, Switzerland; is an industry funded research/investigator for Pfizer AG; and is a consultant for Novartis.
Michael Seitz, MD is an industry funded research/investigator by and is on the Advisory Committee/Board of the Department of Rheumatology, Clinical Immunology & Allergology, University Hospital of Bern, Switzerland.
Peter M. Villiger, MD is on the Advisory Committee/Board for Essex, Wyeth, Roche, Abbott and BMS; and is an industry funded research/investigator and for Essex, Wyeth, and Roche.

Disclosure of Discussion of Non-FDA Approved Uses for Pharmaceutical Products and/or Medical Devices.
The University of Virginia School of Medicine, as an ACCME provider, requires that all faculty presenters identify and disclose any off-label uses for pharmaceutical and medical device products. The University of Virginia School of Medicine recommends that each physician fully review all the available data on new products or procedures prior to clinical use.

TO ENROLL
To enroll in the Medical Clinics of North America Continuing Medical Education program, call customer service at 1-800-654-2452 or visit us online at http://www.theclinics.com/home/cme. The CME program is available to subscribers for an additional fee of USD 228.

FORTHCOMING ISSUES

RECENT ISSUES

THE CLINICS ARE NOW AVAILABLE ONLINE!

Access your subscription at:
www.theclinics.com

Contributors

GUEST EDITOR

WERNER J. PICHLER, MD
Division of Allergology, Clinic for Rheumatology and Clinical Immunology/Allergology,
Inselspital, University of Bern; ADR-AC GmbH, Bern, Switzerland

AUTHORS

JAQUELINE ADAM, MSc
Division of Allergology, Clinic for Rheumatology and Clinical Immunology/Allergology,
Inselspital, University of Bern; ADR-AC GmbH, Bern, Switzerland

ANDREAS J. BIRCHER, MD
Professor; Head of Allergology, Allergy Unit, Department of Dermatology, University
Hospital Basel, Basel, Switzerland

MIGUEL BLANCA, MD, PhD
Allergy Service, Plaza del Hospital Civil s/n, Carlos Haya Hospital, Málaga, Spain

BARBARA DAUBNER, MSc
Division of Allergology, Clinic for Rheumatology and Clinical Immunology/Allergology,
Inselspital, University of Bern, Bern, Switzerland

PASCAL DEMOLY, MD, PhD
Professor, Allergy Department, Hôpital Arnaud de Villeneuve, University Hospital of
Montpellier, Montpellier, France

LARS E. FRENCH, MD
Professor, Department of Dermatology, University Hospital Zurich, Zurich, Switzerland

THOMAS GENTINETTA, MSc
ADR-AC GmbH, Bern, Switzerland

R.M. GUÉANT-RODRIGUEZ, MD, PhD
Laboratoire de Biochimie Biologie Moléculaire Nutrition Métabolisme, CHU de Brabois;
Unité de Pathologie Cellulaire et Moléculaire en Nutrition, Faculté de Médecine,
Vandoeuvre les Nancy, France

THOMAS HARR, MD
Department of Dermatology, University Hospital Zurich, Zurich, Switzerland

OLIVER V. HAUSMANN, MD
Specialist Registrar and Research Fellow, Department of Rheumatology, Clinical
Immunology and Allergology, Inselspital, University of Bern, Bern, Switzerland

KAZUHISA HIRAHARA, MD
Department of Dermatology, Kyorin University School of Medicine, Tokyo, Japan

G. IOHOM, MD, PhD
Department of Anaesthesia and Intensive Care Medicine, Cork University Hospital, University College Cork, Cork, Ireland

TADASHI ISHIDA, MD
Department of Dermatology, Kyorin University School of Medicine, Tokyo, Japan

YOKO KANO, MD, PhD
Department of Dermatology, Kyorin University School of Medicine, Tokyo, Japan

MONIKA KELLER, PhD
ADR-AC GmbH, Bern, Switzerland

M. LAMBERT, MD
Service d'Anesthésie-Réanimation Chirurgicale, CHU de Nancy, Hôpital Central, Nancy Cedex; Faculté de Médecine, Vandoeuvre les Nancy, France

TICHA LIMSUWAN, MD
Instructor, Allergy Immunology and Rheumatology Division, Faculty of Medicine, Ramathibodi Hospital, Mahidol University, Phyathai, Bangkok, Thailand

J.M. MALINOVSKY, MD, PhD
Service d'Anesthésie et Réanimation, CHU de Reims, Pôle URAD, Hôpital Maison Blanche, Reims, France

P.M. MERTES, MD, PhD
Service d'Anesthésie-Réanimation Chirurgicale, CHU de Nancy, Hôpital Central, Nancy Cedex; Faculté de Médecine, Vandoeuvre les Nancy, France

MAURO PAGANI, MD
Allergology and Oncology Service, Medicine Department, Asola Hospital; Azienda Ospedaliera C. Poma, Mantova, Italy

WERNER J. PICHLER, MD
Division of Allergology, Clinic for Rheumatology and Clinical Immunology/Allergology, Inselspital, University of Bern; ADR-AC GmbH, Bern, Switzerland

M.A. REGNIER-KIMMOUN, MD
Service d'Anesthésie-Réanimation Chirurgicale, CHU de Nancy, Hôpital Central, Nancy Cedex; Faculté de Médecine, Vandoeuvre les Nancy, France

MARIO SÁNCHEZ-BORGES, MD
Department of Allergy and Clinical Immunology, Centro Médico-Docente La Trinidad, Carretera La Trinidad-El Hatillo, Estado Miranda; Clínica El Avila, Sexta Transversal Urbanización, Altamira, Caracas, Venezuela

KATHRIN SCHERER, MD
Allergy Unit, Department of Dermatology, University Hospital Basel, Basel, Switzerland

BENNO SCHNYDER, MD
Division of Allergology, Clinic for Rheumatology and Clinical Immunology/Allergology, Inselspital, University of Bern, Bern, Switzerland

CORNELIA S. SEITZ, MD
Assistant Professor, Department of Dermatology, Venereology, and Allergology, University of Göttingen, Göttingen, Germany

MICHAEL SEITZ, MD
Professor of Rheumatology, Department of Rheumatology, Clinical Immunology/
Allergology, Inselspital, University of Bern, Bern, Switzerland

TETSUO SHIOHARA, MD, PhD
Department of Dermatology, Kyorin University School of Medicine, Tokyo, Japan

K. TAJIMA, MD
Service d'Anesthésie-Réanimation Chirurgicale, CHU de Nancy, Hôpital Central,
Nancy Cedex; Faculté de Médecine, Vandoeuvre les Nancy, France

MARIA J. TORRES, MD, PhD
Allergy Service, Plaza del Hospital Civil s/n, Carlos Haya Hospital, Málaga, Spain

AXEL TRAUTMANN, MD
Associate Professor, Allergy Unit, Department of Dermatology, Venereology,
and Allergology, University of Würzburg, Würzburg, Germany

PETER M. VILLIGER, MD
Professor of Rheumatology; Head, Department of Rheumatology, Clinical Immunology/
Allergology, Inselspital, University of Bern, Bern, Switzerland

DANIEL YERLY, PhD
Division of Allergology, Clinic for Rheumatology and Clinical Immunology/Allergology,
Inselspital, University of Bern, Bern, Switzerland

Contents

Drug-induced hypersensitivity syndrome (DIHS) is a severe systemic reaction with several herpesvirus reactivations. Multiple organ failures appear during the course of the disease. The severity of DIHS is determined by the degree of visceral involvement. Autoimmune diseases also develop several months to years after the apparent clinical resolution of DIHS.

The incidence of immune-mediated anaphylaxis during anesthesia ranges from 1 in 10,000 to 1 in 20,000. Neuromuscular blocking agents are most frequently incriminated, followed by latex and antibiotics, although any drug or substance used may be a culprit. Diagnosis relies on tryptase measurements at the time of the reaction and skin tests, specific immunoglobulin E, or basophil activation assays. Treatment consists of rapid volume expansion and epinephrine administration titrated to symptom severity.

Biologicals are proteins used as drugs. Biologicals target clearly defined molecular structures, being part of established pathogenetic pathways. Therefore, their focused mode of action seems to render them superior to classic small molecular drugs regarding "off-target" adverse drug reactions (ADR). Nevertheless, the increasing use of biologicals for the treatment of different diseases has revealed partially unexpected adverse reactions. The often direct interaction of a biological with the immune system provides a clue to most side effects, which have consequently been subclassified, based on pathogenetic principles, into 5 subtypes named α, β, γ, δ, and ϵ, reflecting overstimulation (high cytokine values, type α), hypersensitivity (type β), immune deviation (including immunodeficiency, type γ), cross-reactivity (type δ), and nonimmune mediated side effects (type ϵ). This article presents typical clinical manifestations of these subtypes of ADR to biologicals, proposes general rules for treating them, and provides a scheme for a thorough allergological workup. This approach should help in future handling of these often very efficient drugs.

β-Lactam antibiotics are the drugs most frequently involved in drug hypersensitivity reactions that are mediated by specific immunologic mechanisms. In addition to benzylpenicillin, several chemical structures belonging to 5 major subgroups can induce reactions. The most relevant structure is that of the amoxicillin molecule. Reactions belong to the 4 major mechanisms described by Coombs and Gell, whereby type IV reactions have recently been further subclassified. The most frequent reactions are type I, which are IgE mediated, and type IV, which are nonimmediate and T-cell dependent. IgE-specific antibodies may recognize the benzylpenicilloyl structure or another part of the molecule, such as the side chain, as antigenic determinants. Depending on specific recognition, subjects can be either cross-reactors or selective responders. A variety of entities exist in T-cell reactions, ranging from mild exanthema to life-threatening, severe reactions, such as Stevens-Johnson syndrome or toxic epidermal necrolysis. Diagnostic tests for IgE-mediated reactions can be done in vivo by testing skin with different penicillin determinants or in vitro by quantitating specific IgE antibodies. For nonimmediate reactions, there are also in vitro and in vivo tests, with variable degrees of sensitivity and specificity. The natural history of IgE-mediated reactions indicates that the count of specific IgE antibodies decreases over time and that results of diagnostic tests can become negative.

Inflammatory plaques at injection sites are frequent side effects of heparin treatment and a clinical symptom of delayed-type hypersensitivity (DTH) to heparin. In most cases, changing the subcutaneous therapy from unfractionated to low-molecular-weight heparin or treatment with heparinoids does not provide improvement because of extensive cross-reactivity. Because of their completely different chemical structure, hirudins are a safe alternative for anticoagulation. Despite DTH to subcutaneously injected heparins, patients tolerate heparin intravenously. Therefore, in case of therapeutic necessity and DTH to heparins, the simple shift from subcutaneous to intravenous heparin administration is justified. Skin necrosis is a rare complication of anticoagulation. Heparin-induced skin necrosis is 1 of the symptoms of immune-mediated heparin-induced thrombocytopenia and should result in the immediate cessation of heparin therapy to prevent potentially fatal thrombotic events. This is in contrast to coumarin-induced skin necrosis, where therapy may be continued or restarted at a lower dose.

The number of drugs used for the treatment of different types of cancers is constantly increasing and actually exceeds 100 distinct chemical formulations. The use of most cytotoxic agents is associated with potential hypersensitivity reactions, and the constant increase of their administration has caused an increase in incidence of these adverse effects, thus becoming a relevant problem for clinicians. Hypersensitivity reactions are common with platinum compounds, L-asparaginase, taxanes, procarbazine, and epipodophyllotoxins, whereas they are unusual, but always possible, with the other chemotherapeutic drugs. Reactions associated with individual drugs are discussed in detail. The mechanism underlying these hypersensitivity reactions involves IgE-mediated hypersensitivity reactions, nonallergic hypersensitivity reactions, and a few pathogenetically unclear reactions. More studies are needed to better understand, diagnose, treat, and prevent these reactions. To achieve this goal, a multidisciplinary approach to treat patients with cancer who have potential allergies is needed.

Mario Sánchez-Borges

Adverse reactions to drugs have been classified as predictable (related to the pharmacologic actions of the drug) and unpredictable (related to the individual's immunologic response or genetic susceptibility). The term "drug hypersensitivity" refers to the symptoms or signs initiated by an exposure to a drug at a dose normally tolerated by nonhypersensitive persons. In this article, the current knowledge on hypersensitivity reactions to nonsteroidal antiinflammatory drugs is discussed.

Preface

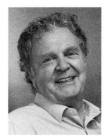

Werner J. Pichler, MD
Guest Editor

Physicians are trained to look for infectious agents and to consider autoimmunity and autoinflammatory disorders, and even rare genetic disorders or paraneoplastic diseases, but are not well prepared to face the fact that drugs given in the best intent to cure or ameliorate diseases and their symptoms may actually be responsible for a new disease suddenly or slowly appearing.

Drug hypersensitivity reactions are embarrassing diseases—not very popular with doctors, the pharmaceutical industry, and others. They are important causes of morbidity and even mortality, however. Moreover, they are the big imitators of diseases, having taken over this role from syphilis, thus causing a lot of confusion in daily clinical medicine. The clinical picture of drug hypersensitivity reactions is far more diverse than most imagine and goes beyond the usual rashes so often encountered in daily clinical practice. Drug hypersensitivity can affect all organ systems: often the skin is involved, but also liver, kidney, lung, and other organs can participate in these systemic immune reactions. If an enigmatic clinical picture is encountered, not fitting well in the usual concepts, always consider a drug hypersensitivity reaction in the differential diagnosis.

The area of drug hypersensitivity has been widely neglected not least because it is a complex area. Pathophysiologic concepts for these reactions were insufficient or lacking and the diseases were difficult to study. In spite of these obstacles, research went on and revealed some interesting and highly relevant practical facts: certain drug hypersensitivity diseases show the highest genetic associations ever found, and abacavir-induced or carbamazepine-induced hypersensitivity reactions can be avoided by prior genotyping for HLA-B alleles. Thus, this somewhat embarrassing area of medicine is now in the forefront of personalized medicine—and the knowledge gained has enormous practical consequences.

This issue tries to reduce the respect/fear of these strange reactions by updating readers on new pathophysiologic concepts and by proposing a rather practical approach to these hypersensitivity reactions; some new concepts of drug hypersensitivity reactions are presented, which may facilitate understanding of the clinical picture and help prevent these disorders. The starting symptoms and danger signs of drug

Med Clin N Am 94 (2010) xv–xvi
doi:10.1016/j.mcna.2010.04.008
0025-7125/10/$ – see front matter

hypersensitivity reactions are discussed, and the clinical picture of severe and imme-diate and also delayed-appearing reactions is described in more detail. Emphasis is also put on side effects encountered with drugs widely used in internal medicine—such as hypersensitivity reactions to biologicals, anticoagulants, and cytostatic drugs, and the frequent reactions to nonsteroidal anti-inflammatory drugs.

I am aware that we are still at the beginning of a better understanding of drug hyper-sensitivity reactions. Nevertheless, the knowledge already gained over the past 20 years is enormous and needs to be spread in the medical community to better recog-nize and avoid these iatrogenic diseases.

I thank the authors for their contributions and for their long-standing interest in this area of medicine. Let us hope that this issue will contribute to better acceptance of this difficult area of medicine and thus may help to prevent some severe or fatal conse-quences of these iatrogenic diseases.

Werner J. Pichler, MD
Division of Allergology
Clinic for Rheumatology and Clinical Immunology/Allergology, Inselspital
University of Bern
CH-3010 Bern, Switzerland

ADR-AC GmbH
Holligenstr 91, CH-3008 Bern, Switzerland

E-mail address:
werner.pichler@insel.ch

Drug Hypersensitivity Reactions: Pathomechanism and Clinical Symptoms

Werner J. Pichler, MD[a,b,*], Jaqueline Adam, MSc[a],
Barbara Daubner, MSc[a], Thomas Gentinetta, MSc[b],
Monika Keller, PhD[b], Daniel Yerly, PhD[a]

KEYWORDS

- Hapten • P-i concept • Gell and Coombs classification
- Specific IgE • Type IV reactions • Exanthema
- Multiple drug hypersensitivity • Flare-up reactions

The immune system has developed to combat infections, which it achieves by a sophisticated interplay between the innate and adaptive immune systems. People are exposed to many infectious agents, but also encounter many (new) chemicals, mostly in very small amounts. Some chemicals, such as drugs, are given consistently and in comparatively high doses. These chemicals can interfere with the immune system in various ways and may lead to somewhat neglected, phenotypically unusual consequences, which are a potential cause of allergic diseases.

Drug-induced adverse reactions are often classified as type A and type B reactions: Type A represent predictable side effects due to a pharmacologic action of the drug, whereas type B reactions are assumed not to be predictable. They comprise so-called idiosyncratic reactions due to some individual predisposition (eg, an enzyme defect), and hypersensitivity reactions.[1] About 1 in 6 adverse drug reactions represents drug hypersensitivity, and are allergic or non–immune-mediated (pseudoallergic) reactions. The latter are common causes of side effects to nonsteroidal antiinflammatory drugs (NSAIDs) (see the article by Mario Sánchez-Borges elsewhere in this issue for further exploration of this topic). It is rare for drugs to cause autoimmunity or immunodeficiency. Such abnormal immune reactions to a drug are a substantial cause of

---

[a] Division of Allergology, Clinic for Rheumatology and Clinical Immunology/Allergology, Inselspital, University of Bern, CH-3010 Bern, Switzerland
[b] ADR-AC GmbH, Holligenstr 91, Bern CH-3008, Switzerland
* Corresponding author. Division of Allergology, Clinic for Rheumatology and Clinical Immunology/Allergology, Inselspital, University of Bern, CH-3010 Bern, Switzerland.
E-mail address: werner.pichler@insel.ch

Med Clin N Am 94 (2010) 645–664
doi:10.1016/j.mcna.2010.04.003
0025-7125/10/$ – see front matter © 2010 Elsevier Inc. All rights reserved.

morbidity, and even mortality, and deserve special attention by the medical community because they represent iatrogenic diseases.

The clinical symptoms and diseases of drug hypersensitivity reactions are heterogeneous and can imitate many different diseases, which often delays a correct diagnosis. Some side effects are mild, but others are severe and even fatal.[2,3] Many allergic reactions affect the skin and can cause a variety of different exanthems. Most common is a maculopapular rash, which is observed in about 2% to 3% of hospitalized patients.[4,5] However, drug hypersensitivity reactions can also affect various internal organs, causing hepatitis, nephritis, carditis, pneumonitis, and so forth.

Any drug is assumed to be able to elicit hypersensitivity reactions. However, the frequency differs widely. Antibiotics and antiepileptics are the most prevalent causes. The risk of sensitization and the severity of clinical symptoms depend on the state of immune activation of the individual, the dose, the duration of treatment, sex (more frequent in women), and the immunogenetic predisposition (in particular human leukocyte antigen B [HLA-B] alleles), whereas a pharmacogenetic predisposition has rarely been detected.

Epicutaneous application of a drug clearly increases the chance of sensitization compared with oral or parental treatments. It may be due to the high density of dendritic cells (DCs) in the skin. Atopy (defined as the genetic predisposition to mount an immunoglobin E [IgE] response to inhaled or ingested innocuous proteins) is normally not associated with a higher risk of drug hypersensitivity. However, an atopic predisposition may prolong the persistence of drug-specific IgE in the serum,[6] and an ongoing IgE-mediated allergic inflammation such as asthma may aggravate the symptoms of an IgE-mediated drug hypersensitivity reaction.

HOW DO SMALL MOLECULES STIMULATE THE IMMUNE SYSTEM?
Hapten and Prohapten Concepts

Small chemical compounds, usually less than 1000 Da, are not immunogenic per se. These compounds are normally degraded, metabolized, and eliminated without stimulating an immune response. However, if the chemical is reactive and able to bind covalently to proteins, DNA, and so forth, a new antigenic determinant arises that can produce a new immune response. This modification can, theoretically, affect any kind of autologous protein, such as soluble extracellular proteins (eg, albumin), membrane proteins (eg, an integrin), and intracellular proteins (eg, enzymes). It can even bind directly to the peptide embedded in the major histocompatibility complex (MHC) molecule itself. The hapten modification may also affect essential proteins or the DNA, which may result in a dose-dependent toxicity (**Fig. 1A**).

A certain toxic effect may also be important for inducing an immune response: the toxicity is sensed by the innate immune system as a danger, and DCs react to so-called danger signals by upregulating costimulatory molecules and cytokines. These danger signals can be generated by a toxic effect on cells, which are then sensed by DCs; or it may occur by activating DCs themselves.

Simultaneously, this drug-protein complex generates new antigenic determinants, which may be recognized by antigen-specific receptors of the immune system. This combined stimulation of innate (DCs and other cells) and adaptive immunity (T and B cells) results in a new, antigen-specific immune response, which is based on T cells and antibody production, both specific to the drug-protein complex (ie, hapten-carrier complex). The ensuing immune response is variable, because it uses against the drug

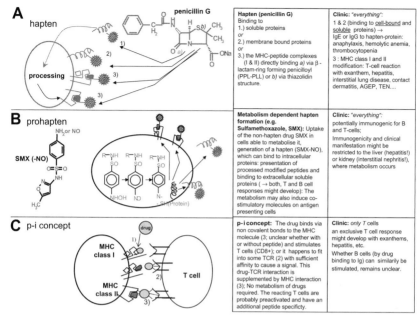

Hapten (penicillin G) Binding to 1.) soluble proteins or 2.) membrane bound proteins or 3.) the MHC-peptide complexes (I & II) directly binding a) via β-lactam-ring forming penicilloyl (PPL-PLL) or b) via thiazolidin structure.	**Clinic:** *"everything"*: 1 & 2 (binding to cell-bound and soluble proteins) → IgE or IgG to hapten-protein: anaphylaxis, hemolytic anemia, thrombocytopenia 3 : MHC class I and II modification: T-cell reaction with exanthem, hepatitis, interstitial lung disease, contact dermatitis, AGEP, TEN....
Metabolism dependent hapten formation (e.g. Sulfamethoxazole, SMX): Uptake of the non-hapten drug SMX in cells able to metabolise it, generation of a hapten (SMX-NO), which can bind to intracellular proteins: presentation of processed modified peptides and binding to extracellular soluble proteins (→ both, T and B cell responses might develop): The metabolism may also induce co-stimulatory molecules on antigen presenting cells	**Clinic:** *"everything"*: potentially immunogenic for B and T-cells; Immunogenicity and clinical manifestation might be restricted to the liver (hepatitis!) or kidney (interstitial nephritis!), where metabolism occurs
p-i concept: The drug binds via non covalent bonds to the MHC molecule (3; unclear whether with or without peptide) and stimulates T cells (CD8+); or it happens to fit into some TCR (2) with sufficient affinity to cause a signal. This drug-TCR interaction is supplemented by MHC interaction (3); No metabolism of drugs required. The reacting T cells are probably preactivated and have an additional peptide specificty.	**Clinic:** *only T cells* an exclusive T cell response might develop with exanthems, hepatitis, etc. Whether B cells (by drug binding to Ig) can similarly be stimulated, remains unclear.

Fig. 1. Hapten and prohapten concepts and the noncovalent drug presentation to T cells. (*A*) Haptens. Drugs are haptens if they can bind covalently to soluble or cell-bound molecules (eg, penicillin G). They can bind directly to the immunogenic major histocompatibility complex (MHC)/peptide complex on antigen-presenting cells (APC); to the embedded peptide or to the MHC molecule itself. Thus, the chemical reactivity of haptens leads to the formation of many distinct antigenic epitopes that can elicit simultaneous humoral and cellular immune responses. Some examples of B- or T-cell–mediated immune responses are listed on the right of the figure. (*B*) Prohaptens. Other drugs are prohaptens, requiring metabolic activation to become haptens (ie, chemically reactive). The metabolism leads to the formation of a chemically reactive compound (eg, from sulfamethoxazole [SMX] to the chemically reactive form SMX-NO). The resulting intake may lead to modification of cell-bound or soluble proteins by the chemically reactive metabolite, similar to a hapten. (*C*) The p-i concept (pharmacologic interaction with immune receptors). Drugs are often designed to fit into certain proteins/enzymes to block their function. Some drugs may also bind to some of the available T-cell receptors (TCR) or MHC molecules (plus or minus embedded peptide). Under certain conditions (see text) this drug interaction with the TCR or MHC molecule may lead to an immune response of the T cell. For a full T-cell stimulation by such an inert drug, an interaction with a particular TCR is required, or the drug interacts with the MHC molecule that is stimulating the TCR/T cells. This p-i type of drug stimulation results in an exclusive T-cell stimulation. (*From* Pichler WJ. Drug hypersensitivity: classification and relationship to T-cell activation. In: Pichler WJ, editor. Drug hypersensitivity. Basel (Switzerland): Karger; 2007. p. 168–89; with permission.)

all of the tools generated to eliminate infections agents. Consequently the clinical situation is variable.

Many drugs are not chemically reactive but are still able to elicit immune-mediated side effects. The prohapten hypothesis tries to reconcile this phenomenon with the hapten hypothesis by stating that a chemically inert drug may become reactive on metabolism.[1,7,8] Sulfamethoxazole (SMX) is a prototype prohapten. It is not chemically reactive but gains reactivity, and thus antigenicity, by intracellular metabolism. A cytochrome P450–dependent metabolism (CYP2C9) in the liver leads to sulfamethoxazole-hydroxylamine (SMX-NHOH), which can be found in the urine and which is easily converted to sulfamethoxazole-nitroso by oxidation. The latter is highly chemically reactive and easily binds to intracellular proteins, creating neoantigenic determinants.[9] Toxic effects of SMX occur when it exceeds a threshold level. Thus, SMX seems to have indirect antigenic and immunogenic features (see **Fig. 1**B).

The p-i Concept

A new possibility of drug interaction with immune receptors has recently been developed by our group: It is called the p-i concept (pharmacologic interactions of drugs with immune receptors). It is a simple concept that postulates that drugs may directly interact with immune receptors, as they do with other receptors, and that this interaction may stimulate the immune cells: This concept contradicts the original belief that the immune-stimulatory capacity of most chemicals and drugs is based on covalent binding and may be predicted by their protein reactivity.[10–12] According to the p-i concept, chemically inert drugs, unable to covalently bind to peptides or proteins, can nevertheless activate certain T cells if they fit with a sufficient affinity into some of the many different T-cell receptors (TCR) or MHC molecules. This reversible interaction is similar to that of a drug ligand to its receptor, and is not based on covalent interaction but only on reversible van der Waals interactions. In vivo, p-i–activated T cells expand and subsequently infiltrate the skin and other organs, resulting in a T-cell–orchestrated inflammation.

Evidence for the p-i mechanism lies in various experimental data:

1. Aldehyde-fixed antigen-presenting cells (APC; unable to process antigen or to convert a prohapten to a hapten) are still able to activate specific terminal complement complex (TCC) if incubated together with the (inert) drug
2. The drug binding to proteins is more labile than the covalent interactions of haptens and can be washed away
3. Calcium influx in TCC happens within seconds after the addition of the drug; before drug uptake, metabolism, and processing can occur.

Second (danger) signal in the p-i concept

To initiate an immune response, in addition to the antigenic feature (signal 1, sensed by specific TCR), DCs provide costimulatory signals after having been activated. This response may be toll-like receptor signaling, or other danger signaling, connected to the antigen presented. This stimulation of DCs is transmitted by many means, and is well documented for haptens, contact sensitizers, and so forth.

In contrast to haptens, p-i–acting drugs do not covalently interact with proteins or with intracellular proteins: thus, these drugs are less toxic. There are 3 hypotheses to explain how the second (danger) signal , which is believed to be essential to starting an immune response, is delivered by p-i–acting drugs (these may also work in combination):

1. The p-i–stimulating drugs are not proinflammatory, and the innate immune system may not be stimulated.[13] Consequently, it is assumed that no generation of an own drug (hapten)-specific immune response occurs. The p-i–stimulated T cells would not arise from naive T cells, but from previously primed effector-memory T cells, which were primed by some prior peptide contact. Consequently, p-i–stimulated T cells have an additional (peptide) specificity. Effector-memory cells have a substantially lower threshold for activation than naive T cells. Thus, only preactivated T cells may be susceptible for the p-i stimulations, which may explain why

concomitantly occurring massive immune stimulations of T cells, as occur during generalized herpes or human immunodeficiency virus infections, are well-known risk factors for drug hypersensitivity reactions. Exacerbations of autoimmune diseases or an ongoing drug hypersensitivity (see later discussion) may represent risk factors for further drug hypersensitivities. Such immune processes correspond with high cytokine levels (eg, interleukin 2 [IL-2], interferon γ [IFNγ]) in the circulation and in the tissues, and an increased expression of MHC and costimulatory molecules in cells of the immune system. Consequently, T cells of patients with generalized immune activations due to virus infections, ongoing autoimmunity, or drug allergies are already preactivated and able to react to a minor signal such as the binding of a small drug to a certain TCR. This theory would explain the high occurrence of drug hypersensitivities in these diseases.

2. The p-i–stimulating drugs have an additional intrinsic activity that somehow activates DCs: for example, some drugs may bind to toll-like receptors (eg, imiquimod and TLR8); others may bind to other receptors linked to cell activation. Such intrinsic activity of a drug, which occurs aside of the normal target structure, may substitute for other danger signals and thus provide the necessary second signal for T-cell activation.

3. Although the p-i concept has been documented for many drugs (SMX, lidocaine, lamotrigine, carbamazepine, p-phenylendiamine, radiocontrast media),[11,14–17] metabolites of these drugs are also implicated in hypersensitivities to these drugs. Detailed analysis of affected patients shows that many T-cell clones react to the parent compound, but others react to metabolites. Thus, hapten and p-i responses occur together. A cross-reactivity can occasionally be observed, indicating that the T-cell clone reacts via p-i and hapten recognition. The common occurrence raises the question of whether the hapten characteristic of a drug (with its immune-stimulatory consequences on innate immunity, as described earlier) is a prerequisite for p-i stimulations to (also) occur. In this scheme, the danger signal may come from the processed, haptenlike drug.

p-i for CD4+ and CD8+ T cells

Full T-cell activation by the drug (measured by immediate Ca^{2+} influx into specific T cells, and cytokine synthesis or proliferation) requires the interaction of the TCR with MHC on APC.[11,18] This finding raises the question of whether the drug binds first to the MHC molecule, modifying its structure, which is sensed by the TCR, and thus leading to specific TCR activation, or whether the drug binds primarily to specific TCR, rendering the MHC interaction only a supplementing signal.

Both concepts are possible: initial data with drug-specific, CD4+ T-cell clones suggest that the interaction of the drug happens first with the TCR, because the MHC-bound peptide could be exchanged or removed without affecting CD4+ T-cell activation (see **Fig. 1**B).[18] Some TCC reacted to the drug even if presented by allogeneic MHC molecules, indicating that no strict HLA restriction for drug presentation exists.[19] However, this may be different for the less well-analyzed CD8+ TCC. Some severe drug hypersensitivity reactions caused by certain drugs have a high HLA-B-allele association.[20–26] In the case of abacavir hypersensitivity (a drug hypersensitivity syndrome strongly associated with the HLA-B*5701 allele[23,24]) key interacting residues in the HLA-B*5701 peptide-binding cleft could be identified, which allow the formation of noncovalent interactions with the drug abacavir.[24] Recent in silico data published by Yang and colleagues[25] suggest that drugs could also fit in empty, non–peptide-bearing MHC class I molecules. Thus, the strong MHC allele; drug specificity can be explained by a steric complementarity together with other strong noncovalent interactions between the drug molecule and the antigen presentation groove. It is tempting to speculate that the interaction of abacavir with empty MHC class I molecules may stabilize these MHC molecules, because MHC molecules without peptides are unstable.

This and other strong MHC class I–associated drug hypersensitivity reactions were among the first examples of personalized medicine; nowadays HLA-B*5701 typing is regularly done before abacavir is prescribed, which has almost eliminated severe abacavir-related drug hypersensitivity reactions. Similarly, among Han Chinese, HLA-B*1502 typing greatly reduces the incidence of Stevens-Johnson syndrome (SJS)/toxic epidermal necrolysis (TEN) in carbamazepin-treated patients.

Based on these findings, 2 types of p-i mechanism may occur. In the case of MHC class I restricted drug hypersensitivity reactions, the drug may first bind to the MHC class I molecules, and subsequently elicit a strong (CD8+ T cell) immune response. Whether this drug binding affects empty MHC I molecules, or whether the MHC-embedded peptide could influence the interaction, is still not clear. Nevertheless, the direct binding of the drug to the MHC molecule itself (and not to the peptide) could explain the extremely strong association with the MHC class I molecule (see **Fig. 1**C), and that eluting peptides from the MHC molecule failed to identify (covalently) drug-peptide complexes.[26]

Alternatively, a more polymorphic CD4+ T-cell response would occur if the drug interacts primarily with the TCR. Full stimulation of these CD4 cells would still require an interaction with the MHC class II molecules; however, probably just by binding to common determinants of the MHC structure, as various MHC class II molecules do, seems to be sufficient to provide T-cell stimulation. Therefore, in CD4 cell reactions, no MHC-associations have been found for these clinically mostly mild reactions (mainly maculopapular exanthems, rarely drug rash with eosinophilia and systemic symptoms [DRESS]). Some clinical features of the p-i concept are as follows:

- Positive skin test reactions to inert drugs, although no cutaneous metabolism of this peculiar drug is known
- Immune reactivity at the first encounter, without time of sensitization.[7] In this case, the drug may already interact with many T cells.
- Generalized reaction to a drug without local danger signs
- Fulminant course of a T-cell–mediated hypersensitivity (as with superantigen stimulations)[7,27]
- Flare-up reactions to a novel drug (?)
- It reflects an abnormal T-cell stimulation with massive/fatal self-destruction as seen in SJS/TEN and DRESS/drug-induced hypersensitivity syndrome (DiHS) (?)

The p-i concept represents a new way to explain drug-induced hypersensitivity reactions. It suggests that certain drug hypersensitivities are also pharmacologic reactions, because the drug interacts not only with the target for which it is designed but also with some immune receptors. The enormous diversity of immune receptors facilitates this possibility of additional drug interactions outside the original scope. The dogma that small chemicals are not full antigens is still valid and must not be rejected, but drugs are able to interfere with the human immune system in additional ways. Related to this finding of pharmacologic stimulation of the immune system by drugs is the development that some of the so-called unpredictable type B drug reactions become the most predictable drug reactions and a paradigm for personalized medicine. It seems that the belief that type B reactions are bizarre reactions is becoming outdated.

CLASSIFICATION OF DRUG HYPERSENSITIVITY REACTIONS

Coombs and Gell[28] classified drug hypersensitivity, as well as other immune reactions, into 4 categories termed type I-IV reactions: This classification relies on the formation of IgE antibodies that bind to high-affinity IgE receptors on mast cells and basophilic leukocytes, on complement-fixing antibodies, and in T-cell reactions. Because recent immunologic data reveal that T cells orchestrate different forms of inflammation, which may result in different symptoms, the classification of Coombs and Gell[28] has been refined[7] into IVa, IVb, IVc, and IVd reactions, to better accommodate this heterogeneity of T-cell functions.

The extended Coombs and Gell[28] classification is a simplification of complex events occurring in vivo. The immune system combines different approaches to defend against a real or presumed pathogen, even if the pathogen is not dangerous, as in allergy. Nevertheless, a certain type of immune reaction may dominate the clinical situation: for example, in anaphylaxis to β-lactam antibiotics, there may not only be drug-specific IgE but also a T-cell reaction to the drug. However, the formation of drug-specific IgE is the relevant clinical event. In patients with an exanthem and hepatitis, an eosinophilic infiltrate may be found in the skin biopsy, but the liver cell destruction by cytotoxic T cells may be the more dangerous event. For the diagnosis of a drug allergy, the skin event may be sufficient.

Type I (IgE-mediated) Allergies

The IgE system reacts to small amounts of antigen. It achieves this sensitivity by the ubiquitous presence of mast cells armed with high-affinity fragment crystallizable IgE receptors (Fc-IgE RI), to which allergen- or drug-specific IgE is bound. On cross-linking the Fc-IgE RI, various mediators (histamine, tryptase, leukotriens, prostaglandins, TNFα, and so forth) are released, which cause the immediate symptoms and may start and facilitate late-appearing allergic inflammations.

IgE-mediated reactions to drugs are believed usually to depend on the prior development of an immune response to a hapten/carrier complex: B cells, able to interact via their surface Ig receptors with the hapten-carrier complex, mature into IgE-secreting plasma cells. This maturation is helped by hapten-carrier complex–specific T cells, which interact with B cells (ie, via CD40-CD40L interaction) and which release IL-4/IL-13, which are switch factors for IgE synthesis. This sensitization phase is normally asymptomatic. On renewed contact with the drug, a hapten-carrier complex is formed again, which then cross-links preformed drug-specific IgE on mast cells and causes mast cell degranulation and immediate allergic symptoms (**Fig. 2**).

Peculiar features of IgE-mediated reactions to drugs

IgE-mediated reactions to drugs have some features that need to be considered to better understand these reactions:

1. Very small amounts of a drug seem to be sufficient to allow interaction and cross-linking of receptor-bound IgE molecules. Even intradermal (ID) skin tests with drugs may elicit systemic reactions, and fatal reactions to ID testing have been described.[29] What is the difference to protein-specific reactions? Why are drug-induced anaphylactic reactions often so severe?

The drug itself is normally too small to cross-link 2 adjacent IgE molecules, and it needs to bind covalently to proteins to cross-link specific IgE bound to Fc-IgE receptors (see **Fig. 2**). If a protein does not consist of repetitive determinants, it needs at least 2 distinct IgE-binding sites (epitopes) that can bind and cross-link 2 distinct

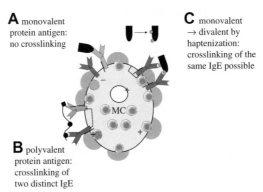

A monovalent protein antigen: no crosslinking

B polyvalent protein antigen: crosslinking of two distinct IgE

C monovalent → divalent by haptenization: crosslinking of the same IgE possible

Fig. 2. IgE cross-linking is facilitated by hapten binding to proteins. A protein usually contains a few different epitopes, to which IgEs with the appropriate specificities bind. These IgEs are cross-linked by the protein if the epitopes are localized far enough away to allow binding of separate IgEs. If the protein contains only 1 epitope, or if the epitope is too close and thus prevents binding of a second IgE, no cross-linking can ensue (*A, B*). The potent allergenicity of haptens may be related to their ability to generate new hapten epitopes on a protein: with hapten modification, not 1, but several identical epitopes appear on the protein (*C*). Not only different IgEs, specific for distinct protein epitopes (*B*), but even IgEs with identical (hapten) specificity can be cross-linked (*C*). This may accelerate mast cell degranulation. For details, see the text.

IgE molecules. If the protein contains only 1 epitope, no cross-linking can occur, because the IgE molecules can only bind to a single epitope, making cross–linking impossible.[30]

The situation is different for haptens. A hapten may modify a protein at various positions. Consequently, different new epitopes arise (see **Fig. 2**, position A, B, and so forth). If these new epitopes are spacially distinct enough to allow binding of distinct IgE molecules, at least 2 or more IgE could bind. Even IgE with the same hapten specificity could bind, and cross-linking Fc-IgE receptors would no longer depend on the proximity of at least 2 distinct IgE molecules. Consequently, hapten formation is the main facilitator of IgE cross-linking, as a single hapten-modified protein can cross-link IgE molecules with the same (or different) specificity. This enhanced cross-linking ability may result in rapid and fulminant mast cell degranulations, and may explain the severity of drug-induced anaphylaxis (see schematic representation in **Fig. 2**).

2. A second feature of drug-induced anaphylaxis is that 50% or more of patients with immediate reactions to various drugs deny any prior contact with the drug; 4/5 of the patients with lethal anaphylaxis had no prior contact with the drug.[31] This was previously interpreted as sign of a non–immune-mediated anaphylaxis (pseudoallergy), because prior contact with the drug was believed to be essential for specific IgE formation. However, IgE specific to neuromuscular blocking agents (NMBAs) could be detected in perioperative anaphylaxis by skin tests and by serology even at the first encounter with these drugs,[32] and, similarly, a substantial proportion of patients with radiocontrast media–elicited anaphylaxis had positive immediate skin tests.[33]

This raised the question that perhaps other chemical compounds had sensitized these patients. Observation of the distinct use of the antitussive drug pholcodein in Norway and Sweden may have shed some light on this issue: peripoerative anaphylaxis was found to be sixfold more frequent in Norway than in Sweden.[34] Pholcodein was licensed in Norway, but not in Sweden. Pholcodein use stimulated the production of pholcodein- and morphin-specifc IgE molecules, which also reacted with tertiary and quaternary ammonium groups contained in NMBA.[35] Thus, in Norway many people were silently sensitized to a cross-reactive compound contained in an antitussive.[34] Their reactions were clearly IgE mediated and pholcodein/NMBA/quarternary ammonium specific, but not elicited by NMBA.

3. Anaphylactic reactions were often considered to be dose independent, as sometimes very small amounts can cause severe reactions. However, all drug-induced reactions are dose dependent. However, the reaction due to IgE is often caused by minute amounts. Further diminishing the dose, as is done in desensitization procedures, shows that even these reactions are dose dependent.[36]

Clinical features of IgE-mediated reactions

IgE-mediated reactions can cause mild to severe, even lethal, diseases: in sensitized individuals, the reaction can start within seconds after contact with the parentally applied drug, and minutes after oral drug uptake. Symptoms may start with palmar, plantar, genital, and axillar itch, and facial and thoracal redness. These symptoms should be considered an alarm sign, as they often herald a severe, anaphylactic reaction, developing rapidly within minutes (**Fig. 3**). The symptoms rapidly generalize and, within approximately 10 to 20 minutes, a generalized urticaria may develop. The patient becomes restless and anxious. Laryngeal swelling may be suspected if he/she has difficulty speaking or swallowing, because the tongue is swollen. He or she may also complain about chest tightness and dyspnea; signs of acute bronchospasm. Periorbital and perioral swellings often occur later. More severe and complex reactions are called anaphylaxis,[37] and, in most cases with anaphylaxis, some circulatory events with decrease of blood pressure and (transient) unconsciousness are observed, together with a generalized redness, itch, or urticaria.

Anaphylactic shock occurs often within 10 to 15 minutes, and asphyxia due to laryngeal edema often occurs between 15 and 60 minutes. Asphyxia may account for 60% of anaphylaxis-related deaths.[38] Some patients develop gastrointestinal symptoms (nausea, cramps, vomiting, and fecal incontinence). The reduction in blood pressure may be due to a shift of intravascular volume into the extravascular space or to the development of a cardiac arrhythmia, which is more serious. The full syndrome is anaphylactic shock, which is lethal in approximately 1% to 2% of all anaphylaxis cases. The more rapidly it appears, the more serious it is likely to be. Risk factors for a severe course are high-dose, preexisting (undertreated) asthma, and older age, because myocardial infarction, cerebral hypoxia, and brain damage can lead to death days after the acute event. Patients with recurrent anaphylactic reactions to various triggers (eg, food, drugs, hymenoptera stings) may have mastocytosis.

Although most patients show the involvement of different organs, in perioperative anaphylaxis the symptoms may initially affect only 1 organ system (eg, the cardiovascular system with arrhythmia); skin symptoms may not be visible but can appear later. Anaphylaxis is a severe event, and survivors often have some cognitive or intellectual impairment. **Table 1** summarizes the main drugs causing anaphylaxis.

Most IgE-mediated reactions to drugs are less severe, and often only an urticaria, angioedema, or a local wheal may develop. However, any IgE-mediated drug allergy can be potentially life threatening, because the mild symptoms might be due to a low dose, and each treatment might boost the drug-specific IgE response.

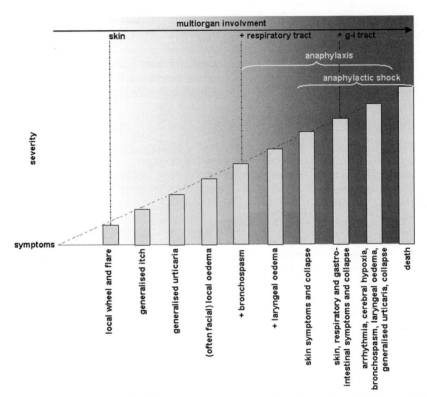

Fig. 3. Anaphylaxis. Anaphylaxis is a complex and severe allergic reaction affecting multiple organs. It can be seen as the sum of different, severe allergic manifestations in various organs. Symptoms resemble mild to moderate allergic reactions (urticaria, angioedema, bronchospasm). In many, but not all, cases, the cardiovascular system is involved, as a result of relative hypovolemia, due to a shift of intravascular volume to extravascular space (less dangerous), or due to arrhythmia. The most severe form is anaphylactic shock, which can result in death in 1% to 2% of affected persons (see text). (*From* Pichler WJ. Drug hypersensitivity: classification and relationship to T-cell activation. In: Pichler WJ, editor. Drug hypersensitivity. Basel (Switzerland): Karger; 2007. p. 168–89; with permission.)

PSEUDOALLERGY (NON–IMMUNE-MEDIATED HYPERSENSITIVITY)

So-called pseudoallergic reactions (non–immune-mediated hypersensitivities) to drugs, which are as frequent as true IgE-mediated reactions, are a pathogenetically poorly defined problem.

Most of these reactions resemble the clinical features of milder forms of immediate, IgE-mediated reactions (erythema, urticaria), but some reactions cause anaphylaxis and can be lethal. Detection of specific immune mechanism is negative. NSAID-induced pseudoallergic reactions seem to arise less rapidly (often >15 minutes after intake) than true IgE-mediated allergies, and they may require higher drug doses than true IgE-mediated reactions. Increased tryptase levels in the acute stage underline the role of mast cell degranulation in some of these reactions (see **Table 1**).

Pseudoallergic reactions can be elicited by many drugs, but some drugs seem to elicit them more often (see **Table 1**). Some drugs might elicit either pseudoallergic, or presumably true allergic reactions, because positive prick skin tests can be

Table 1	
The main drugs causing anaphylaxis	
Drugs Involved in IgE-mediated Allergies[a]	**Drugs Causing Pseudoallergic Reactions[a]**

• Foreign proteins (chimeric antibodies)
• Immunoglobulin preparations (IgE anti-IgA)
• β-Lactam antibiotics
    Penicillin
    Cephalosporin
• Pyrazolones
• Quinolones
• NMBAs[b]
	• (Radio) contrast media[c]
	• Plasma expanders
	• NSAID: acetylsalicylic acid, diclophenac, mefenamic acid, ibuprofen
	• Vancomycin
	• Pyrazolones
	• Quinolones
	• NMBAs

[a] Not complete; only the main groups are mentioned.
[b] The main cause of perioperative anaphylaxis is NMBAs, followed by antibiotics (mainly intravenous cephalosporins) and latex. Skin tests may be positive even if the drug was given the first time.[32]
[c] Some patients with immediate reactions to contrast media have positive immediate skin tests to contrast media.[33]

detected (contrast media, NMBAs). In vitro, these drugs do not spontaneously release mediators from basophils.

Some people seem to show a higher tendency to react in this way (urticaria), because they develop similar, mostly mild symptoms to a heterogeneous panel of drugs, with clearly distinct chemical and pharmacologic features. Neither IgE nor T-cell reactions are evident, the reactions are recurrent, but provocation tests often remain negative, which makes this disease hard to diagnose and to understand. Additional cofactors are probably needed for patients to develop clinical symptoms after receiving a drug. A few patients may have slightly increased tryptase levels, but further diagnostic workup does not reveal mastocytosis. Some milder reactions can be suppressed by pretreatment with antihistamines, but it is doubtful whether pretreatment with antihistamines and corticosteroids can prevent more severe reactions, such as to contrast media.[39] The most common form of such reactions is related to NSAIDs (see the article by Mario Sánchez-Borges elsewhere in this issue for further exploration of this topic).

IGG-MEDIATED REACTIONS (CYTOTOXIC MECHANISM AND IMMUNE COMPLEX DEPOSITION, TYPES II AND III)

Type II and type III reactions rely on the formation of complement-fixing IgG antibodies (IgG1, IgG3). IgM is occasionally involved. They are similar, in that both depend on the formation of immune complexes and interaction with complement and Fc-IgG receptor (Fc-IgGI, IIa, and IIIa)–bearing cells (on macrophages, natural killer [NK] cells, granulocytes, and platelets), but the target structures and physiologic consequences are different.

In type II reactions, the drug-specific antibodies formed lead to cell destruction or sequestration. Affected target cells include erythrocytes, leukocytes, platelets, and probably hematopoietic precursor cells in the bone marrow. The antibody-coated cells will be sequestrated to the reticuloendothelial system in the liver and spleen by Fc- or complement-receptor binding. More rarely, intravascular destruction may occur by complement-mediated lysis.

Hemolytic anemia has been attributed to penicillin and its derivatives, cephalosporins, levodopa, methyldopa, quinidine, and some antiinflammatory drugs. Cephalosporins are currently the main cause. The clinical symptoms of hemolytic anemia are insidious and may be restricted to symptoms of anemia and jaundice with dark urine. Occasionally a positive direct and (if the drug is present during the test) indirect Coombs test can be found.

Thrombocytopenia is a common side effect of drug treatment, in particular following quinine, quinidine, and sulfonamide antibiotics. It is a common complication of treatments with certain biologicals (mainly monoclonal antibodies). Drug-induced immune thrombocytopenia usually develops after 5 to 8 days of exposure to the sensitizing medication, or after a single exposure in patients previously exposed to the same drug. Patients with this condition often present with widespread petechial hemorrhages in the skin and buccal mucosa, sometimes accompanied by urinary tract or gastrointestinal bleeding. Intracranial hemorrhage is rare. After discontinuation of the provoking medication, platelet counts usually return to normal within 3 to 5 days. (See the article by Trautmann and Seitz elsewhere in this issue for further exploration of this topic).

Formation of immune complexes is a common event in a normal immune response and does normally not cause symptoms. It is not clear why, under certain circumstances, an immune complex disease develops: Very high immune complex levels; a relative deficiency of some complement components, and thus lower capacity to eliminate immune complexes; or an aberrant Fc-IgG-R function might be considered.[40] Thus, reduced removal of immune complexes may lead to inappropriate deposition of immune complexes and recruitment of inflammatory cells, in particular polymorphonuclear cells (PMNs), because of immune complex binding to Fc-IgG-R on PMNs. In addition, anaphylatoxins C3a and C5a, generated as a result of local complement activation, may attract PMNs.

A type III reaction may result in a small vessel as vasculitis or serum sickness: In serum sickness, antibodies are generated within 4 to 10 days. Complement (C1q)-containing immune complexes are deposited in the postcapillary venules and attract neutrophilic leukocytes by interacting with their Fc-IgG-RIII,[41] which thereby release proteolytic enzymes that can mediate tissue damage.

Nonprotein and protein drugs (biologicals) are responsible for serum sickness. Hypersensitivity vasculitis reportedly has an incidence of 10 to 30 cases per million people per year. Most reports concern cefaclor, followed by trimethoprim-SMX, cephalexin, amoxicillin, NSAID, and diuretics. Biologicals such as rituximab, infliximab, and natalizumab have increasingly been associated with serum sickness[42] (see the article by Hausmann and colleagues elsewhere in this issue for further exploration of this topic). Vasculitis may be localized, mainly to the skin, as palpable purpura; purplish red spots, usually found on the legs. In children, it is often referred to as Henoch-Schönlein purpura, sometimes appearing in combination with an arthritis. The prognosis is good when no internal involvement is present. Histology can reveal IgA-containing immune complexes, and the histology of kidney lesions is identical to IgA nephropathy, a main cause of chronic renal failure (**Fig. 4**).

T-CELL–MEDIATED, DELAYED DRUG HYPERSENSITIVITY REACTIONS
Subclassification of Type IV Reactions

The detailed analysis of T-cell subsets and functions in the last 30 years has revealed that T cells play a major role in most immune reactions: as helper T cells, which regulate B-cell maturation to antibody-producing cells; as drug-specific T cells, which

Antibody mediated hypersensitivity reactions (I-III) and delayed type hypersensitivity reactions (IV a-d)

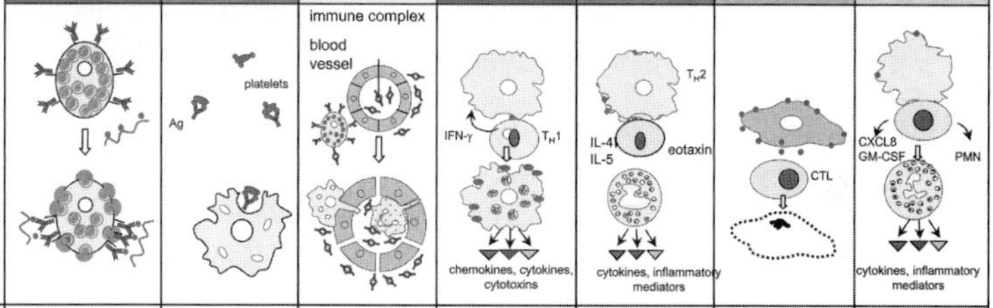

	Type I	Type II	Type III	Type IV a	Type IV b c	Type IV c	Type IV d
Immune reactant	IgE	IgG	IgG	IFN-γ, TNFα (Th1 cells)	IL-5, IL-4/IL-13 (Th2 cells)	Perforin/ GranzymeB (CTL)	CXCL-8, IL-17 (?) GM-CSF (T-cells)
Antigen	Soluble antigen	Cell- or matrix-associated antigen	Soluble antigen	Antigen presented by cells or direct T cell stimulation	Antigen presented by cells or direct T cell stimulation	Cell-associated antigen or direct T cell stimulation	Soluble antigen presented by cells or direct T cell stimulation
Effector	Mast-cell activation	FcR⁺ cells (phagocytes, NK cells)	FcR⁺ cells Complement	Macrophage activation	Eosinophils	T cells	Neutrophils
	(diagram: mast cell activation)	(diagram: platelets, Ag)	(diagram: immune complex, blood vessel)	(diagram: IFN-γ, Th1 → chemokines, cytokines, cytotoxins)	(diagram: Th2, IL-4 IL-5 → eotaxin; cytokines, inflammatory mediators)	(diagram: CTL)	(diagram: CXCL8, GM-CSF → PMN; cytokines, inflammatory mediators)
Example of hypersensitivity reaction	Allergic rhinitis, asthma, systemic anaphylaxis	Some drug allergies (e.g., penicillin)	Serum sickness, Arthus reaction	Tuberculin reaction contact dermatitis (with IVc)	Chronic asthma, chronic allergic rhinitis Maculopapular exanthema with eosinophilia	Contact dermatitis Maculopapular and bullous exanthema hepatitis	AGEP Behçet disease

Fig. 4. Revised Gell and Coombs classification of drug reactions. Drugs can elicit many different immune reactions. All reactions are T-cell–regulated, but the effect or function relies mainly on antibody-mediated effector functions (types I–III) or more T-cell/cytokine-dependent functions (types IVa–IVd).[7] Type I are IgE-mediated reactions. Cross-linking IgE molecules on high-affinity IgE receptors (Fc-IgE RI) on mast cells and basophilic leukocytes leads to degranulation and release of mediators, which cause a variety of symptoms (vasodilatation, increased permeability, bronchoconstriction, itch, and so forth.). Type II reactions are IgG mediated, and cause cell destruction due to complement activation or interaction with Fc-IgG receptor–bearing killer cells. Type III reactions are also IgG mediated: complement deposition and activation in small vessels and recruitment of neutrophilic granulocytes via Fc-IgG receptor interaction leads to a local vascular inflammation. Type IVa reactions correspond to Th1 reactions with high IFNγ/TNFα secretion, and involve monocyte/macrophage activation. CD8 cell recruitment (type IVc reaction) often occurs. Type IVb reactions correspond to eosinophilic inflammation and to a Th2 response with high IL-4/IL-5/IL-13 secretion; they are often associated with an IgE-mediated type I reaction. Type IVc reactions: the cytotoxic reactions (by CD4 and CD8 cells) rely on cytotoxic T cells as effector cells (type IVc). They seem to occur in all drug-related delayed hypersensitivity reactions. Type IVd reactions correspond to a T-cell–dependent, sterile neutrophilic inflammatory reaction. It is distinct from the rapid influx of polymorphonuclear cells (PMN) in bacterial infections. It seems to be related to high CXCL-8/GM-CSF production by T cells (and tissue cells). (From Pichler WJ. Drug hypersensitivity: classification and relationship to T-cell activation. In: Pichler WJ, editor. Drug hypersensitivity. Basel (Switzerland): Karger; 2007. p. 168–89; with permission.)

orchestrate different forms of inflammation; or as effector T cells mediating cytotoxicity. Based on these findings, as well as studies of immune reactions to drugs in vitro and in vivo, a refined subclassification of T-cell–meditated type IV reactions was developed. It considers the distinct cytokine production by T cells, and thus incorporates the well-accepted Th1/Th2 distinction of T cells; it includes the cytotoxic activity of CD4 and CD8 T cells (IVc); and it emphasizes the participation of different effector cells such as monocytes (IVa), eosinophils (IVb), or neutrophils (IVd), which are the cells causing inflammation and tissue damage.[7]

Type IVa reactions correspond to Th1-type immune reactions: Th1-type T cells activate macrophages by secreting large amounts of interferon-γ, drive the production of complement-fixing antibody isotypes involved in type II and III reactions (IgG1, IgG3), and are costimulatory for proinflammatory responses (tumor necrosis factor, IL-12) and CD8+ T-cell responses. The T cells promote these reactions by IFNγ secretion and possibly other cytokines (eg, TNFα, IL-18). An in vivo correlate would be a monocyte activation (eg, in skin tests to tuberculin or even granuloma formation, as seen in sarcoidosis), but Th1 cells are also known to help in the activation of CD8 cells, which might explain the common combination of IVa and IVc reactions (eg, in contact dermatitis).

Type IVb corresponds to the Th2-type immune response. Th2 T cells secrete the cytokines IL-4, IL-13 and IL-5, which promote B-cell production of IgE and IgG4, macrophage deactivation, and mast cell and eosinophil responses: The high production of the Th2 cytokine IL-5 leads to an eosinophilic inflammation, which is the characteristic inflammatory cell type in many drug hypersensitivity reactions.[7] In addition, there is a link to type I reactions, as Th2 cells boost IgE production by IL-4/IL-13 secretion. An in vivo correlate might be an eosinophil-rich maculopapular exanthem but also infestations with nematodes, or an allergic inflammation of the bronchi or nasal mucosa (asthma and rhinitis).

In type IVc reactions, T cells can themselves act as effector cells. They emigrate to the tissue and can kill tissue cells such as hepatocytes or keratinocytes in a perforin/granzymeB-, granulysin-, and FasL-dependent manner (**Fig. 5**).[27,43,44] Such reactions occur in most drug-induced delayed hypersensitivity reactions, usually together with other type IV reactions (monocyte, eosinophil, or PMN recruitment and activation). Cytotoxic T cells thus play a role in maculopapular or bullous skin diseases (with high granulysin production) as well as in neutrophilic inflammations (eg, acute generalized exanthematous pustulosis [AGEP]), and in contact dermatitis. Type IVc reactions seem to be dominant in bullous skin reactions, in which activated CD8+ T cells kill keratinocytes,[7,43,44] but they may also be the dominant cell type in hepatitis or nephritis.[27]

Type IVd reactions involve the new concept that T cells can also coordinate (sterile) neutrophilic inflammations.[45] Typical examples would be sterile neutrophilic inflammations of the skin, in particular AGEP. In this disease, CXCL8 and granulocyte-macrophage colony-stimulating factor (GM-CSF)–producing T cells recruit neutrophilic leukocytes via CXCL8 release, and prevent their apoptosis via GM-CSF release.[46] In addition to AGEP, such T-cell reactions are also found in Behçet disease and pustular psoriasis.[47] To what extent the cytokine IL-17, associated with neutrophilic inflammations, is involved in these reactions is not yet clear.

Tolerance Mechanism

Most patients can take drugs without developing immune-mediated side effects. It could be argued that these patients lack precursor cells able to interact with the drug. However, the great heterogeneity of the immune response to drugs,[7] a high precursor frequency in sensitized patients,[48] and the finding that 2% to 4% of the normal population, but 30% to more than 50% of human immunodeficiency virus–infected patients may react with SMX suggest that, rather than a lack of precursor cells, other factors such as the underlying immune status (preactivation of memory

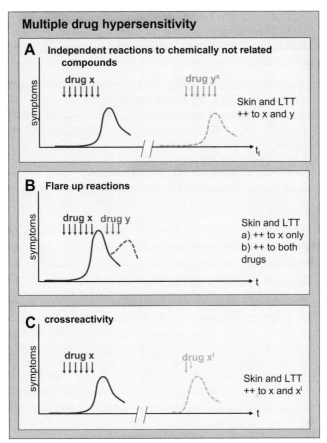

Fig. 5. True multiple drug hypersensitivities, flare-up reactions, and cross-reactivities. Immune-mediated multiple drug hypersensitivities can be attributed to different mechanisms: (*A*) 2 structurally distinct drugs elicit a separate immune response and sometimes also different clinical symptoms. The sensitization may occur separately or during the same time span and simultaneous treatments. This response corresponds to a true multiple drug hypersensitivity. (*B*) so-called flare-up reactions are due to massive immune stimulation during a drug allergy: the preexisting drug allergy is a risk factor for a second reaction: if, because of the prior drug hypersensitivity, the drug is changed, the second drug may cause a transient aggravation of preexisting symptoms. This reaction is often interpreted as second drug allergy, but the second drug is usually (but not always) tolerated again later. (*C*) Structurally related drugs can cause reappearance of symptoms due to cross-reactivity. The second reactions occur more rapidly. (*From* Pichler WJ. Drug hypersensitivity: classification and relationship to T-cell activation. In: Pichler WJ, editor. Drug hypersensitivity. Basel (Switzerland): Karger; 2007. p. 168–89; with permission.)

T cells) and regulatory mechanisms may be important. Thereby regulation may occur on different levels. At present, these regulatory mechanism in immune responses to small molecules are not yet well understood: in DRESS and SJS/TEN, Treg cells were investigated: they were expanded during acute DRESS, but contracted after resolution, leading to an enhanced response to more drugs, as well as to autoimmunity.[49] In contrast, the functional defects of Tregs in TEN were restored on recovery. Further work is needed, but the frequently observed multiple-drug hypersensitivity syndrome after DRESS may be explained by this Treg defect. Tolerance mechanisms to drugs are[c]

1. Ignorance: even if drugs bind to immune receptors, the interaction (affinity, surface contact) is too weak to elicit a significant reaction
2. Lack of danger signals and preactivation: the hapten-carrier complexes do not sufficiently stimulate the innate immunity, which is necessary to develop a primary immune response. Or, in the case of the p-i concept, TCR stimulation by the drug is not sufficient to induce cytokine production and proliferation, because the T cells are not sufficiently preactivated to react to this signal
3. Regulatory T cells may be insufficiently activated in some patients, making them prone to react to small chemical compounds. These patients may have multiple drug allergies and may also suffer from autoimmunity
4. The liver as a tolerogenic organ: the generation of reactive metabolites in the liver may induce tolerance, which might prevent the development of an immune reaction to the drug in the periphery.

Clinical Symptoms of T-cell–mediated Reactions

The most frequent manifestations of drug allergies are delayed cutaneous reactions; so-called rashes. Rashes comprise a broad spectrum of clinical and distinct histopathological features that usually appear between 6 hours and 10 days after drug intake. The skin is most often affected during drug hypersensitivity, but liver involvement is common if moderate elevations of liver enzymes are considered (they are often attributed to a toxic effect of the drug, but may be immune mediated). Other organs such as kidney, lung, and pancreas may also be involved. (For details of the clinical symptoms see the articles by Harr and colleagues and Scherrer and colleagues elsewhere in this issue for further exploration of this topic).

Multiple drug hypersensitivity syndrome and flare-up reactions
The term multiple drug hypersensitivity is widely used for different side effects to various drugs: it is used to characterize patients with multiple drug intolerance (pseudoallergy to various, structurally distinct NSAID, and so forth); others reserve this term for well-documented repeated immune-mediated reactions to structurally unrelated drugs.[50] Cross-reactivity due to structural similarity is not included.

In our experience, about 10% of patients with well-documented drug hypersensitivity (positive skin or lymphocyte transformation test) have multiple drug allergies[51]: they may have reacted to an injected lidocain with a massive angioedema; years later the same patient develops an allergy to corticosteroids. Both drugs are positive in skin and lymphocyte transformation tests. Alternatively, a patient reacts to amoxicillin, phenytoin, and SMX within a few months, but with different symptoms (maculopapular exanthema [MPE], drug-induced hypersensitivity syndrome [DiHS]/DRESS, erythrodermia). Most patients with multiple drug hypersensitivity have had severe reactions to at least 1 drug. An IgE-mediated reaction might be followed by a T-cell–mediated reaction. The pathomechanism of this syndrome is unknown, but it

---

[c] *From* Pichler WJ. Drug hypersensitivity: classification and relationship to T cell activation. In: Pichler WJ, editor. Drug hypersensitivity. Basel (Switzerland): Karger; 2007. p. 168–89; with permission.

is tempting to speculate that the tolerance mechanism to small molecular compounds fail in these patients (see **Fig. 5**).

An immune reaction to a drug, via a hapten or p-i mechanism, can be seen as a failure of tolerance, and the same patient might not only develop other drug allergies but also autoimmunity.[49] Preliminary data suggest that a previous drug allergy might be a risk factor for the development of a delayed hypersensitivity reaction to contrast media.[33]

Multiple drug hypersensitivity should be differentiated from flare-up reactions and true cross-reactivity (see **Fig. 5**). Flare-up reactions are clinically important and frequent: patients with systemic drug allergies show a massive activation of their immune system,[52] similar to acute viral infections. This immune activation may make existing drug allergies risk factors for future drug allergies (see earlier discussion). Flare-up reactions occur when, as a result of an existing drug allergy, drug therapy is changed to a new drug: the second drug may then exacerbate the existing drug allergy (more symptoms of exanthema, increased alanine aminotransferase [ALAT], and fever after 1 or 2 days), and it is often confused with a new drug allergy. Such flare-up reactions are common in severe reactions such as DiHS/DRESS (see earlier discussion). With some exceptions,[27] they are normally not dangerous. The mechanism is unclear, but possibly related to the p-i concept explained earlier: the second drug may not have caused its own, specific immune reaction, but the drug may still bind to the immune receptors of preactivated T cells, and thus briefly augment the symptoms. However, later, in remission, the second drug may again be tolerated, as the costimulatory conditions no longer exist. However, there are also accounts of sensitizations to the second drug, which occurred during the DRESS/DiHS disease.

SUMMARY

Small chemical compounds can interact with the immune system in 2 ways: by forming hapten-carrier complexes, which can stimulate innate and adaptive immunity (T and B cells) and cause localized or systemic reactions due to an immune response against the hapten-carrier complex; alternatively, chemicals that are unable to form covalent bonds can directly interact with proteins by van der Waals and other forces. Some of these labile interactions occur with immune receptors (pharmacologic interaction with immune receptors, p-i concept). Because the immune system offers more than 10^{12} different TCR and a few hundred MHC molecules, some of these drug-protein interactions are affine enough to elicit signaling in the receptor-bearing T cell. The type of immune response may differ as a function of the primary interaction of the drug with a particular MHC class I molecule or with the TCR. Full activation of the reactive T cell always requires TCR interaction with the MHC molecule. The consequence of the hapten and p-i mechanisms are drug-allergic diseases, which can appear within minutes to hours. They are mainly caused by mast cell degranulation due to drug-specific IgE or by a direct effect of the drug on mast cells. Delayed reactions start after 6 hours; some even after many days. Delayed reactions become manifest as different types of exanthems, with or without internal involvement, in which the function of drug-specific T cells and their cytokines regulate the type of allergic reaction. This process leads to the further subclassification of type IV reactions as types IVa, IVb, IVc, and IVd, corresponding to T-cell reactions with monocyte/DC (IVa), eosinophil (IVb), cytotoxic T cell (IVc), and neutrophil (IVd) activations.

662   Pichler et al

REFERENCES

1. Naisbitt DJ, Gordon SF, Pirmohamed M, et al. Immunological principles of adverse drug reactions: the initiation and propagation of immune responses elicited by drug treatment. Drug Saf 2000;23:483–507.
2. Lazarou J, Pomeranz BH, Corey PN. Incidence of adverse drug reactions in hospitalized patients: a meta-analysis of prospective studies. JAMA 1998;279:1200–5.
3. Roujeau JC, Stern RS. Severe adverse cutaneous reactions to drugs. N Engl J Med 1994;331:1272–85.
4. Bigby M, Jick S, Jick H, et al. Drug-induced cutaneous reactions. A report from the Boston Collaborative Drug Surveillance Program on 15,438 consecutive inpatients, 1975 to 1982. JAMA 1986;256:3358–63.
5. Hunziker T, Kunzi UP, Braunschweig S, et al. Comprehensive hospital drug monitoring (CHDM): adverse skin reactions, a 20-year survey. Allergy 1997;52:388–93.
6. Manfredi M, Severino M, Testi S, et al. Detection of specific IgE to quinolones. J Allergy Clin Immunol 2004;113:155–60.
7. Pichler WJ. Drug hypersensitivity: classification and relationship to T cell activation. In: Pichler WJ, editor. Drug hypersensitivity. Basel (Switzerland): Karger; 2007. p. 168–89.
8. Griem P, Wulferink M, Sachs B, et al. Allergic and autoimmune reactions to xenobiotics: how do they arise? Immunol Today 1998;19:133–41.
9. Sanderson JP, Naisbitt DJ, Farrell J, et al. Sulfamethoxazole and its metabolite nitroso sulfamethoxazole stimulate dendritic cell costimulatory signaling. J Immunol 2007;178:5533–42.
10. Schnyder B, Mauri-Hellweg D, Zanni M, et al. Direct, MHC-dependent presentation of the drug sulfamethoxazole to human alphabeta T cell clones. J Clin Invest 1997;100:136–41.
11. Zanni MP, von Greyerz S, Schnyder B, et al. HLA-restricted, processing- and metabolism-independent pathway of drug recognition by human alpha beta T lymphocytes. J Clin Invest 1998;102:1591–8.
12. Pichler WJ. Pharmacological interaction of drugs with antigen-specific immune receptors: the p-i concept. Curr Opin Allergy Clin Immunol 2002;2:301–5.
13. Pichler WJ. Direct T-cell stimulations by drugs–bypassing the innate immune system. Toxicology 2005;209:95–100.
14. Sieben S, Kawakubo Y, Al Masaoudi T, et al. Delayed-type hypersensitivity reaction to paraphenylenediamine is mediated by 2 different pathways of antigen recognition by specific alphabeta human T-cell clones. J Allergy Clin Immunol 2002;109:1005–11.
15. Naisbitt DJ, Britschgi M, Wong G, et al. Hypersensitivity reactions to carbamazepine: characterization of the specificity, phenotype, and cytokine profile of drug-specific T cell clones. Mol Pharmacol 2003;63:732–41.
16. Wu Y, Farrell J, Pirmohamed M, et al. Generation and characterization of antigen-specific CD4+, CD8+, and CD4+CD8+ T-cell clones from patients with carbamazepine hypersensitivity. J Allergy Clin Immunol 2007;119:973–81.
17. Keller M, Lerch M, Britschgi M, et al. Processing-dependent and -independent pathways for recognition of iodinated contrast media by specific human T cells. Clin Exp Allergy 2010;40(2):257–68.

18. Burkhart C, Britschgi M, Strasser I, et al. Non-covalent presentation of sulfame-thoxazole to human CD4+ T cells is independent of distinct human leucocyte antigen-bound peptides. Clin Exp Allergy 2002;32:1635–43.
19. von Greyerz S, Bultemann G, Schnyder K, et al. Degeneracy and additional allor-eactivity of drug-specific human alpha beta(+) T cell clones. Int Immunol 2001; 13:877–85.
20. Tassaneeyakul W, Jantararoungtong T, Chen P, et al. Strong association between HLA-B*5801 and allopurinol-induced Stevens-Johnson syndrome and toxic epidermal necrolysis in a Thai population. Pharmacogenet Genomics 2009;19: 704–9.
21. Man CB, Kwan P, Baum L, et al. Association between HLA-B*1502 allele and anti-epileptic drug-induced cutaneous reactions in Han Chinese. Epilepsia 2007;48: 1015–8.
22. Hetherington S, Hughes AR, Mosteller M, et al. Genetic variations in HLA-B region and hypersensitivity reactions to abacavir. Lancet 2002;359:1121–2.
23. Mallal S, Nolan D, Witt C, et al. Association between presence of HLA-B*5701, HLA-DR7, and HLA-DQ3 and hypersensitivity to HIV-1 reverse-transcriptase inhibitor abacavir. Lancet 2002;359:727–32.
24. Chessman D, Kostenko L, Lethborg T, et al. Human leukocyte antigen class I-restricted activation of CD8+ T cells provides the immunogenetic basis of a systemic drug hypersensitivity. Immunity 2008;28:822–32.
25. Yang L, Chen J, He L. Harvesting candidate genes responsible for serious adverse drug reactions from a chemical-protein interactome. PLoS Comput Biol 2009;5:e1000441.
26. Yang CW, Hung SI, Juo CG, et al. HLA-B*1502-bound peptides: implications for the pathogenesis of carbamazepine-induced Stevens-Johnson syndrome. J Allergy Clin Immunol 2007;120:870–7.
27. Mennicke M, Zawodniak A, Keller M, et al. Fulminant liver failure after vancomycin in a sulfasalazine-induced DRESS syndrome: fatal recurrence after liver trans-plantation. Am J Transplant 2009;9:2197–202.
28. Coombs PR, Gell PG. Classification of allergic reactions responsible for clinical hypersensitivity and disease. In: Gell RR, editor. Clinical aspects of immunology. Oxford (UK): Oxford University Press; 1968. p. 575–96.
29. Riezzo I, Bello S, Neri M, et al. Ceftriaxone intradermal test-related fatal anaphy-lactic shock: a medico-legal nightmare. Allergy 2010;65:130–1.
30. Christensen LH, Holm J, Lund G, et al. Several distinct properties of the IgE repertoire determine effector cell degranulation in response to allergen chal-lenge. J Allergy Clin Immunol 2008;122:298–304.
31. Pumphrey R. Anaphylaxis: can we tell who is at risk of a fatal reaction? Curr Opin Allergy Clin Immunol 2004;4:285–90.
32. Mertes PM, Lambert M, Gueant-Rodriguez RM, et al. Perioperative anaphylaxis. Immunol Allergy Clin North Am 2009;29:429–51.
33. Brockow K, Romano A, Aberer W, et al. Skin testing in patients with hypersensi-tivity reactions to iodinated contrast media - a European multicenter study. Allergy 2009;64:234–41.
34. Florvaag E, Johansson SG. The pholcodine story. Immunol Allergy Clin North Am 2009;29:419–27.
35. Baldo BA, Fisher MM, Pham NH. On the origin and specificity of antibodies to neuromuscular blocking (muscle relaxant) drugs: an immunochemical perspec-tive. Clin Exp Allergy 2009;39:325–44.

36. Castells M. Rapid desensitization for hypersensitivity reactions to medications. Immunol Allergy Clin North Am 2009;29:585–606.

37. Sampson HA, Munoz-Furlong A, Campbell RL, et al. Second symposium on the definition and management of anaphylaxis: summary report–Second National Institute of Allergy and Infectious Disease/Food Allergy and Anaphylaxis Network symposium. J Allergy Clin Immunol 2006;117:391–7.

38. Pumphrey RS. Fatal anaphylaxis in the UK, 1992–2001. Novartis Found Symp 2004;257:116–28 [discussion: 28–32, 57–60, 276–85].

39. Tramer MR, von Elm E, Loubeyre P, et al. Pharmacological prevention of serious anaphylactic reactions due to iodinated contrast media: systematic review. BMJ 2006;333:675.

40. Aitman TJ, Dong R, Vyse TJ, et al. Copy number polymorphism in Fcgr3 predisposes to glomerulonephritis in rats and humans. Nature 2006;439:851–5.

41. Stokol T, O'Donnell P, Xiao L, et al. C1q governs deposition of circulating immune complexes and leukocyte Fcgamma receptors mediate subsequent neutrophil recruitment. J Exp Med 2004;200:835–46.

42. Pichler WJ. Adverse side-effects to biological agents. Allergy 2006;61:912–20.

43. Nassif A, Bensussan A, Dorothee G, et al. Drug specific cytotoxic T-cells in the skin lesions of a patient with toxic epidermal necrolysis. J Invest Dermatol 2002;118:728–33.

44. Schnyder B, Frutig K, Mauri-Hellweg D, et al. T-cell-mediated cytotoxicity against keratinocytes in sulfamethoxazol-induced skin reaction. Clin Exp Allergy 1998;28: 1412–7.

45. Britschgi M, Steiner UC, Schmid S, et al. T-cell involvement in drug-induced acute generalized exanthematous pustulosis. J Clin Invest 2001;107:1433–41.

46. Schaerli P, Britschgi M, Keller M, et al. Characterization of human T cells that regulate neutrophilic skin inflammation. J Immunol 2004;173:2151–8.

47. Keller M, Spanou Z, Schaerli P, et al. T cell-regulated neutrophilic inflammation in autoinflammatory diseases. J Immunol 2005;175:7678–86.

48. Beeler A, Engler O, Gerber BO, et al. Long-lasting reactivity and high frequency of drug-specific T cells after severe systemic drug hypersensitivity reactions. J Allergy Clin Immunol 2006;117:455–62.

49. Takahashi R, Kano Y, Yamazaki Y, et al. Defective regulatory T cells in patients with severe drug eruptions: timing of the dysfunction is associated with the pathological phenotype and outcome. J Immunol 2009;182:8071–9.

50. Sullivan T. Studies of the multiple drug allergy syndrome. J Allergy Clin Immunol 1989;83:270.

51. Gex-Collet C, Helbling A, Pichler WJ. Multiple drug hypersensitivity–proof of multiple drug hypersensitivity by patch and lymphocyte transformation tests. J Investig Allergol Clin Immunol 2005;15:293–6.

52. Hari Y, Frutig-Schnyder K, Hurni M, et al. T cell involvement in cutaneous drug eruptions. Clin Exp Allergy 2001;31:1398–408.

Table 2
Classifying drug hypersensitivity: immediate reaction or non–immediate reaction

	Immediate Reaction (Presumably Mast Cell Meditated)	Nonimmediate Reaction (Presumably T-cell Meditated)
Time Between Exposure and Onset of the Reaction	≤1 h (in special conditions like intolerance to acetylsalicylic acid, ≤3 h)	≥6 h (in the case of strong T-cell sensitization, earlier)
Time of Recovery	Few hours	Several days to weeks
Clinical Nature of the Reaction	Urticaria, angioedema, anaphylaxis	Maculopapular exanthema and other skin manifestations including late-appearing urticarial rash and angioedema, disorders of blood cells, systemic reactions such as drug rash with eosinophilia and systemic symptoms (DRESS), conditions such as hepatitis, nephritis

(nonimmune mediated hypersensitivities). Pseudoallergic reactions tend to arise later after drug administration (within 1–3 hours) and do require a higher dose than IgE-mediated allergies. In susceptible persons, many active drug substances can elicit such reactions. Typical inducers are mentioned in **Table 4**.

It has been a dogma that allergic reactions to drugs are only those that are observed on reexposure or on longer-lasting exposure (at least 3 days). However, more recent data suggest that a previous contact to the causative drug is not an obligatory prerequisite for immune-mediated drug hypersensitivity. In patients with cetuximab-induced anaphylaxis, IgE antibodies were found already in pretreatment samples.[9] The antibodies were shown to be specific for galactose-α-1,3-galactose, which is present on the Fab portion of the cetuximab heavy chain and is also very similar to substances in the ABO blood group. Further examples are anaphylaxis to neuromuscular blocking agents (NMBAs) in anesthesia, which occurs in more than 50% of the events at first exposure, but is still often skin test positive, compatible with an IgE-mediated mechanism.[10] Quarternary ammonium compounds in antitussives (pholcodin) or cosmetics have been implied in silently occurring sensitizations to these NMBA.[11] Even

Table 3
Differential diagnosis of the most frequent cutaneous drug eruptions

IgE-Mediated Urticaria	• Pseudoallergy and other nonimmune-mediated mast cell degranulations (eg, Aspirin, opiates) • Viral infections • Connective tissue disease
T-cell Meditated Maculopapular Exanthema	• Viral and bacterial infections (eg, syphilis) • Generalized eczema • Connective tissue disease • Cutaneous lymphoma • Graft-versus host disease • Skin toxicity (eg, chemotherapy) • Cytokine dysbalance (eg, tumor necrosis factor blockers) • Superantigen stimulations (Kawasaki syndrome, staphylococcal scaled skin syndrome)

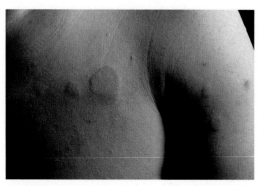

Fig. 1. Drug-induced urticaria.

anaphylaxis to contrast media may also sometimes be IgE mediated,[12,13] although the cross-reactive sensitizing compound is unknown.

Nonimmediate Type Hypersensitivity Reactions

Nonimmediate reactions are those that occur more than 1 hour after the last drug administration. However, there is a certain overlap in the time of manifestations; some IgE-mediated reactions may occur after 1 hour, whereas some nonimmediate reactions may start before 1 hour. Nonimmediate drug allergies are most frequently T-cell mediated, whereas IgG-mediated responses are rare. Nonimmediate drug allergies may clinically manifest as a broad spectrum of diseases.

The most frequent type B reactions are maculopapular or morbilliform exanthema, accounting for up to 90% of all drug-induced cutaneous eruptions.[4] The lesions often appear initially on the trunk and subsequently spread to the extremities in a symmetric fashion. Lesions consist of erythematous macules and infiltrated papules and are often morbilliform, rubelliform, or scarlatiniform (**Fig. 2**). Pruritus and mild fever may be present. Skin lesions usually appear more than 2 days after the drug has been started, mainly around day 8 to 11, and occasionally persists 2 to 3 days after having stopped the drug. The rash usually lasts for 1 to 2 weeks and clears with cessation of the causative drug. Typically, a more or less pronounced desquamation occurs after clearing of the lesions. A large body of experimental and clinical data indicate that such rashes often correspond to T-cell mediated (type IV) hypersensitivities.

Other less frequent nonimmediate type cutaneous hypersensitivity reactions include fixed drug eruption, symmetric drug-related intertriginous and flexural exanthema, acute generalized exanthematous pustulosis, and bullous exanthema (see the article

| Table 4 | | |
Immediate reactions and typically involved drugs		
IgE-Mediated Reaction	β-Lactam antibiotics, quinolones, sulfonamide antibiotics, macrolides, pyrazolones, chlorhexidine, neuromuscular blocking agents,[a] contrast medium,[a] protein-based therapeutics, including biologicals	
Pseudoallergic Reactions	Acetylsalicylic acid and other nonsteroidal antiinflammatory drugs, plasma volume expander (colloids), neuromuscular blocking agents,[a] contrast medium[a]	

[a] Drugs which can induce IgE-mediated or pseudoallergic reactions.

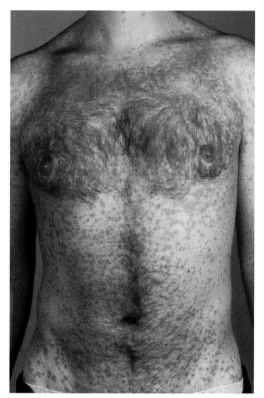

Fig. 2. Maculopapular or morbilliform exanthema.

by Harr and French in this issue for further exploration of this topic). There are other various nonimmediate type hypersensitivity reactions in which skin involvement is not predominant or is even absent. Drugs which are typically involved in such infrequent nonimmediate reactions are mentioned in **Table 5**.

Drug-induced hypersensitivity syndrome

This term is synonymous with drug-related eosinophilia with systemic symptoms (DRESSs) or drug hypersensitivity syndrome. It is a severe systemic disease. Typical signs and symptoms are a macular exanthema, an erythematous centrofacial swelling, fever, general malaise, lymph-node swelling, and involvement of other organs: hepatitis (50%), nephritis (10%), and more rarely pneumonitis, colitis, and pancreatitis.[14] The type of organ involvement seems to depend on the type of drug causing DRESS.[15] For example, minocycline-induced DRESS is associated with lymphadenopathy, whereas allopurinol-induced DRESS has renal insufficiency. More than 70% of patients with DRESS show a marked eosinophilia (often >1 g/L), and activated T cells are often found in the circulation. Importantly, signs and symptoms can start up to 12 weeks after start of the treatment, often after increasing the dose. Signs and symptoms may persist and recur for many weeks even after cessation of drug treatment. The lethality is about 10% and is mainly because of liver failure. A recurrence of symptoms, often in the third week, is typical. It is related to reactivation of herpes viruses, in particular human herpes virus 6, Epstein-Barr virus, or cytomegalovirus.

Table 5
Nonimmediate reactions and typically involved drugs

Hemolytic Anemia	Methyldopa, levodopa, interferon-α, cyclosporin, and fludarabine
Leucopenia	Aminopyrine and dipyrone, thyroid inhibitors, co-trimoxazole, sulfasalazine, clomipramine
Thrombopenia	Heparin, quinine, quinidine, therapeutic antibodies (biologicals)
Serum Sickness Syndrome	β-Lactam antibiotics
Drug-Induced Lupus	Hydralazine, procainamide, quinidine, minocycline, anti-TNF-α agents, carbamazepine, terbinafine, and isoniazid
Vasculitis	Sulfonamide antibiotics and diuretics
MPE	β-Lactam antibiotics, sulfonamide antibiotics, macrolides, quinolones, diuretics and others
Fixed Drug Eruption	Phenytoin, sulfonamide antibiotics, tetracycline, barbiturates
SDRIFE	β-Lactam antibiotics, mercury
AGEP	Aminopenicillins, cephalosporins, macrolides sulfonamide antibiotics, celecoxib, diltiazem, quinolone, diltiazem, terbinafine, corticosteroids
SJS and TEN	Allopurinol, phenytoin, carbamazepine, lamotrigine, co-trimoxazole, barbiturate, NSAID (oxicams), sertraline, pantoprazole, tramadol, nevirapine
DRESS	Carbamazepine, phenytoin, lamotrigine, minocycline, allopurinol, dapsone, sulfasalazine, co-trimoxazole, abacavir (without eosinophilia)

Abbreviations: AGEP, acute generalized exanthematous pustulosis; DRESS, drug rash with eosinophilia and systemic symptoms; MPE, maculopapular exanthema; NSAID, nonsteroidal antiinflammatory drug; SDRIFE, symmetric drug-related intertriginous and flexural exanthema; SJS, Stevens-Johnson syndrome; TEN, toxic epidermal necrolysis; TNF, tumor necrosis factor.

Japanese researchers have proposed diagnostic criteria for the diagnosis of DRESS, a disease often still not recognized[16]:

- Maculopapular rash developing more than 3 weeks after starting with a limited number of drugs
- Prolonged clinical symptoms after discontinuation of the causative drug
- Fever (>38°C)
- Liver abnormalities (alanine aminotransferase >100 U/L) or other organ involvement
- Leukocyte abnormalities (at least 1 present):
  Leukocytosis (>11 × 10^9 cells per liter)
  Atypical lymphocytosis (>5%)
  Eosinophilia (>1.5 × 10^9 cells per liter)
- Lymphadenopathy
- Human herpesvirus 6 reactivation (detected during the second to third week after start of symptoms).

The presence of all these 7 criteria confirms the diagnosis for typical drug-induced hypersensitivity syndrome (DiHS); the presence of 5^{1-5} for atypical DiHS.

Interstitial nephritis
Some drugs, in particular β-lactam antibiotics, proton-pump-inhibitor, sulfonamide antibiotics, disulfiram nonsteroidal antiinflammatory drug (NSAID), can cause

interstitial nephritis.[17] Sometimes manifestations of drug-induced interstitial nephritis are associated with an exanthema, but often the symptoms start insidiously. Lower back pain and malaise may be the only symptoms, until renal insufficiency is discovered.

Cytopenia
Drug-induced cytopenia may be mediated by IgG antibodies and may manifest as hemolytic anemia or an unexpected precipitous fall in the peripheral leukocyte count.

Serum sickness syndrome
Fever, arthralgia, macular and urticarial exanthema, lymphadenopathy, and sometimes edema are the classic clinical manifestations of serum sickness. In the past, the widespread use of heterologous serum frequently produced the full serum sickness syndrome 1 to 3 weeks after antiserum administration. At present, nonprotein drugs such as penicillins and cephalosporins are the most common causes of serum sickness, with a latency period of 6 to 8 hours. Drug-induced serum sickness is usually self-limited, with symptoms lasting 1 to 2 weeks before resolving.

Drug-induced lupus erythematosus
Typical clinical symptoms of drug-induced lupus erythematosus (DILE) are sudden onset of fever, malaise, myalgia, arthralgia and arthritis, several weeks after drug initiation. The skin is affected in about 25% of cases. Characteristic is an erythematous eruption occurring often on light-exposed surfaces. The average age of patients with DILE is nearly twice that of patients with idiopathic systemic lupus erythematosus (SLE). Approximately half the patients with drug-induced SLE are women compared with 90% of patients with idiopathic SLE. Similar to idiopathic lupus, DILE can be divided into systemic, subacute cutaneous and chronic cutaneous lupus. The clinical and laboratory manifestations of drug-induced SLE are similar to those of idiopathic SLE, but central nervous system and renal involvement are rare in DILE. Recognition of DILE is important because it usually reverts spontaneously within a few weeks after stopping the drug.[18]

Vasculitis
Drugs may rarely elicit cutaneous or systemic vasculitis with an incidence of 10 to 30 cases per million people per year. Typical clinical manifestations are palpable purpuric papules predominantly of the legs. However, sometimes drug-induced vasculitis manifests as clinical syndromes indistinguishable from classic systemic forms of vasculitis, such as Wegener granulomatosis, polyarteritis nodosa, or Churg-Strauss syndrome. Withdrawal of the offending agent alone is often sufficient to induce prompt resolution of clinical manifestations, without need for systemic therapy.[19]

DIAGNOSIS AND MANAGEMENT DURING THE FLORID PHASE OF AN ADR
Diagnosis

Whenever a patient treated with a drug develops an exacerbation or a new medical problem, an ADR should be included in the differential diagnosis. In case of a hypersensitivity reaction, it is essential to identify the underlying mechanism and the causative drug. Immune-mediated drug hypersensitivity reactions and their causative drugs can be suspected by the constellation of exposure, timing, the previously described patterns of organ manifestations, and underlying conditions. There is no single standardized diagnostic test that allows confirming a drug allergy. For the diagnostic approach regarding drug-induced type B reactions, a comprehensive investigation is important. This investigation includes the evaluation for fever, lymphadenopathy, and manifestations of the skin and mucous membranes and laboratory investigations.

Initial questions on clinical assessment include the following:

- Which active drug substances and xenobiotics are involved (including phytodrugs)?
- What is the temporal relationship between exposure to each drug and onset of the reaction?
- Since when has the drug been taken? Most drug allergies occur in the first 2 weeks; some drugs, particularly those causing internal involvement, cause symptoms within the first 2 to 3 months of treatment. Drugs taken for years are very improbable causes for drug allergies. However, some reactions may appear after intermission or dose increase.
- What is the nature of the reaction? Does it correspond to known adverse reactions to (one of) the involved drugs?
- Are other drugs administered concurrently that could have caused the reaction?
- Are there any underlying conditions of the patient that could explain the reaction (eg, infections, food)?
- If the reaction occurred in the past, did the reaction resolve after cessation of the drug (and if so, how long did the recovery take)?
- Has a similar reaction occurred to the same drug in the family? What is the genetic background of the patient? Recent findings show a strong genetic association between HLA alleles and the susceptibility to drug-specific immune-mediated hypersensitivity: HLA-B5701 is associated with abacavir hypersensitivity; HLA-B5801 with allopurinol-induced severe cutaneous adverse reactions, including the DRESS, Stevens-Johnson syndrome (SJS), and toxic epidermal necrolysis (TEN); and HLA-B1502 with carbamazepine-induced SJS and TEN, but not with maculopapular exanthema (MPE). Carbamazepine-SJS/TEN associated with HLA-B1502 is seen in Southeast Asians but not in Caucasians.[20]

The answers to these questions may allow speculation regarding mechanism and causative drugs. The suspected diagnosis can be supported by laboratory investigations. In immediate reactions and especially anaphylactic episodes, measurements of total tryptase in serum 60 to 240 minutes after onset of symptoms is helpful. An increase in the level of tryptase can be quantified as soon as 30 minutes after onset of symptoms. The half-life of tryptase is about 120 minutes. To enable comparison with baseline levels, a new sample should be collected more than 2 days after the reaction.[21] A transient increase of serum tryptase (even only doubling of baseline values, but still below the cut-off value) indicates an involvement of mast cells. However, the sensitivity of determining the serum tryptase is still rather low, and normal values can neither exclude an anaphylaxis nor allow differentiating between immunologic and nonimmunologic mast cell activation.

During the acute phase of nonimmediate reactions, the finding of an eosinophilia supports the diagnosis of an immune-mediated hypersensitivity reaction. Additional laboratory investigations may determine the severity of reaction and the involvement of internal organs (eg, increased level of liver enzymes). For atypical skin lesions, a biopsy with histologic examination may help to recognize or exclude an important differential diagnosis.

In the rare cases in which an IgG-mediated mechanism (type II or III reaction) is suspected, the direct antiglobulin test (Coombs test) may support diagnosing immune hemolytic anemia, leading to further detailed analyses, often requiring close collaboration of different disciplines.[22] Assessment of complement levels (C3, C4, CH50), possibly of complement split products reflecting a complement activation, and of immune complexes (C1q binding or Raji cell assays) can support the diagnosis in cases with serum sickness syndrome, but negative values are frequent and do not rule out immune hemolytic anemia.

Various signs and symptoms of drug allergy are described as potential early danger signals.[23] They are listed in **Table 6**. Even though the predictive value of these signs have not been investigated prospectively, it is prudent to take heed of them.

Treatment

Treatment for immediate type hypersensitivity reactions

The causative or presumably causative drugs should immediately be withdrawn. In mild reactions with urticaria only, slow intravenous administration of antihistamines are the primary recommended treatment. However, antihistamines cannot antagonize histamine that has already been bound to H1 receptors, and they do not have an effect on other mediators such as leukotrienes and platelet activating factor.[24] Thus in immediate reactions with danger signals (see **Table 6**), angioedema, respiratory symptoms, or circulatory signs indicating an anaphylaxis, epinephrine (10 µg/kg) should be administered promptly via the intramuscular route in the anterolateral thigh. Glucocorticoids, when given in pharmacologic quantities, have an antiinflammatory effect and may reduce the risk of late relapse.[25] However, the onset of action of glucocorticoids is slow (>45 minutes), as it depends on new gene products.

Treatment for nonimmediate type hypersensitivity reactions

During systemic T-cell mediated drug allergies, patients are more susceptible to react nonspecifically to different xenobiotics. Thus, withdrawal of the causative, potentially causative, and not urgently needed drug is prudent. However, there are some exceptions to this rule. In late-occurring MPE in the absence of cutaneous danger signals (see **Table 6**), urgently required treatment may be continued. Such "treating through" requires monitoring for mucosal or systemic involvement (fever, eosinophilia, lymphadenopathia, hepatitis).

Mild nonimmediate drug reactions are self-limited diseases, and treatment is symptomatic. In clinical praxis, corticosteroids (topical, sometimes systemic) and/or

Table 6 Signs of severity	
Immediate Onset Reactions	Involvement of extradermal organs like rhinoconjunctivitis, obstructive respiratory symptoms, nausea, vomiting, and so on Sudden onset of generalized pruritus Itching of the perioral area, the inguinae, palms or soles Sudden flush if accompanied by conjunctivitis or rhinitis
Delayed Onset Reactions	Fever, malaise Prolonged clinical symptoms after discontinuation of the causative drug Lymphadenopathy Burning or painful skin Bullous lesions, epidermal detachment (Nikolsky sign) Mucosal involvement Facial edema or diffuse erythematous swelling Confluent lesions of extended body surfaces Eosinophilia >1.5 × 10^9 cells per liter Liver involvement

antihistamines are used to block or reduce prolonged or late phase reactions. However, there are no randomized trials for their use.

The management of patients with SJS/TEN is described in another article by Harr and French elsewhere in this issue for further exploration of this topic. Considering the familiar occurrence of severe drug hypersensitivity reactions, avoidance of the responsible drug and chemically related compounds is essential for the patient and may be advisable for first-degree relatives.[26]

For the treatment of DRESSs, corticosteroids are used. Occasionally, even liver transplantation is necessary. Recurrence of the disease in the transplanted liver has been suspected in 1 case.[27]

DIAGNOSIS AND MANAGEMENT AFTER THE FLORID REACTION

Reexposure to the causative drug has to be avoided to prevent the recurrence of hypersensitivity reactions. Thus the identification of the causative drug and underlying mechanism is required. Clinical and laboratory investigations during the florid phase may be useful, but in most instances they do not provide sufficient evidence for a reliable diagnosis. If the identification of the underlying mechanism and causative drug, are important for the further management of the patient, an allergologic workup is required. Available drug allergy tests have only limited diagnostic accuracy. Therefore, an allergologic workup may not always provide a clear-cut diagnosis. Nevertheless, positive results are mostly meaningful and reduce the need of challenge tests. Therefore, allergologic workup is recommended at least in the following situations:

- Severe hypersensitivity reaction: all cases with a suspicion for an IgE-mediated reaction (as the next reaction may be anaphylaxis). DRESSs/DiHS, SJS/TEN, severe MPE (with longer lasting infiltration, confluence of lesions), internal organ involvement (interstitial nephritis, pancreatitis, pneumonitis) with or without skin involvement.
- The incriminated active substances cannot easily be omitted or replaced
- There are uncertainties about cross-reaction or tolerability of alternative treatment options
- Requirement of graded challenge, provocation tests and desensitization (see later section).

After the diagnosis, patients should be informed carefully about their drug allergy, whereby symptoms, drug that elicits reaction, modes of diagnosis of drug allergy, and possible alternatives should be indicated in their "allergy passport" (**Fig. 3**).

Allergologic Workup

The workup encompasses a detailed case history and an accurate determination of the reaction type, followed by appropriate skin and in vitro tests.

Skin tests

Skin tests (prick, intradermal) are quite easy to perform and may provide some help in the identification of the causative drug in both immediate and nonimmediate reactions. However, concentrations to be used for prick or intradermal testing have only been evaluated for selected drugs, especially antibiotics and NMBAs.[28,29]

Patch testing is widely done in Europe, with some success,[30] but the test procedures and concentrations still need further investigation to be generally recommended. Multicenter studies are on the way. For nonimmediate reactions, late reading and thus multiple consultations are required.

Name:

Prename:

Date of birth:

Diagnosis established by:

(stamp of medical office)

Allergy to the following active substance(s)		Severity and type of reaction a) Severe (e.g. anaphylaxis) b) Mild to moderate (e.g. exanthema)		Sensitization established by H = History and clinical pattern, S= Skin testing P = Provocation test, O = Others			Alternative active substance(s) P = Provocation test , S= Skin testing R = Recommendation only	
Trade name	Generic name	Severity and type	Date of reaction	Date of diagnosis	Established by	Remarks	Generic name	Based on

Fig. 3. Example of "allergy passport" (modified according to the allergy passport of Swiss Society of Allergology and Immunology).

Most researchers recommend performing skin tests 1 to 6 months after the acute event, as effector cells may be exhausted immediately after the reaction. Because the sensitivity of the tests might decrease over time, they should best be performed in the first year after the reaction.[31]

For various drugs, skin tests have an acceptable specificity to confirm the suspicion of a causative drug. However, negative skin tests do not have sufficient sensitivity to exclude an immune-mediated hypersensitivity in the case of a suggestive history.

Specific IgE

For immediate reactions of a few drugs, in vitro IgE assays are available. Such in vitro tests have a low sensitivity for drugs such as amoxicillin, penicillin G, suxamethonium, rocuronium, morphine, and sulfamethoxazole, but seem to be good for chlorhexidine.

Basophil activation test

The basophil activation test (BAT) may be another in vitro test to identify the relevant drug in immediate hypersensitivity reactions. It is based on flow cytometric quantification of drug-induced CD63 expression or CD203c upregulation or measurement of sulfoleukotriene release by enzyme-linked immunosorbent assay. The sensitivity of IgE-meditated reactions also depends on the drug tested; in some instances it appears to be even superior to Radioallergosorbent-based IgE determinations (RAST)[32] and comparable to the skin tests. A role of BAT in the diagnosis of pseudoallergic reaction has not been established, although some investigators postulate that basophils of patients with NSAID hypersensitivity show some increased reactivity in NSAID-stimulated BAT.[33]

The lymphocyte transformation test

The lymphocyte transformation test (LTT) is an in vitro test for the investigation of nonimmediate hypersensitivity reactions or severe IgE-mediated reactions, in which T cells are also involved. The test measures the drug-specific stimulation of cells by assessing proliferation or expression of activation markers. LTT is a rather complex test and requires pure drug substance and skilled personnel. Thus its availability is limited to specialized centers. The specificity of the test is good (>90%). The sensitivity depends on the type of reaction and is overall low (about 30%) but good in DRESSs/DiHS (>90%). This test is usually performed 1 to 6 months after the acute event. However, data from Japan suggest that in bullous skin diseases tests are more frequently positive in the first weeks of disease.[34]

Graded challenge and drug provocation

If skin and in vitro tests remain inconclusive and the clinician has reason to believe that the patient is unlikely to be allergic, a graded challenge may be performed. A graded challenge corresponds to a cautious titrated administration of an active substance. Another option is a drug provocation test, which is currently the gold standard in the diagnosis of immediate hypersensitivity reactions. However, use of this test is limited by the possibility of severe relapse of the reaction.[35] Furthermore false negative results are possible[36] Therefore a drug provocation test should be reserved for situations in which the identification of the causative drug is important. More frequently, tests are performed with alternative drugs to establish a safe substitution. Provocation tests in nonimmediate type hypersensitivity reactions are not well standardized—neither the dose nor the time of treatment is established. Thus, no data on sensitivity or specificity are available. At present, these tests cannot be recommended as a routine procedure for the identification of the culprit drug.

Recommendation of Alternative Drugs

If a patient requires continued or a new treatment, cross-reactivity among drugs should be taken into consideration.

β-Lactams

Based on early reports and because of similarities in their β-lactam ring structures of penicillins, it has been believed that these drugs cross-react with cephalosporins, carbapenems, and monobactams. Therefore, it has been a paradigm that in patients with immediate penicillin allergy other β-lactams should not be given. However, more recent data show only little or even no cross-reactivity between penicillins and cephalosporins of the second or higher generation.[37] Also the practice of avoiding carbapenems and monobactam in penicillin-allergic patients should be reconsidered. With regard to monobactams, the administration of aztreonam in ceftazidime allergic patients may have an increased risk for immediate hypersensitivity.[38]

There are only few data available for nonimmediate hypersensitivity reactions. In vitro data indicate that cross-reactivity of T cells between penicillins and cephalosporins are very rare,[39] and are in agreement with our clinical experience. However, clinical data on this topic in the literature are scarce.

Sulfonamides

A common clinical problem is the putative cross-reactivity among sulfonamides. Recent data have demonstrated that IgE-mediated and T-cell–mediated cross-reactivity between sulfonamide antibiotics (which share the immunologic determinant of the *N*1 heterocyclic ring) and nonantibiotics are unlikely.[40,41] Thus in patients allergic to sulfanilamide-antibiotics, other sulfonamide-derived drugs (eg, diuretics, sulfonylureas, celecoxib, and sumatriptan) must not be excluded. However cross-reactions do occur with the antiinflammatory compound sulfasalazine, which is broken down in the gastrointestinal tract into sulfapyridine (an aromatic sulfonamide) and aminosalicylic acid. There is no relationship between sulfonamide allergy and intolerance to sulfite preservatives in food.

Heparins

The most common hypersensitivity reactions are local delayed type allergies to subcutaneously injected low-molecular-weight heparins. There is an extensive cross-reactivity among heparins and heparinoids (see the article by Trautmann and Seitz elsewhere in this issue for further exploration of this topic). However, patients with delayed type hypersensitivity to subcutaneously injected heparins often tolerate intravenous heparin application.

Desensitization

Desensitization may be a treatment option for patients with drug allergy for whom no alternative drug exists. Starting at a suballergenic dose with gradual increase may allow the application of full therapeutic doses with minimal risk for anaphylaxis.[42] The desensitized state is not permanent and is sustained only with a daily maintenance dose of the drug. Classically, the procedure is applied in IgE-mediated reactions, but its use has been extended to other drug reactions.[43] Drugs for which desensitization may be successful include allopurinol, co-trimoxazole, β-lactam antibiotics, and cisplatin. Patients with intolerance to acetylsalicylic acid can also be desensitized, with occasional beneficial effect in asthma and polyposis symptoms.[44] The mechanism of drug desensitization is not well understood.

REFERENCES

1. Gomes ER, Demoly P. Epidemiology of hypersensitivity drug reactions. Curr Opin Allergy Clin Immunol 2005;5:309–16.
2. Greenberger PA. 8. Drug allergy. J Allergy Clin Immunol 2006;117(2 Suppl): 464–70.
3. Johansson SG, Bieber T, Dahl R, et al. Revised nomenclature for allergy for global use. Report of the Nomenclature Review Committee of the World Allergy Organization, October 2003. J Allergy Clin Immunol 2004;113:832–6.
4. Bigby M. Rates of cutaneous reactions to drugs. Arch Dermatol 2001;137:765–70.
5. Weiss ME, Adkinson NF. Immediate hypersensitivity reactions to beta-lactam antibiotics. Ann Intern Med 1987;107:204–15.
6. El-Shanawany T, Williams PE, Jolles S. Clinical immunology review series: an approach to the patient with anaphylaxis. Clin Exp Immunol 2008;153:1–9.
7. Mertes PM, Laxenaire MC. Allergic reactions occurring during anaesthesia. Eur J Anaesthesiol 2002;19:240–62.
8. Ellis AK, Day JH. Diagnosis and management of anaphylaxis. CMAJ 2003;169: 307–11.
9. Chung CH, Mirakhur B, Chan E, et al. Cetuximab-induced anaphylaxis and IgE specific for galactose-alpha-1,3-galactose. N Engl J Med 2008;358(11): 1109–17.
10. Mertes PM, Laxenaire MC. Adverse reactions to neuromuscular blocking agents. Curr Allergy Asthma Rep 2004;4:7–16.
11. Harboe T, Johansson SG, Florvaag E, et al. Pholcodine exposure raises serum IgE in patients with previous anaphylaxis to neuromuscular blocking agents. Allergy 2007;62(12):1445–50.
12. Brockow K, Romano A, Aberer W, et al. Skin testing in patients with hypersensitivity reactions to iodinated contrast media – a European multicenter study. Allergy 2009;64:234–41.
13. Kvedariene V, Martins P, Rouanet L, et al. Diagnosis of iodinated contrast media hypersensitivity: results of a 6-year period. Clin Exp Allergy 2006;36(8):1072–7.
14. Knowles SR, Shapiro LE, Shear NH. Anticonvulsant hypersensitivity syndrome: incidence, prevention and management. Drug Saf 1999;21:489–501.
15. Peyrière H, Dereure O, Breton H, et al. Variability in the clinical pattern of cutaneous side-effects of drugs with systemic symptoms: does a DRESS syndrome really exist? Br J Dermatol 2006;155(2):422–8.
16. Shiohara T, Inaoka M, Kano Y. Drug induced hypersensitivity syndrome (DIHS): a reaction induced by a complex interplay among herpesvirus and antiviral and antidrug immune responses. Allergol Int 2006;55(1):1–8.
17. Spanou Z, Keller M, Britschgi M, et al. Involvement of drug-specific T cells in acute drug-induced interstitial nephritis. J Am Soc Nephrol 2006;17(10):2919–27.
18. Sarzi-Puttini P, Atzeni F, Capsoni F, et al. Drug-induced lupus erythematosus. Autoimmunity 2005;38(7):507–18.
19. Doyle MK, Cuellar ML. Drug-induced vasculitis. Expert Opin Drug Saf 2003;2: 401–9.
20. Chung WH, Hung SI, Chen YT. Human leukocyte antigens and drug hypersensitivity. Curr Opin Allergy Clin Immunol 2007;7(4):317–23.
21. Ebo DG, Fisher MM, Hagendorens MM, et al. Anaphylaxis during anaesthesia: diagnostic approach. Allergy 2007;62:471–87.
22. Pruss A, Salama A, Ahrens N, et al. Immune hemolysis-serological and clinical aspects. Clin Exp Med 2003;3(2):55–64.

23. Bircher AJ. Symptoms and danger signs in acute drug hypersensitivity. Toxicology 2005;209:201–7.
24. Evans C, Tippins E. Emergency treatment of anaphylaxis. Accid Emerg Nurs 2005;13(4):232–7.
25. Ewan PW. Anaphylaxis. BMJ 1998;316:1442–5.
26. Ghislain PD, Roujeau JC. Treatment of severe drug reactions: Stevens-Johnson syndrome, toxic epidermal necrolysis and hypersensitivity syndrome. Dermatol Online J 2002;8:5.
27. Mennicke M, Zawodniak A, Keller M, et al. Fulminant liver failure after vancomycin in a sulfasalazine-induced DRESS syndrome: fatal recurrence after liver transplantation. Am J Transplant 2009;9(9):2197–202.
28. Empedrad R, Darter AL, Earl HS, et al. Nonirritating intradermal skin test concentrations for commonly prescribed antibiotics. J Allergy Clin Immunol 2003;112: 629–30.
29. Mertes PM, Laxenaire MC, Lienhart A, et al. Reducing the risk of anaphylaxis during anaesthesia: guidelines for clinical practice. J Investig Allergol Clin Immunol 2005;15(2):91–101.
30. Barbaud A. Skin testing in delayed reactions to drugs. Immunol Allergy Clin North Am 2009;29:517–35.
31. Brockow K, Romano A. Skin tests in the diagnosis of drug hypersensitivity reactions. Curr Pharm Des 2008;14(27):2778–91.
32. Sanz ML, Gamboa PM, Garcia-Aviles C, et al. Drug hypersensitivities: which room for biological tests? Eur Ann Allery Clin Immunol 2005;37:230–5.
33. Nizankowska-Mogilnicka E, Bochenek G, Mastalerz L, et al. EAACI/GA2LEN guideline: aspirin provocation tests for diagnosis of aspirin hypersensitivity. Allergy 2007;62(10):1111–8.
34. Kano Y, Hirahara K, Mitsuyama Y, et al. Utility of the lymphocyte transformation test in the diagnosis of drug sensitivity: dependence on its timing and the type of drug eruption. Allergy 2007;62:1439–44.
35. Aberer W, Kränke B. Provocation tests in drug hypersensitivity. Immunol Allergy Clin North Am 2009;29:567–84.
36. Demoly P, Romano A, Botelho C, et al. Determining the negative predictive value of provocation tests with beta-lactams. Allergy 2010;65:327–32.
37. Pichichero ME. Use of selected cephalosporins in penicillin-allergic patients: a paradigm shift. Diagn Microbiol Infect Dis 2007;57:13–8.
38. Frumin J, Gallagher JC. Allergic cross-sensitivity between penicillin, carbapenem, and monobactam antibiotics: what are the chances? Ann Pharmacother 2009;43:304–15.
39. Mauri-Hellweg D, Zann M, Frei E, et al. Cross-reactivity of T cell lines and clones to beta-lactam antibiotics. J Immunol 1996;157:1071–9.
40. Brackett CC. Likelihood and mechanisms of cross-allergenicity between sulfonamide antibiotics and other drugs containing a sulfonamide functional group. Pharmacotherapy 2004;24(7):856–70.
41. Strom BL, Schinnar R, Apter AJ, et al. Absence of cross-reactivity between sulfonamide antibiotics and sulfonamide nonantibiotics. N Engl J Med 2003;349:1628–35.
42. Castells M. Desensitization for drug allergy. Curr Opin Allergy Clin Immunol 2006; 6:476–81.
43. Solensky R. Drug desensitization. Immunol Allergy Clin North Am 2004;24:425–43.
44. Stevenson DD. Aspirin and NSAID sensitivity. Immunol Allergy Clin North Am 2004;24(3):491–505.

Danger Signs in Drug Hypersensitivity

Kathrin Scherer, MD*, Andreas J. Bircher, MD

KEYWORDS

- Drug hypersensitivity • Adverse drug reaction
- Clinical danger signs • Immediate-type hypersensitivity
- Delayed-type hypersensitivity

Adverse drug reactions (ADRs) are a frequent problem in clinical routine; 10% to 15% of all patients receiving pharmacotherapy are affected. Predictable pharmacologic side effects (type A [eg, nonsteroidal anti-inflammatory drugs (NSAIDs) and ventricular ulcer]) are distinguished from chronic side effects that are associated with the duration of therapy (type C [eg, nephropathy caused by analgesics]) and from long-term side effects (type D [eg, carcinogenicity or teratogenicity]). Unpredictable side effects (type B, allergies/pseudoallergies/idiosyncrasia) are immunologic reactions, classified according to Gell and Coombs into 4 main pathophysiologic subtypes, or nonimmunologic intolerance reactions. They encompass approximately one-fifth to one-seventh of all ADRs.

In allergic adverse reactions, IgE-mediated immediate-type reactions (Gell and Coombs type I) as well as T-cell–mediated delayed-type reactions (Gell and Coombs type IV) are most frequent.

The skin is involved in approximately 20% of all ADRs in the sense of clinical findings or subjective symptoms on skin, mucosae, or adnex structures. Adverse cutaneous reactions to drugs affect 2% to 3% of hospitalized patients,[1,2] which are frequently not severe, but some are fatal. The skin is not only a main target of drug allergies but also an important herald organ: it may reveal signs of a more severe cutaneous reaction or may point to the possible involvement of internal organs, or of a systemic hypersensitivity reaction.[3] The early recognition of such herald signs may initiate immediate actions with the aim of preventing the development to more severe or even life-threatening reactions[4] or a specific treatment may be started in some cases.[5]

This article discusses risk factors, early symptoms, and danger signs indicating a possibly severe course of an ADR and advises on early actions. In clinical situations, however, there may be a combination of overlapping symptoms and signs, some of which may be drug related, whereas others are related to the underlying disease.

Allergy Unit, Department of Dermatology, University Hospital Basel, Petersgraben 4, CH-4031 Basel, Switzerland
* Corresponding author.
E-mail address: schererk@uhbs.ch

Med Clin N Am 94 (2010) 681–689
doi:10.1016/j.mcna.2010.04.007
0025-7125/10/$ – see front matter © 2010 Elsevier Inc. All rights reserved.

medical.theclinics.com

Particularly in the acute stage, ADRs, which can mimic many diseases, are always an important differential diagnosis.[6]

PATIENTS AT RISK FOR DRUG HYPERSENSITIVITY REACTIONS

Some patients have an increased risk of developing a drug-hypersensitivity reaction. These patients need to be identified early and in some cases precautions may be taken.

Prior Drug Reaction

A reliable history of a prior ADR, or even a documentation of such or a proved sensitization to a specific drug molecule, have to be noted. Drug-specific antibodies or drug-specific lymphocytes may already be present, potentially resulting in a fast recurrence (more or less severe) of the earlier reaction on accidental or intentional re-exposure. Potential cross-reactivity between related drug molecules has to be considered.

Multiple Drug Therapy

Treatment with multiple drugs seems to elevate the risk for a hypersensitivity reaction, although the exact mechanism is unclear. Excessive demands on enzyme systems for oxidation or acetylation of multiple drugs may interfere with metabolism, lead to accumulation of drugs, and result in accumulation of reactive metabolites and drug interactions. The balance of metabolic bioactivation of a drug and detoxification is an important component of individual susceptibility for drug hypersensitivity.[7] Also, intermittent or repeated administration of the same drug increases the likelihood of a patient developing a sensitization to the drug or one of its metabolites compared with continuous treatment.

Route of Administration

The route of administration is relevant because immunogenicity decreases from the topical > subcutaneous > intramuscular > oral > intravenous route. Topical administration of a drug is an important mode of sensitization, especially for antibiotics.

Apart from drug- and treatment-related risk factors, patient-related risks have to be considered.

Concomitant Illness

Concomitant illnesses or an underlying disease may have an important influence on the likelihood of developing a drug-related hypersensitivity reaction. This is well known and has been shown repeatedly for viral infections, such as HIV,[8] Epstein-Barr virus, cytomegalovirus, and other human herpesviruses as well as autoimmune disorders and blood cell malignancies. Current understanding of these reactions is based on the danger hypotheses, which state that a drug signal by itself is not sufficient to cause an immune response, but a second signal is mandatory, such as a danger signal or costimulatory signal.[8] This would be provided by the generalized virus infection. Drug allergies themselves may also represent risk factors for subsequent drug allergies, and in severe forms a reactivation of virus-infections of the herpes group may occur.[9]

Dose Changes

Elevation of drug doses during treatment may contribute to the elicitation of ADRs to a previously well-tolerated drug. Diseases of liver and kidney may interfere with transformation or elimination of potentially harmful reactive drugs or metabolites.[10]

Immunogenetic Factors

A breakthrough for risk factor analysis was the observation that in severe drug hypersensitivity reactions, certain HLA-B alleles predispose for drug allergies. This is already used routinely, as abacavir treatment is given only to HLA-B*5701–negative persons because a strong predictive association between carriage of HLA-B*5701 and abacavir hypersensitivity reactions in Caucasian and Hispanic ethnic groups has been demonstrated.[11] Because HLA-B*1502 is a risk factor in Han Chinese for carbamazepine-induced severe hypersensitivity reactions, Taiwan has also installed HLA-B*1502 typing before carbamazepine is given.[12]

Aggravating Factors

Patients with a history of bronchial asthma are more likely to develop bronchospasm in immediate-type allergic reactions and have a poorer outcome. Patients with coronary heart disease or hypertension are more likely to suffer from complications from anaphylaxis or its treatment with epinephrine. β-Blocking agents or angiotensin-converting enzyme inhibitors may aggravate immediate-type reactions or complicate treatment. Long-term preventive measures to reduce the risk of fatality in patients with anaphylaxis include optimal management of relevant comorbidities, such as asthma, cardiovascular disease, and mastocytosis as well as awareness of other concomitant factors.[13]

CUTANEOUS DANGER SIGNS IN IMMEDIATE-TYPE REACTIONS

One of the most important prodromal symptoms in anaphylaxis is sudden onset of pruritus, particularly in the paraoral region, palms, and plantae and on the scalp. A flush reaction of the face and upper thorax, sometimes accompanied by conjunctivitis and rhinitis, heralds a severe course and rapid evolution of the anaphylaxis (**Box 1**). In a retrospective analysis of 266 patients with anaphylaxis, the spectrum of symptoms encompassed pruritus, urticaria, and angioedema (90%); dyspnea and bronchospasm (60%); dizziness and syncope (29%); flush (28%); abdominal colics and diarrhea (26%); swelling of the tongue; edema of the larynx, dysphonia, and dysphagia (24%); nausea and vomiting (20%); hypotension (20%); rhinitis (16%); conjunctivitis (12%) and and headaches, and pruritus without skin changes (<5% each).[14] Webb and Lieberman[15] reported similar percentages in 2006 in 601 patients.

Typical early symptoms of angioedema of the tongue and larynx that may develop into asphyxia and hypoxia are the urge to clear the throat, hoarseness, tightness of the throat, blurred speech and salivation (**Fig. 1**). Further unspecific early symptoms of impending anaphylaxis are agitation, excitation, feeling of impending doom, and

---

Box 1
Danger signs for severe immediate-type reactions

Sudden onset of extensive pruritus, in particular palmoplantar and scalp

Flush on face and neck with conjunctivitis and rhinitis

Angioedema of the oral mucosa, in particular pharynx and larynx

Severe urticaria

Dyspnea and bronchospasm, especially in known asthmatics

Hypotension

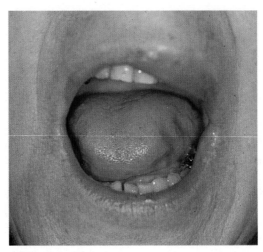

Fig. 1. Angioedema of the lips and tongue.

mortal fear.[16] Other signs that should alert and result in therapeutic interventions are the development of extensive urticaria, especially if it evolves quickly; dyspnea and bronchospasm, especially in known asthmatics; and hypotension.

An anaphylactoid reaction with pruritus, flush and erythema of the trunk, angioedema, and hypertension—the so-called red man syndrome—has been ascribed to too rapid infusions of high doses of vancomycin. A direct histamine release has been shown.[17] Early recognition of these symptoms and immediate action (drug withdrawal and treatment) are mandatory.

CUTANEOUS DANGER SIGNS IN DELAYED-TYPE REACTIONS

The disease entities mentioned below are discussed in more detail in the articles by Bischer; Harr and French elsewhere in this issue for further exploration of this topic.

Delayed-type, T-cell–mediated reactions frequently manifest on the skin with erythema, macules, and infiltrated papules and plaques predominantly on the trunk and the proximal extremities. For the interpretation of the severity of such a reaction, the type of putative causative drug and the time point of the first appearance of symptoms during the treatment course have to be taken into account, because some drugs are more likely to cause severe reactions (eg, allopurinol) than others (eg, amoxicillin). Infiltrated, palpable lesions are potential heralds of the severe drug-induced syndromes, such as drug rash with eosinophilia and systemic symptoms (DRESS) or drug-induced hypersensitivity syndrome (DIHS), used synonymously with DRESS for the purpose of this article. Atypical target lesions or widespread erythema, particularly in the upper chest and back, and development of epidermolysis or bullae are heralds of Stevens-Johnson syndrome (SJS) and toxic epidermal necrolysis (TEN).

Not all infiltrated lesions herald severe hypersensitivity reactions, however. The general condition of a patient see below usually allows a decisive differentiation because patients with impending severe reactions are usually sicker, have higher temperatures, and complain about malaise compared with patients with mild cutaneous reactions. Such general symptoms should prompt a search for internal organ involvement (differential blood count, liver and eventually kidney parameters) (discussed later). Uncomplicated pruritic maculopapular exanthems (MPEs) also do not normally develop into SJS/TEN. The primary lesions of MPEs are macules or papules, which, even in case of coalescence, are usually visible at the rims in contrast to atypical target lesions or plane erythemas in SJS/TEN. Patients with MPEs also do not exhibit severe mucosal involvement.

Important cutaneous alert signs (**Box 2**) for these severe drug hypersensitivity reactions are a central facial erythematous edema (**Fig. 2**) which is different from the usually pale asymmetric angioedema, as well as involvement of extended body surfaces with confluent lesions and diffuse erythematous swellings developing into erythroderma. Atypical target lesions (**Fig. 3**)[2] are a sign of impending development of severe bullous drug reactions, such as SJS and TEN.[18] Another typical and early sign of SJS/TEN in patients with confluent macular exanthema is burning of the skin or painfulness of the skin on touch. Bullous lesions may be about to develop[19]; if lateral, tangential pressure on macular lesions leads to epidermal detachment—the so-called Nikolsky sign (**Fig. 4**)—it is an indication for intraepidermal blister formation.[5] Confluent vesicles, bullous lesions, and even widespread detachment of necrolytic epidermis are signs of an advanced stage.

Mucosal involvement, in particular stomatitis or balanitis, could represent isolated, localized drug reactions, such as fixed drug eruptions but have to be taken seriously if more than one mucosal area is extensively affected and erosions and ulcerations occur (**Fig. 5**). In SJS/TEN, severe mucositis of more than one mucosa usually appears early and is followed by epidermal blister formation and necrolysis. Conjunctival involvement, in particular, warrants early cooperation with ophthalmologists because persistent ocular complications are frequent.

Exanthematic purpura (nonblanchable erythematous lesions) represents vasculitis of cutaneous blood vessels (**Fig. 6**) or a problem in the coagulation cascade. Hemorrhagic or palpable lesions are a sign of perivascular inflammation after destruction of blood vessels and should prompt a search for systemic vasculitis with involvement of internal organs or thrombocytopenia. Bullous transformation and necrosis may follow, which can be extensive and deep, depending on the size of vessel affected. Drug-induced thrombocytopenia (eg, from heparin) or warfarin necrosis presents with a black deep-reaching necrosis of extended skin areas.[20]

Drug-induced pseudolymphoma typically has a late onset, has a less severe course, and presents with protracted infiltrated lesion.[21]

Box 2
Cutaneous danger signs for severe delayed-type reactions

Centrofacial edema (diffuse erythematous swelling)

Involvement of large body surfaces or erythroderma

Painful skin, skin tender to touch

Atypical target lesions

Nikolsky sign positive, vesiculobullous lesions, epidermolysis

Erosive stomatitis; mucositis, especially if affecting more than one mucosa

Hemorrhagic necrotizing lesions

Purpura

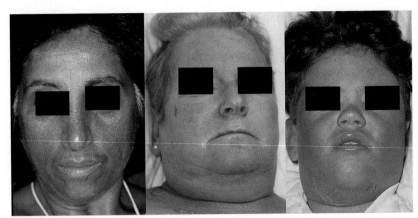

Fig. 2. Central facial erythematous swelling in DRESS syndrome (*left*), SJS (*middle*), and toxic epidermal necrolysis (*right*).

GENERAL SIGNS AND INTERNAL ORGAN INVOLVEMENT

Sudden onset of high fever (>39°C), otherwise unexplained, disseminated lymphadenopathy, arthralgias, and arthritides may present herald signs for severe hypersensitivity reactions, such as DRESS or serum sickness–like reactions. Facial edema (discussed previously) is also typical of DRESS (see **Fig. 2**). Lymphadenopathy, however, may appear late in the course of events. Drug hypersensitivity reactions may manifest in almost any organ, with liver, kidney, and lung the most frequently involved. Hepatopathy, nephropathy, and pneumonitis need to be looked for repeatedly and may be the first or only organs affected. In a laboratory, eosinophilia and presence of activated lymphocytes are typical danger signs for DRESS/DIHS, whereas cytopenia may be found in SJS/TEN. Isolated drug fever is rare.

WHAT TO ASSESS

Recognition, description, and documentation of the skin lesions are essential in establishing the correct diagnosis. With respect to a single lesion, it is not sufficient to call it a rash. The exact morphology needs to be recognized (eg, erythema, macule, papule or plaque, edema, vesicle, blister, bulla, pustule, and the presence of the Nicolsky sign at various time points). Not only the type of skin lesion but also the distribution on the body is important to facilitate the differential diagnosis, especially in flexural

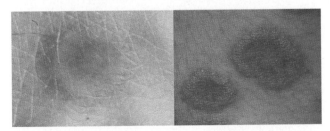

Fig. 3. Typical target lesions (*left*) are less than 3 cm in diameter with a regular round shape, well-defined border, and at least 3 different zones (2 concentric rings around a central disk). Atypical (*right*) target lesions have only 2 zones, are mostly flat, and have irregular shape and darker color and sometimes a central blister. Atypical targets are heralds for SJS/TEN.

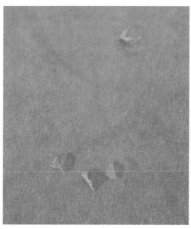

Fig. 4. Positive Nikolsky sign in edematous, erythematous skin indicating necrolytic detachment of the epidermis in SJS/TEN.

exanthemas (systemic drug-related intertriginous and flexural exanthema syndrome [SDRIFE-syndrome],[22] erythema multiforme, and acute, generalized exanthematous pustulosis [AGEP]). The speed of the evolution of the symptoms over time allows an estimate of the severity of an ADR, because rapidly developing exanthems are more dangerous. For more details see the article by Bircher elsewhere in this issue for further exploration of this topic.

TO DO IN THE ACUTE PHASE

If an acute ADR of type B is suspected, all substances consumed, prescription drugs, over-the-counter drugs, herbal medicine, and food supplements should be assessed with regard to the likelihood of being the causative agent, even if not taken on a regular basis. If the drugs have been taken for a long period of time (>4–12 weeks), their involvement in drug hypersensitivity is unlikely. The latency between start of intake of the drug and first signs of an ADR, however, may be up to 12 weeks in DRESS/DIHS, depending on the drug. For SJS/TEN, the usual time interval between start of treatment with the culprit drug and the onset of an adverse reaction is on average 1 to 3 weeks; more

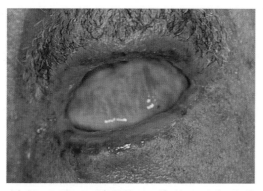

Fig. 5. Severe mucositis in a patient with TEN, manifesting >1 day before epidermolysis of the skin was detectable.

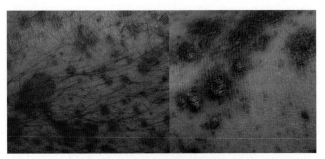

Fig. 6. Hemorrhagic, macular purpura (*left*), bullous lesions, and necrosis (*right*) have to be looked for as signs for cutaneous or systemic vasculitis or thromobocytopenia.

than 90% of the reactions occur within the first 63 days of drug use. There are, however, drug-specific differences in the mean latency between start of intake and first symptoms (eg, 15 days for carbamazepine, 24 days for phenytoin, 17 days for phenobarbital, and 20 days for allupurinol). For others, the latency can be much longer.[23,24] All medication and the putative culprit should be stopped except the most essential drugs. Attention must be paid to danger signs (see **Boxes 1** and **2**) because heralds of a potential severe course and patients need to be monitored closely with respect to vital signs and general condition as well as the development of involvement of organs other than the skin (eg, pneumopathy, lymphadenopathy, and nephropathy).

Exact documentation of the sequence of drug intake, especially if more than 1 drug has been taken, and the appearance of the first symptoms, the exact morphology of skin and mucosal lesions, and the evolution of the symptoms are essential for a later allergological work-up. A skin biopsy may be helpful. Photodocumentation of the rash is often useful.

Early involvement of other specialists, such as ophthalmologists or otorhinolaryngologist, is helpful in correctly assessing the mucosal situation and the involvement of other organs. Treatment is managed according to recommendations and the individual situation of a patient as discussed in the article by Bischer and colleagues and Kano and colleagues elsewhere in this issue.

SUMMARY

ADRs are frequently considered iatrogenic complications and, therefore, pose a specific challenge for the physician-patient relationship. Early recognition of a potential ADR is possible, especially on the skin, in addition to characteristic clinical danger signs. Cutaneous manifestations are variable, depending on the causative pathomechanism. It is impossible to conclude the causative agent from the morphology of the cutaneous lesions. The intake of several drugs in the time before the elicitation of the drug reaction usually poses a diagnostic challenge. It is crucial for the precision of any further allergological work-up to document the type of rash precisely as well as the time course of drug intake and appearance of the first symptoms.

REFERENCES

1. Demoly P, Bousquet J. Epidemiology of drug allergy. Curr Opin Allergy Clin Immunol 2001;1(4):305–10.
2. Wolf R, Orion E, Marcos B, et al. Life-threatening acute adverse cutaneous drug reactions. Clin Dermatol 2005;23(2):171–81.

3. Bircher AJ. Arzneimittelallergie und Haut. Stuttgart (Germany): Georg Thieme; 1996. New York.
4. Garcia-Doval I, LeCleach L, Bocquet H, et al. Toxic epidermal necrolysis and Stevens-Johnson syndrome: does early withdrawal of causative drugs decrease the risk of death? Arch Dermatol 2000;136(3):323–7.
5. Bachot N, Roujeau JC. Physiopathology and treatment of severe drug eruptions. Curr Opin Allergy Clin Immunol 2001;1(4):293–8.
6. Bachot N, Roujeau JC. Differential diagnosis of severe cutaneous drug eruptions. Am J Clin Dermatol 2003;4(8):561–72.
7. Naisbitt DJ, Gordon SF, Pirmohamed M, et al. Immunological principles of adverse drug reactions: the initiation and propagation of immune responses elicited by drug treatment. Drug Saf 2000;23(6):483–507.
8. Vilar FJ, Naisbitt DJ, Park BK, et al. Mechanisms of drug hypersensitivity in HIV-infected patients: the role of the immune system. J HIV Ther 2003;8(2):42–7.
9. Shiohara T, Kano Y. A complex interaction between drug allergy and viral infection. Clin Rev Allergy Immunol 2007;33(1–2):124–33.
10. Bonnetblanc JM, Vaillant L, Wolkenstein PH. [Facteurs prédisposants des réactions cutanées aux médicaments]. Ann Dermatol Venereol 1995;122(8): 484–6 [in French].
11. Hughes AR, Mosteller M, Bansal AT, et al. Association of genetic variations in HLA-B region with hypersensitivity to abacavir in some, but not all, populations. Pharmacogenomics 2004;5(2):203–11.
12. Chung WH, Hung SI, Chen YT. Human leukocyte antigens and drug hypersensitivity. Curr Opin Allergy Clin Immunol 2007;7(4):317–23.
13. Simons FE. Anaphylaxis: recent advances in assessment and treatment. J Allergy Clin Immunol 2009;124(4):625–36.
14. Kemp SF, Lockey RF, Wolf BF, et al. Anaphylaxis. a review of 266 cases. Arch Intern Med 1995;155(16):1749–54.
15. Webb L, Lieberman P. Anaphylaxis: a review of 601 cases. Ann Allergy Asthma Immunol 2006;97(1):39–43.
16. Yunginger JW. Anaphylaxis. Ann Allergy 1992;69(2):87–96.
17. Renz CL, Thurn JD, Finn HA, et al. Antihistamine prophylaxis permits rapid vancomycin infusion. Crit Care Med 1999;27(9):1732–7.
18. Tas S, Simonart T. Management of drug rash with eosinophilia and systemic symptoms (DRESS Syndrome): an update. Dermatology 2003;206(4):353–6.
19. Bircher AJ. Symptoms and danger signs in acute drug hypersensitivity. Toxicology 2005;209(2):201–7.
20. Scherer K, Tsakiris DA, Birches AJ. Hypersensitivity reactions to anticoagulant drugs. Curr Pharm Des 2008;14:2863–73.
21. Bocquet H, Bagot M, Roujeau JC. Drug-induced pseudolymphoma and drug hypersensitivity syndrome (drug rash with eosinophilia and systemic symptoms: DRESS). Semin Cutan Med Surg 1996;15(4):250–7.
22. Hausermann P, Harr T, Bircher AJ. Baboon syndrome resulting from systemic drugs: is there strife between SDRIFE and allergic contact dermatitis syndrome? Contact Derm 2004;51(5–6):297–310.
23. Guillaume JC, Roujeau JC, Dever J, et al. The culprit drugs in 87 cases of toxic epidermal necrolysis (Lyell's syndrome). Arch Dermatol 1987;123(9):1166–70.
24. Mockenhaupt M. Epidemiology and causes of severe cutaneous adverse reactions to drugs. In: Pichler WJ, editor. Drug hypersensitivity. Basel (Switzerland): Karger; 2007. p. 18–31.

Acute Symptoms of Drug Hypersensitivity (Urticaria, Angioedema, Anaphylaxis, Anaphylactic Shock)

Ticha Limsuwan, MD[a], Pascal Demoly, MD, PhD[b],*

KEYWORDS

- Urticaria • Angioedema • Anaphylaxis • Anaphylactic shock
- Drug hypersensitivity

Drug hypersensitivity reactions (HSRs) are the adverse effects of drugs which, when taken at doses generally tolerated by normal subjects, clinically resemble allergy.[1] Although they occur in a small percentage of patients (about one-third of all adverse drug reactions, which affect 10% to 20% of the hospitalized patients and more than 7% of the general population), these reactions are often unpredictable and can be life threatening.[2,3] Only when a definite immunologic mechanism (either drug-specific antibody or T-cell) is demonstrated should these reactions be classified as drug allergy. For general communication, when a drug allergic reaction is suspected, "drug HSR" is the preferred term, because true drug allergy and nonallergic drug HSR[4] may be difficult to differentiate from the clinical presentation alone, especially in situations of acute severe HSR, such as anaphylaxis. However, for a long-term plan of treatment and prevention, referral to an allergist-immunologist for confirmation of diagnosis is needed to offer specific preventive measurements.

The European Network for Drug Allergy (ENDA), working under the aegis of the European Academy of Allergy and Clinical Immunology (EAACI), has simplified the clinical classification of drug HSRs into 2 types, according to the delay of onset of the reaction after the last administration of the drug[5,6]: (1) *immediate reaction,* occurring less than 1 hour after the last drug intake, usually in the form of urticaria, angioedema, rhinitis, conjunctivitis, bronchospasm, and anaphylaxis or anaphylactic shock;

Conflict of interest: The authors have nothing to disclose.

[a] Allergy Immunology and Rheumatology Division, Faculty of Medicine, Ramathibodi Hospital, Mahidol University, 270, Rama 6th Road, Phyathai, Bangkok 10400, Thailand

[b] Allergy Department and INSERM U657, Hôpital Arnaud de Villeneuve, University Hospital of Montpellier, Avenue du Doyen Gaston Giraud, 34295 Montpellier Cedex 5, France

* Corresponding author.

E-mail address: pascal.demoly@inserm.fr

Med Clin N Am 94 (2010) 691–710

doi:10.1016/j.mcna.2010.03.007

medical.theclinics.com

and (2) *nonimmediate reaction*, with variable cutaneous symptoms occurring after more than 1 hour and up to several days after the last drug intake, such as late-occurring urticaria, maculopapular eruptions, fixed drug eruptions, vasculitis, toxic epidermal necrolysis, Stevens-Johnson syndrome, or drug reaction with eosinophilia and systemic symptoms (DRESS). The first category is mostly mediated through specific IgE, whereas the latter is specifically T-cell–mediated.

Acute urticarial and angioedema reactions are common clinical problems frequently encountered by internists and general practitioners. Although most are benign and self limiting, a mucocutaneous swelling of the upper respiratory tract could be life threatening by itself or a feature of anaphylaxis.[7–9] By contrast, urticaria and angioedema alone are not specific to drug allergic reaction, and can be caused by various pathogenic mechanisms.[10] In this article, the authors review acute symptoms of drug HSRs, especially urticaria, angioedema, anaphylaxis, and anaphylactic shock, and how to approach these problems in general.

URTICARIA AND ANGIOEDEMA

Acute urticaria and angioedema are common clinical problems with an estimated lifetime incidence of 15% to 25% in the general population.[10,11] Acute urticaria is more common in children, young adults, and people with atopic diseases, whereas the chronic form is more prevalent in middle-aged women, with peak incidence during the third and fourth decades.[10,12] Isolated angioedema is still a poorly understood clinical issue and a difficult subject to approach for both internists and specialists.[13]

Clinical Features of Urticaria and Angioedema

Urticaria (or "hives") gives rise to blancheable, raised (edematous), smooth, pink to red papules, although classically it produces pale wheals surrounded by an erythematous flare and is characteristically intensely pruritic. These lesions are usually discrete, round or oval in shape, can vary in size from 1 mm to many centimeters, and may occur anywhere on the body (**Fig. 1**). In the vast majority of cases the wheals are transient, lasting for only a few hours in any one place, but with new wheals appearing in other places. Most urticarial eruptions therefore "move" around the body—a useful pointer from clinical history that the eruption is urticarial.[10,11,14,15]

Angioedema, also called Quincke edema, is characterized by an acute, transient, nonpitting, red to skin-colored, well-demarcated, edematous swelling that involves deeper layers of skin (deep dermis, or subcutaneous and submucosal layers); it occurs in an asymmetric distribution, and has no predilection for dependent areas. Angioedema usually affects the face (particularly the lips, tongue, perioral, and periorbital areas) (**Fig. 2**), extremities, genitalia, scalp, as well as the upper respiratory airways and the intestinal epithelial lining. Pruritus is characteristically absent or minimal, but can be accompanied by a sense of burning, pressure or tightness, or by a dull ache in the affected area. Moreover, whereas most urticarial lesions regress within 24 hours, angioedema may last for several days.[10,13]

Differentiation Between Urticaria and Angioedema

Identifying and distinguishing angioedema from urticaria is important. First, along with anaphylaxis, angioedema is the only truly potentially life-threatening aspect of acute immediate hypersensitivity reactions, if the airway is affected. Patients should maintain ready access to epinephrine, because laryngeal edema is a cause of death if

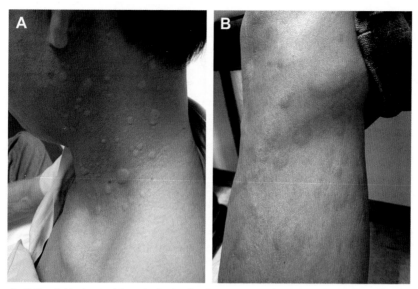

Fig. 1. Urticarial lesions with typical raised, edematous, pink, smooth papules and classically surrounded by erythematous flare (*A*), and gyrate pattern of urticaria (*B*).

unrecognized and/or inadequately treated.[16–18] Second, patients with urticaria and angioedema tend to have more severe disease, more prolonged disease, and symptoms that are less responsive to therapy as compared with patients with urticaria alone.[7,11,19] Finally, although about half of the patients with urticaria also have angioedema, as there is often a continuum spectrum of manifestations ranging from superficial wheals in the upper dermis merging with angioedema of the subcutaneous and submucosal tissues,[8] 40% of the patients have urticaria alone and 10% have isolated angioedema.[7] Thus for angioedema with urticaria the approach scheme is the same as for urticaria, whereas isolated angioedema is a separate entity requiring a different clinical approach.[13]

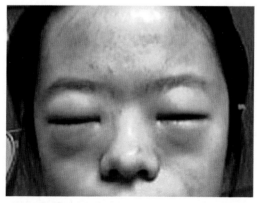

Fig. 2. Angioedema presenting as bilateral eyelid swelling, from nonsteroidal anti-inflammatory drug–induced angioedema.

Differential Diagnosis of Urticaria

Although urticaria is generally not difficult to diagnose, classifying patients with drug-induced urticaria is crucial for developing a meaningful differential diagnosis, identifying specific triggers, and choosing allergy tests. The following conditions should be ruled out:

1. Dermatographism represents the most common physical urticaria, affecting 2% to 5% of the population. In contrast to the normal urticarial lesions, which are usually round or oval in shape, dermatographism consists of linear pruritic wheals appearing on areas of skin within 2 to 5 minutes of stroking and resolves after 30 minutes or up to 3 hours. Only a small portion of affected patients are symptomatic and require treatment with antihistamines. Systemic symptoms are absent. Common triggers include scratching the skin and contact with clothing, towels, or sheets. Dermatographism may follow an acute viral infection or drug reaction, and the duration is variable.[10]

2. Urticarial vasculitis should be suspected when the lesions are painful (more than pruritic), last more than 24 hours, leave permanent pigmentary change, are non-blancheable, form vesicles, or are accompanied by purpura. Questions regarding systemic (vasculitis) symptoms including fever, arthralgia or arthritis, renal disease with proteinuria or hematuria, gastrointestinal manifestations of nausea and abdominal pain, and pulmonary disease with cough, dyspnea, or hemoptysis should be addressed. Frequently the provoking antigen cannot be found, but diagnostic tests classically reveal elevated acute-phase proteins, including an erythrocyte sedimentation rate and low complement serum levels (CH50 or C1q, C2, or C4). Skin biopsies help confirmation of diagnosis by revealing the classic features of leukocytoclastic vasculitis; this can be associated with systemic lupus erythematosus, rheumatic fever, juvenile rheumatoid arthritis (Still disease), or other connective tissue diseases. It is a rule of thumb to perform skin biopsies of urticarial lesions if they persist at the same site for more than 24 hours.[10,11]

3. Contact urticaria, in which contact of the skin with an allergen causes immediate hives at the site of contact, can be either allergic, such as allergy to natural rubber latex, or nonallergic, due to, for example, certain chemicals in foods and cosmetics. The disease can be complicated by angioedema and even severe anaphylaxis, especially in IgE-mediated allergic contact urticaria.[12,15]

4. Erythema multiforme is an acute disorder characterized by persistent targetlike lesions, which are symmetric, round, red or purple, with characteristically dark cyanotic centers that are typically less pruritic than urticaria. Also, these lesions are usually found on the extremities, including the palms and soles, dorsa of the hands and the feet, forearms, and lower legs. These lesions are self limiting with a recovery phase of approximately 3 weeks.[10] In the absence of severity criteria such as the widespread distribution of skin lesion or cutaneous detachment, the reaction is usually associated with herpes simplex or mycoplasma infection, and mostly affects children and young adults.[20] It is not uncommon for these virus-triggered reactions to recur.

5. Primary mast cell disorders, although rare, account for a few cases of urticaria; physicians should recognize these disorders. Solitary mastocytomas are more common in children, with the classic lesion of hyperpigmented macule or papule, which when mechanically irritated by rubbing the skin develop a wheal and flare (Darier's sign). More than half of childhood mastocytomas resolve during puberty. In contrast, urticaria pigmentosa is rarely confused with urticarial

lesions, given the distinctive pigmented cutaneous lesions for which it is named. Even less common is systemic mastocytosis, a highly symptomatic but rarely malignant clonal disorder of the mast cell and its CD34+ precursors. This condition is almost always accompanied by other symptoms, including prominent gastrointestinal symptoms, neuropsychiatric symptoms, and recurrent anaphylaxis, as a result of increased total numbers of mast cells deposited in various organs, especially skin, bone marrow, gastrointestinal tract, liver, spleen, or lymph nodes, and elevations of the constitutively expressed α-form of tryptase in the serum. A bone marrow biopsy is needed for the diagnosis.[11,21]

Differential Diagnosis of Angioedema

Angioedemas are frequently erroneously labeled when there are clinical manifestations of swollen skin or mucosa around the facial area. Many conditions may mimic angioedema.[13]

1. Edema refers to the swelling of tissue due to excess fluid in an interstitial space. Edema and angioedema show a predilection for areas where the skin is lax rather than taut (especially the eyelids and genitalia), but only edema occurs predominantly in dependent areas such as the buttocks and lower extremities.
2. Facial cellulitis, caused by an infectious process of adjacent organs, is often painful, lasts for several days, is associated with fever and followed by peeling.
3. Superior vena cava syndrome is caused by a progressive obstruction or narrowing of the superior vena cava vein frequently by tumor invasion or mass effect, resulting in the gradual swelling of eyelids, lips, and venous engorgement at the face, neck, and upper part of the thorax.
4. Swelling of the oropharynx should be differentiated from tonsillitis, peritonsillar abscess, and pharyngeal foreign body.
5. Acute (facial) eczema is caused by the direct contact of certain sensitizers with the skin, leading to a pruritic papulovesicular dermatitis characterized early by erythema and edema.
6. Facial swelling as an early manifestation of DRESS (**Fig. 3**) is accompanied by lymphadenopathy, hypereosinophilia, lymphocytosis, and hepatitis.
7. Dermatomyositis presents with heliotrope (violaceous edema of the eyelids), which is persistent and associated with systemic symptoms and characteristic musculocutaneous symptoms such as muscular weakness from myositis and cutaneous eruptions (**Fig. 4**).

ANAPHYLAXIS AND ANAPHYLACTIC SHOCK

Anaphylaxis is the most serious systemic immediate hypersensitivity reaction, often but not always IgE-dependent, is rapid in onset, and can cause death.[22] Although the true prevalence of anaphylaxis is unknown, it is not as rare as generally believed; rather, it seems to be underrecognized and undertreated. In children, adolescents, and young adults, foods are the most common trigger. In middle-aged and older adults, drugs and stinging insect venoms are important causes, as is idiopathic anaphylaxis.[23] An estimated incidence of anaphylaxis is 50 to 2000 episodes per 100,000 person-years with a possible lifetime prevalence of 0.05% to 2%.[24] Although death from anaphylaxis is considered rare (< about 1%), some drugs have been associated with these fatalities, such as β-lactams, radiocontrast media (RCM), and muscle relaxants.[25]

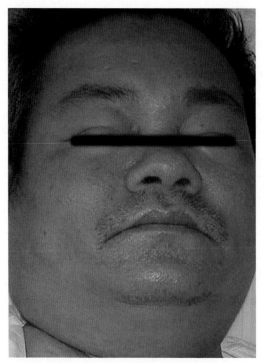

Fig. 3. Face swelling in early manifestation of DRESS syndrome.

Clinical Presentation and Diagnosis of Anaphylaxis and Anaphylactic Shock

In the diagnosis of anaphylaxis, the clinical history and physical examination are the most important instruments. Although recently a multidisciplinary group of experts in the United States has suggested clinical criteria for diagnosing anaphylaxis by the division into 3 categories[22] according to the previous history of allergic reaction and known exposure, in order to include atypical presentation, here the authors

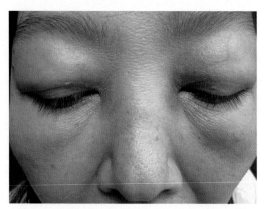

Fig. 4. Heliotrope sign in dermatomyositis, showing swelling and violaceous discoloration of eyelids.

have simplified the procedure by presenting only the first category, in which the diagnosis is based on a combination of clinical signs and symptoms of at least 2 organ involvements (**Table 1**). Skin (urticaria and/or angioedema) is involved in almost 90% of the episodes. Conjunctivitis is part of an acute mucosal allergic reaction to drugs (**Fig. 5**).[16,26] Other organ involvements include the lower respiratory system (dyspnea, wheezing, hypoxemia) in more than half of the patients, the upper respiratory airway system (laryngeal or tongue swelling) in up to 20%, gastrointestinal manifestations (nausea, vomiting, diarrhea, abdominal pain), and cardiovascular manifestations (dizziness, syncope, hypotension, or collapse) in about one-third of the patients.[16,25–27] The presence of hypotension and shock are not always necessary in the diagnosis of anaphylaxis.[22] However, when there is a drop in blood pressure of more than 30% from the patient's baseline or the systolic blood pressure is lower than the standard value, the term "anaphylactic shock" is used; this can be an isolated manifestation in rare patients who experience an acute hypotensive episode after exposure to a known allergen or in a specific situation such as perioperative anaphylaxis.[22] In these situations where diagnosis of anaphylaxis poses difficulties, laboratory tests such as plasma histamine or total tryptase may be helpful. However, these tests do have certain limitations: (1) suboptimal specificity and sensitivity; (2) plasma histamine not available worldwide and requiring special handling (eg, centrifuging and freezing the plasma promptly); (3) limited timing for taking the blood sample (30–60 minutes after the onset of the episode). Although plasma or serum total tryptase levels are more practical (ie, increased from 15 minutes to 3 hours after symptom onset and requiring no special handling), they are seldom increased except in anaphylactic shock triggered by an injected agent, such as an injectable antibiotic or anesthetic agent.[23]

Symptom onset varies widely but generally occurs within seconds or minutes after exposure. The intravenous route of drug administration is usually associated with

Table 1 Clinical diagnosis of anaphylaxis	
Anaphylaxis is highly likely when there is an acute onset of clinical symptoms involving *at least 2* organ systems together with skin and mucosal tissue involvement	
Skin and mucosal tissue	Urticaria, angioedema, generalized pruritus or flushing, rhinitis, conjunctivitis
Respiratory system	Lower airway: dyspnea, wheezing, bronchospasm, reduced peak expiratory flow, hypoxemia Upper airway: stridor or upper airway obstruction from laryngeal edema or tongue swelling, together with hypersialorrhea, dysphonia, or dysphagia
Gastrointestinal symptoms	Crampy abdominal pain, nausea, vomiting, diarrhea
Cardiovascular system	Dizziness, syncope, hypotension (collapse)
Anaphylactic shock is defined as anaphylaxis accompanied by reduced blood pressure. On rare occasions, patients can present with isolated acute hypotensive episodes	
Infants and children	Low systolic blood pressure (age specific) or >30% decrease in systolic blood pressure
Adults	Systolic blood pressure <90 mm Hg or >30% decrease from patient's baseline

Data from Sampson HA, Munoz-Furlong A, Campbell RL, et al. Second symposium on the definition and management of anaphylaxis: summary report—Second National Institute of Allergy and Infectious Disease/Food Allergy and Anaphylaxis Network Symposium. J Allergy Clin Immunol 2006;117(2):391–7; and Kemp SF, Lockey RF, Wolf BL, Lieberman P. Anaphylaxis. A review of 266 cases. Arch Intern Med 1995;155(16):1749–54.

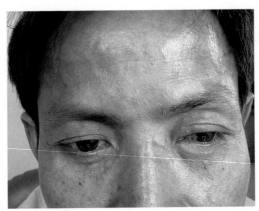

Fig. 5. Urticaria and angioedema involving eyelids, forehead, and face, associated with conjunctivitis and bronchospam, after positive oral aspirin challenge.

a rapid onset of reaction, whereas symptoms associated with the ingestion of an allergen may be more delayed (within the first 2–3 hours and exceptionally even up to several hours). It should be noted, however, that the onset of symptoms can occur immediately after ingestion, and such rapidly occurring events can be fatal. There is a direct relationship between the time of onset of the symptoms after antigen administration and their severity: the more rapid the onset, the more severe the episode.[28] In rare cases, an episode can be protracted, lasting for more than 24 hours, or can recur after initial resolution (biphasic anaphylaxis).[22]

Differential Diagnosis of Anaphylaxis

When the history of exposure to an offending agent is elicited, the diagnosis of anaphylaxis is often obvious because anaphylaxis is a dynamic continuum, usually characterized by a definable exposure to a potential trigger and by rapid onset, evolution, and resolution of symptoms within minutes to hours after treatment. Skin symptoms and signs such as itching, flushing, urticaria, and angioedema are extremely helpful in the diagnosis of allergic reaction,[23] but might be absent or unrecognized in 10% or more of all episodes, especially in severe episodes.[22,25] When gastrointestinal symptoms or respiratory symptoms predominate, or cardiopulmonary collapse makes obtaining a history impossible, anaphylaxis may be confused with other entities. Some of these differential diagnoses are listed in **Table 2**. Common diagnostic dilemmas involve acute asthma, syncope, and panic attacks.[23] These conditions, however, usually lack typical cutaneous signs and symptoms, and vasovagal reaction is associated with nausea, sweating, and bradycardic hypotension whereas anaphylaxis is almost always associated with tachycardic hypotension.

TRIGGERS OF ACUTE URTICARIA, ANGIOEDEMA, AND ANAPHYLAXIS
Mechanisms Involved

Acute urticaria/angioedema or anaphylactic reactions occurring within a few hours following the last administration of the drug may be due to allergic mechanisms (either IgE-dependent or other antibodies such as IgM or IgG) or nonallergic mechanisms (**Table 3**). An allergic mechanism involves the cross-linking of IgE and aggregation of the IgE receptors on mast cells and basophils. Nonallergic reactions include

Table 2
Differential diagnosis for anaphylaxis and anaphylactic shock

Presentation	Differential Diagnosis
Hypotension	Septic shock Vasovagal reaction Cardiogenic shock (sudden asystole may be a sign of anaphylactic shock as well) Hypovolemic shock
Respiratory distress with wheezing or stridor	Airway foreign body, especially in small children Asthma and chronic obstructive pulmonary disease exacerbation
Postprandial syndromes	High monosodium glutamate ingestion Sulfite ingestion Scrombroid fish poisoning[a]
Flush syndromes	Carcinoid syndrome Postmenopausal hot flushes Alcohol-induced flush Red man syndrome (vancomycin injection)
Excess endogenous production of histamine syndromes	Systemic mastocytosis[a] Basophil leukemia[a] Acute promyelocytic leukemia (tretinoin treatment)[a]
Nonorganic diseases	Panic attacks Vocal cord dysfunction syndrome Munchausen stridor
Miscellaneous	Cardiovascular (myocardial infarction)[a] Neurologic events (seizure, cerebrovascular event)

[a] May include hypotension.

Data from Lieberman PL. Anaphylaxis. In: Adkinson NF, Busse WW, Bochner BS, et al, editors. Middleton's allergy: principles and practice. 7th edition. Elsevier; 2009. p. 1027–50; and Tang AW. A practical guide to anaphylaxis. Am Fam Physician 2003;68(7):1325–32.

nonspecific histamine release (eg, opiates, RCM, plasma volume expander, and vancomycin), induction of leukotriene synthesis (nonsteroidal anti-inflammatory drugs [NSAIDs]), or bradykinin accumulation (angiotensin-converting enzyme [ACE] inhibitors).[5,6] Regardless of the initiating trigger and mechanism, cellular events in mast cells and basophils result in the rapid release of granule-associated preformed mediators, particularly histamine and tryptase. Moreover, the downstream production of arachidonic acid metabolites (including prostaglandins, leukotrienes, and synthesis of platelet-activating factor) and array of cytokines and chemokines lead to the development of immediate anaphylactic symptoms and a late-phase reaction.[22,23] It is of interest that some drugs can trigger acute allergic symptoms via both allergic and nonallergic mechanisms, such as NSAIDs, RCM, opiates, and some chemotherapeutic agents.[29–31]

Urticaria should be regarded as a symptom that can be triggered by a wide range of exogenous factors or endogenous diseases with allergic, inflammatory, or infectious mechanisms, and not uniquely the allergic reaction in nature.[10] The common causes of acute urticaria/angioedema are acute infections.[32] Acute viral infection, and especially upper respiratory tract infections (URI), appear to be the most common cause of acute urticaria, which are usually present a few days before the onset of wheal formation. The prevalence of URI in acute urticaria varies between 28% and 62%.[12,32,33] Because the drugs commonly prescribed during the treatment of these infections such as antibiotics and NSAIDs can also elicit acute urticaria, they are frequently

Table 3
Common triggers of acute urticaria, angioedema, and anaphylaxis

Nonallergic Triggers	Allergic Triggers
Acute urticaria/Angioedema	Food
Viral infections	Mostly peanuts, tree nuts, shellfish,
Physical stimuli	fish, milk, and egg
Certain food like strawberries	Food-dependent exercise induced
(unknown reason)	anaphylaxis (often associated with
Chemical substances: RCM,[a] volume	sensitization to omega5-gliadin)
expanders, aspirin, NSAIDs[a]	Drug
Drug causing direct mast cell	–Common: Antibiotics (β-lactams,
degranulation: opiates,[a] vancomycin	fluoroquinolone[a])
paclitaxel, docitaxel and doxorubicin,	NSAIDs[a]
quinolones[a]	RCM[a]
Acute manifestation of autoimmune	Myorelaxant
disease, connective tissue disease, or	Platinum compounds
malignancy	–Less common: opiates[a]
Isolated angioedema	Insect stings
ACE-inhibitor	Hymenoptera (bee, wasp, hornet, yellow
Aspirin, other NSAIDs[a]	jacket, sawfly), fire ant, or other biting
C1 INH deficiency (hereditary	insects (eg, flies, mosquitoes, kissing
angioedema or acquired form)	bugs)
Factor XII mutation and estrogen intake	Latex
Anaphylaxis	
Physical	
Idiopathic	

Abbreviations: NSAIDs, nonsteroidal anti-inflammatory drugs; RCM, radiocontrast media.
[a] Drugs capable of triggering acute HSRs either by nonallergic or allergic (IgE-specific) mechanism (see text).

accused wrongly. Unfortunately, there are no clinical predictors to differentiate between acute urticaria from infection and that from drug allergy, except the circumstantial evidence of resolution of infection and hives at the same time.[10] A significant proportion of physical stimuli (such as exposure to sun, water, or temperature extremes, pressure from, eg, wearing a heavy backpack, vibration), foods, chemical substances, and drugs (such as aspirin, NSAIDs, vancomycin, opiates, RCM, some chemotherapeutic agents, and volume expanders) can cause urticaria and angioedema by nonimmune-mediated mechanism (see **Table 3**).[9,11] Aspirin- and NSAID-induced urticaria and angioedema are common. Their prevalence in the general population has been reported to be 0.1% to 0.3%.[34] However, in selected populations, such as atopics, young adults, and 21% to 30% of patients with chronic urticaria, the risk of developing wheal and flare after the ingestion of this agent is increased.[35,36] Pathogenesis is believed to be the inhibition of cyclooxygenase (COX)-1, leading to a shunting of arachidonic acid metabolism toward the 5-lipooxygenase pathway, which results in an increased synthesis and release of cysteinyl leukotrienes.[37] The intake of aspirin and NSAIDs can also elicit adverse respiratory symptoms, such as asthmatic attacks and nasoocular symptoms (eg, conjunctivitis and rhinosinusitis) through the same pathomechanism, particularly in up to 10% of asthmatic patients and some atopic individuals.[38,39] Most sensitive persons who experience urticaria, angioedema, or respiratory symptoms may have similar reactions to chemically different conventional NSAIDs (antigenically unrelated to aspirin), so-called cross-reactivity, and must take low-dose acetaminophen or specific COX-2 inhibitors for treatment of fever, pain, or inflammation.[40–42] Other agents capable of the direct stimulation of histamine release from mast cells include opioids (such as codeine and morphine), vancomycin (red man syndrome), RCM, and certain chemotherapeutic agents (such as paclitaxel, docetaxel, and doxorubicin).[11,31] Volume expanders, particularly gelatin and dextran, are responsible for a few cases of acute HSR during operation.[29,43] These agents, particularly via intravenous administration, can produce symptoms identical to IgE-mediated immediate type reactions, including urticaria, angioedema, bronchospasm, and anaphylaxis (formerly termed "anaphylactoid reactions"). Other triggers are allergic, such as drug, food, insect sting, and latex (see **Table 3**). Exacerbations of chronic urticaria may be regarded as acute urticaria and allergens may be suspected. These conditions include autoimmune diseases (eg, thyroiditis and autoantibody to IgE receptor) and other systemic diseases (eg, connective tissue diseases, neoplastic conditions, and some chronic infections).[44]

Angioedema is classified as angioedema associated with mast cell degranulation from allergic reaction or nonallergic mechanism, and angioedema mediated by the accumulation of bradykinin. The first category is usually associated with urticaria and is caused by similar allergic and nonallergic triggers (see **Table 3**). The latter is usually associated with isolated angioedema and is caused by certain medications (eg, ACE inhibitors), C1 esterase inhibitors (C1 INH), or other deficiencies (hereditary or acquired angioedema, eg, lymphoma, autoimmune connective diseases).[13] *ACE inhibitor–induced angioedema* is not dose related, and is a class-specific mediated angioedema. Apart from the catalysis of the transformation of angiotensin I to angiotensin II, ACE also inactivates bradykinin. Thus, ACE inhibitors have the potential to keep bradykinin levels elevated. As bradykinin is a powerful vasoactive substance, excess levels may cause vasodilatation and increased vascular permeability. The overall incidence of ACE-induced angioedema is reported to be around 0.1% to 0.5%,[45–48] but it is the most common cause of acute angioedema cases referred to emergency hospital departments (23%–38%), in which up to 20% may be life threatening, especially when upper airway involvement occurs.[49] Furthermore, although 50% of ACE inhibitor–induced angioedema may occur during the first week of therapy, some patients may have taken the ACE inhibitor without any problem for weeks, months, or even years before the development of angioedema.[29,45] The face and oral mucosa, including the larynx and subglottal area, are most often affected, but isolated visceral angioedema, causing abdominal pain, has also been reported. Emergency treatment as well as hospitalization for observation may be necessary in severe cases. Angiotensin II receptor antagonists do not actually interfere with bradykinin metabolism; nevertheless, some reports postulate recurrent angioedema after switching to these compounds.[48,50,51]

Aspirin and NSAIDs can induce periorbital angioedema either in isolation or as part of an upper respiratory reaction in "aspirin-sensitive asthma." Isolated periorbital angioedema is a typical manifestation of cutaneous reaction to aspirin and NSAIDs in atopic and young adults (see **Fig. 2**).[29,34,52,53] Most of these patients exhibit cross-reactivity with other NSAIDs, and should receive similar management to those presenting with urticaria and angioedema alone or with respiratory symptoms.[53]

Hereditary angioedema (HAE) is a rare, dominantly inherited disease that affects about 1 in 50,000 persons, representing approximately 1% of all cases of angioedema. HAE is mediated by bradykinin.[54] It is a result of deficiency (type 1) or dysfunction (type 2) of the plasma inhibitor of the first component of complement C1 INH. Recently a new, estrogen-dependent form, characterized by a mutation in factor XII, has been described,[55] This form of HAE affects women, and angioedematous attacks are often triggered by intake of anticonceptive hormones or pregnancy. HAE is characterized clinically by recurrent bouts of painless, nonpruritic, nonpitting edema involving the face, larynx, gastrointestinal tract, and extremities. Attacks are triggered by emotional stress, vigorous exercise, alcohol consumption, hormonal changes, and minor trauma such as dental maneuvers, and lasts 1 to 4 days. Facial and extremity edema resolve gradually without harm, whereas untreated laryngeal edema is progressive and can result in death by asphyxiation.[10,13,54] Patients with mutations in factor XII have laryngeal edema less frequently than patients with classic C1 INH deficiency. Treatment with H1 antihistamines and corticosteroids has little effect, while CI INH reconstitution or the bradykinin receptor antagonist icatibant reduces swelling.[54]

Acquired C1 INH deficiency. C1 INH deficiency may also be acquired as a result of immune complex-mediated depletion or antibody directed against C1 INH, associated with lymphoproliferative disease, particularly B-cell lymphoma, carcinoma, or connective tissue diseases such as systemic lupus erythematosus.[10,13]

Anaphylaxis' common causes include allergic triggers such as foods, drugs, insect stings, and latex, as well as physical factors/exercise and idiopathic anaphylaxis (where no cause is identified) (see **Table 3**). Approximately one-third of anaphylactic episodes are triggered by foods such as shellfish, peanuts, eggs, milk, fish, and tree nuts. Another common cause of anaphylaxis is a sting from a fire ant or hymenoptera (bee, wasp, hornet, yellow jacket, and sawfly).[22,23] The incidence of latex allergy has stabilized after educational campaigns and the substitution of power-free latex and nonlatex gloves in hospitals. However, latex allergy still incorporates an unpredictable risk affecting the general population, in both occupational and nonoccupational settings exposed to latex (gloves, condoms, and urinary catheters).[25]

The drugs that most often cause anaphylaxis include antibiotics, NSAIDs, RCM, and muscle relaxants.

- Antibiotics: In most studies, antibacterial agents were responsible for the highest number of reports of anaphylaxis, including β-lactams (penicillins and cephalosporins) and fluoroquinolones. At one time, penicillin was probably the most common cause. Between 1 and 5 per 10,000 patient-courses with penicillin result in allergic reactions, with 1 in 50,000 to 1 in 100,000 courses having a fatal outcome.[56,57] However, it appears that during recent years the incidence of anaphylaxis to cephalosporins as well as fluoroquinolones is increasing.[43,58–63]
- Aspirin and NSAIDs: Some NSAIDs can cause anaphylaxis in the outpatient setting.[16,26,64] Propyphenazone and pyrazolone were mainly responsible for this reaction. The mechanism was thought to be allergic in nature.[43,52,53,65] However, other NSAIDs have also been reported to be associated with anaphylaxis, such as the diclofenac and oxicam groups, and celecoxib, although drug-specific IgE could not be identified.[25,29,64,66–69]
- RCM can result in severe adverse reaction at a rate of 0.2% for ionic agents and 0.04% for lower osmolarity, nonionic agents. Although they were previously thought to induce acute HSR by a nonallergic mechanism, IgE antibody–mediated mechanisms have recently been identified in some patients.[29,30,70]
- Muscle relaxants are one of the major causes of anaphylaxis during general anesthesia. IgE antibodies against quarternary ammonium ions have been identified and cross-reactivity to other muscle relaxants have been frequently observed. Patients were successfully treated with test-negative agents.[60]
- Chemotherapeutic agents, particularly platinum salts such as carboplatin, cisplatin, and oxaliplatin, are associated with acute HSR after several courses of treatment and usually with a positive skin test. Cross-reactivity to other platins

has been reported, and desensitization offers an effective means for continuation of therapy in cancer patients requiring these agents.[31]

- Other substances: Opioids have been reported to be a cause of anaphylaxis during general anesthesia in a small fraction of patients.[60] Rare, but important causes of anaphylaxis are also chlorhexidin (particularly in urology) and dyes such as patent blue (used in surgery to trace draining lymph nodes).[71,72]

MANAGEMENT OF ACUTE URTICARIA, ANGIOEDEMA, AND ANAPHYLAXIS
Pharmacologic Treatment

As with the treatment of any critically ill patient, the treatment of anaphylaxis begins with a rapid assessment and maintenance of the airway, breathing, and circulation. When a patient fulfills criteria for anaphylaxis, even with symptoms involving nonvital organs, the patient should receive adrenaline/epinephrine immediately intramuscularly, in an attempt to prevent more severe anaphylaxis (self-injectable epinephrine preparations normally contain 0.3 mg epinephrine for adults and 0.15 mg for children; higher doses may be required in adults or overweight persons). Delaying treatment until the development of multiorgan symptoms may be risky because the ultimate severity of anaphylaxis is difficult or impossible to predict at the time of onset of the episodes.[22,73] Subsequent management strategies are determined on the basis of the clinical course and response to adrenaline/epinephrine (**Box 1**).[22,73,74]

For urticaria and angioedema however, H1 antihistamines are the mainstay of treatment. Both first- and second-generation H1 antihistamines are effective in controlling symptoms. Second-generation H1 antihistamines are generally considered the first choice in treatment, because of the lower sedative effects.[76] The addition of a relatively brief use of systemic corticosteroids (0.5–1 mg/kg/d) may be considered in patients with severe symptoms, particularly in the presence of angioedema, to achieve better symptomatic control. These medications have serious potential side effects and may be associated with a significant flare of symptoms after tapering or withdrawal, and thus are not routinely indicated.[11,21]

Observation

After treatment of an anaphylactic reaction, an observation period should be considered for all patients, given that the reaction might recur as the effect of the adrenaline/epinephrine wears off (intramuscular injection results in increased serum levels for an hour or more) and due to the risk of a biphasic reaction (around 1%–20% of the reactions).[77] A reasonable length of time is 4 to 6 hours for most patients, with a prolonged period or hospital admission for those with severe or refractory symptoms.[22]

Evaluation and Long-Term Plan of Management of Acute Urticaria, Angioedema, and Anaphylaxis

The first step is a thorough history taking to identify the cause of urticaria, angioedema, and anaphylaxis, and to determine those at risk for future attacks. In contrast to anaphylaxis, most patients with acute urticaria and angioedema do not require extensive laboratory evaluation except to confirm a causative agent (eg, skin testing for a suspected allergen). Moreover, almost all cases of acute urticaria and angioedema in adults are self limited within 3 weeks.[78]

A complete history and physical examination are the most important tools in the diagnosis and evaluation of urticaria and angioedema. This process is frequently time consuming. Specific questions should address the following: a history of viral infection; recent insect bites or stings; suspected food; skin contact with foreign

---

Box 1
Management of acute anaphylaxis

Immediate intervention

1. Assessment of airway, breathing, circulation, and consciousness

2. Administer adrenaline/epinephrine 1:1000 dilution (1 mg in 1 mL) intramuscularly, 0.2 to 0.5 mg (0.01 mg/kg in children with maximum dose of 0.3 mg) every 5 to 15 minutes, or in a situation of general anesthesia where intravenous access and cardiac monitoring are available, treatment tailored to the severity of symptoms may be used (ie, initial intravenous dose: 10–20 µg in grade II reactions, 100–200 µg in case of grade III reactions, repeated every 1–2 minutes as necessary, to control symptoms and blood pressure).

General measures

1. Place patient in recumbent position and elevate lower extremities.

2. Establish and maintain airway.

3. Administer oxygen.

4. Establish venous access and administer normal saline intravenously for fluid replacement. If severe hypotension exists, rapid infusion of volume expanders (colloid-containing solution) is necessary.

5. Seek help

Specific measures to consider after adrenaline/epinephrine injections, where appropriate

1. H1 antihistamines, such as chlorpheniramine or diphenhydramine 50 mg intravenously.

2. Nebulized β_2 agonist (eg, salbutamol) for bronchospasm resistant to epinephrine.

3. Systemic corticosteroid, such as methylprednisolone 1 to 2 mg/kg per day, are not usually helpful acutely, but might prevent prolonged reactions or relapses.

4. Vasopressor (eg, dopamine) for hypotension refractory to volume replacement and epinephrine.

5. Glucagon for patient taking β-blockers.

6. Atropine for symptomatic bradycardia.

7. Consider transportation to an emergency department or an intensive care facility.

8. For cardiopulmonary arrest during anaphylaxis, high-dose epinephrine and prolonged resuscitation efforts are encouraged.

Data from[22,73,75]

---

material, heat, cold, or water; and drugs. It is crucial to identify all medications (including prescription, over-the-counter, oral, topical, conventional including blood transfusion, RCM, and herbal) that are taken intermittently or regularly, and which the patient is currently using. Questioning about history of latex sensitivity or possible exposures may reveal a potential occult contact allergen.[11,21] Despite extensive evaluation, possible eliciting factors for acute urticaria and angioedema are not always identified.[78] For patients experiencing anaphylactic reaction, the evaluation and management are more complex, and are detailed in **Box 2**. The prescription of self-injectable epinephrine is mandatory until allergy testing, but is of less interest in the case of a drug allergy. A follow-up evaluation with an allergist should be made in all patients to confirm the anaphylaxis trigger and to plan for long-term individualized preventive measures (see **Box 2**).[22,23,73]

Box 2
Long-term management and preventive measures for patients with anaphylaxis

General measures to be taken before discharging a patient from an emergency department

Obtain thorough history to identify potential causes of anaphylaxis and to determine those at risk of future attacks, and organize:

1. Prescription of self-injectable adrenaline/epinephrine for patients experiencing severe anaphylactic symptoms after exposure to a known allergen in the community (such as food or insect sting).

2. Patient education, in particular how to avoid the allergen and its cross-reactive substances or how to recognize and treat anaphylactic episodes promptly if they occur; also how to gain access to emergency medical services and the closest emergency department.

3. Follow-up with an allergist.

Role of allergist-immunologist specialist

- Confirmation of allergic triggers

  Detailed history and physical examination

  Skin tests: prick and intradermal tests with immediate reading

  Laboratory tests: specific IgE, in vitro test for drug allergy

  Controlled administration of suspected allergen: drug provocation test, food challenge

- Individualized preventive measures and long-term management

  Desensitization (in confirmed IgE-mediated allergic reaction and no alternative measures)

  Avoidance of the causative allergen and cross-reactive substance

  Find safe alternative treatment for the patient (particularly in drug allergy)

  Premedication may be useful in nonallergic hypersensitivity reaction

Data from Refs.[6,22,23]

Diagnostic Workup for Drug Allergy

The history of drug allergy alone is in fact often not reliable because different drugs are frequently taken simultaneously, every one of which is capable of accounting for the symptoms, and it may be imprecise. Acute urticaria and angioedema are nonspecific processes and may be caused by multiple factors as described above, while anaphylaxis may be confused with other conditions as well. Depending on history only (without proving the relationship between drug intake and symptoms or clarifying the underlying pathomechanism of the reaction) leads to overdiagnosis and unnecessary elimination of useful drugs. Particularly in cases where essential and/or frequently prescribed drug classes (eg, β-lactams, paracetamol, NSAIDs, local anesthetics, and myorelaxants) are involved, a diagnosis procedure should be performed in a specialist center, which may include repeated detailed clinical history and physical examination, skin tests, laboratory tests and, ultimately, drug provocation tests.[6,79] Only a formal diagnosis of drug HSRs allows one to bring into play the measures required for prevention and treatment. Skin-prick tests and/or intradermal tests with immediate reading (after 20 minutes) are particularly important tools for demonstrating an IgE-dependent mechanism. Unfortunately, reliable skin test procedures and validated test concentrations for drug allergy are often missing. However, some agents have satisfactory high sensitivity and predictive value (eg, penicillins, cephalosporins,[80,81]

24. Lieberman P, Camargo CA Jr, Bohlke K, et al. Epidemiology of anaphylaxis: findings of the American College of Allergy, Asthma and Immunology Epidemiology of Anaphylaxis Working Group. Ann Allergy Asthma Immunol 2006;97(5):596–602.

25. Helbling A, Hurni T, Mueller UR, et al. Incidence of anaphylaxis with circulatory symptoms: a study over a 3-year period comprising 940,000 inhabitants of the Swiss Canton Bern. Clin Exp Allergy 2004;34(2):285–90.

26. Kemp SF, Lockey RF, Wolf BL, et al. Anaphylaxis. A review of 266 cases. Arch Intern Med 1995;155(16):1749–54.

27. Webb LM, Lieberman P. Anaphylaxis: a review of 601 cases. Ann Allergy Asthma Immunol 2006;97(1):39–43.

28. Lieberman PL. Anaphylaxis. In: Adkinson NF, Busse WW, Bochner BS, et al, editors. Middleton's Allergy: principles and practice. 7th edition. China: Elsevier; 2009. p. 1027–50.

29. Bircher AJ. Drug-induced urticaria and angioedema caused by non-IgE mediated pathomechanisms. Eur J Dermatol 1999;9(8):657–63 [quiz: 63].

30. Laroche D, Aimone-Gastin I, Dubois F, et al. Mechanisms of severe, immediate reactions to iodinated contrast material. Radiology 1998;209(1):183–90.

31. Limsuwan T, Castells MC. Outcomes and safety of rapid desensitization for chemotherapy hypersensitivity. Expert Opin Drug Saf 2010;9(1):39–53.

32. Mortureux P, Leaute-Labreze C, Legrain-Lifermann V, et al. Acute urticaria in infancy and early childhood: a prospective study. Arch Dermatol 1998;134(3):319–23.

33. Schuller DE, Elvey SM. Acute urticaria associated with streptococcal infection. Pediatrics 1980;65(3):592–6.

34. Sanchez-Borges M, Capriles-Hulett A, Caballero-Fonseca F. NSAID-induced urticaria and angioedema: a reappraisal of its clinical management. Am J Clin Dermatol 2002;3(9):599–607.

35. Asero R. Risk factors for acetaminophen and nimesulide intolerance in patients with NSAID-induced skin disorders. Ann Allergy Asthma Immunol 1999;82(6):554–8.

36. Sanchez-Borges M, Capriles-Hulett A. Atopy is a risk factor for non-steroidal anti-inflammatory drug sensitivity. Ann Allergy Asthma Immunol 2000;84(1):101–6.

37. Mastalerz L, Setkowicz M, Sanak M, et al. Hypersensitivity to aspirin: common eicosanoid alterations in urticaria and asthma. J Allergy Clin Immunol 2004;113(4):771–5.

38. Stevenson DD, Szczeklik A. Clinical and pathologic perspectives on aspirin sensitivity and asthma. J Allergy Clin Immunol 2006;118(4):773–86 [quiz: 87–8].

39. Szczeklik A, Stevenson DD. Aspirin-induced asthma: advances in pathogenesis, diagnosis, and management. J Allergy Clin Immunol 2003;111(5):913–21 [quiz: 22].

40. Sanchez-Borges M, Caballero-Fonseca F, Capriles-Hulett A. Safety of etoricoxib, a new cyclooxygenase 2 inhibitor, in patients with nonsteroidal anti-inflammatory drug-induced urticaria and angioedema. Ann Allergy Asthma Immunol 2005 Aug;95(2):154–8.

41. Sanchez-Borges M, Caballero-Fonseca F, Capriles-Hulett A. Tolerance of nonsteroidal anti-inflammatory drug-sensitive patients to the highly specific cyclooxygenase 2 inhibitors rofecoxib and valdecoxib. Ann Allergy Asthma Immunol 2005 Jan;94(1):34–8.

42. Settipane RA, Schrank PJ, Simon RA, et al. Prevalence of cross-sensitivity with acetaminophen in aspirin-sensitive asthmatic subjects. J Allergy Clin Immunol 1995;96(4):480–5.

43. Leone R, Conforti A, Venegoni M, et al. Drug-induced anaphylaxis: case/non-case study based on an Italian pharmacovigilance database. Drug Saf 2005; 28(6):547–56.

44. Zuberbier T, Asero R, Bindslev-Jensen C, et al. EAACI/GA(2)LEN/EDF/WAO guideline: management of urticaria. Allergy 2009;64(10):1427–43.

45. Agostoni A, Cicardi M. Drug-induced angioedema without urticaria. Drug Saf 2001;24(8):599–606.

46. Kostis JB, Kim HJ, Rusnak J, et al. Incidence and characteristics of angioedema associated with enalapril. Arch Intern Med 2005;165(14):1637–42.

47. Sabroe RA, Black AK. Angiotensin-converting enzyme (ACE) inhibitors and angio-oedema. Br J Dermatol 1997;136(2):153–8.

48. Warner KK, Visconti JA, Tschampel MM. Angiotensin II receptor blockers in patients with ACE inhibitor-induced angioedema. Ann Pharmacother 2000; 34(4):526–8.

49. Bluestein HM, Hoover TA, Banerji AS, et al. Angiotensin-converting enzyme inhibitor-induced angioedema in a community hospital emergency department. Ann Allergy Asthma Immunol 2009;103(6):502–7.

50. Fuchs SA, Koopmans RP, Guchelaar HJ, et al. Are angiotensin II receptor antagonists safe in patients with previous angiotensin-converting enzyme inhibitor-induced angioedema? Hypertension 2001;37(1):E1.

51. Howes LG, Tran D. Can angiotensin receptor antagonists be used safely in patients with previous ACE inhibitor-induced angioedema? Drug Saf 2002; 25(2):73–6.

52. Quiralte J, Blanco C, Castillo R, et al. Intolerance to nonsteroidal antiinflammatory drugs: results of controlled drug challenges in 98 patients. J Allergy Clin Immunol 1996;98(3):678–85.

53. Quiralte J, Blanco C, Delgado J, et al. Challenge-based clinical patterns of 223 Spanish patients with nonsteroidal anti-inflammatory-drug-induced-reactions. J Investig Allergol Clin Immunol 2007;17(3):182–8.

54. Zuraw BL. Clinical practice. Hereditary angioedema. N Engl J Med 2008;359(10): 1027–36.

55. Bork K, Wulff K, Hardt J, et al. Hereditary angioedema caused by missense mutations in the factor XII gene: clinical features, trigger factors, and therapy. J Allergy Clin Immunol 2009;124(1):129–34.

56. Neugut AI, Ghatak AT, Miller RL. Anaphylaxis in the United States: an investigation into its epidemiology. Arch Intern Med 2001;161(1):15–21.

57. Tang AW. A practical guide to anaphylaxis. Am Fam Physician 2003;68(7): 1325–32.

58. Demoly P, Messaad D, Sahla H, et al. Immediate hypersensitivity to ceftriaxone. Allergy 2000;55(4):418–9.

59. Gibbs MW, Kuczkowski KM, Benumof JL. Complete recovery from prolonged cardio-pulmonary resuscitation following anaphylactic reaction to readministered intravenous cefazolin. Acta Anaesthesiol Scand 2003;47(2):230–2.

60. Mertes PM, Laxenaire MC, Alla F. Anaphylactic and anaphylactoid reactions occurring during anesthesia in France in 1999-2000. Anesthesiology 2003; 99(3):536–45.

61. Novembre E, Mori F, Pucci N, et al. Cefaclor anaphylaxis in children. Allergy 2009; 64(8):1233–5.

62. Romano A, Quaratino D, Venemalm L, et al. A case of IgE-mediated hypersensitivity to ceftriaxone. J Allergy Clin Immunol 1999;104(5):1113–4.

63. Warrington RJ, McPhillips S. Independent anaphylaxis to cefazolin without allergy to other beta-lactam antibiotics. J Allergy Clin Immunol 1996;98(2):460–2.

64. Berkes EA. Anaphylactic and anaphylactoid reactions to aspirin and other NSAIDs. Clin Rev Allergy Immunol 2003;24(2):137–48.

65. Himly M, Jahn-Schmid B, Pittertschatscher K, et al. IgE-mediated immediate-type hypersensitivity to the pyrazolone drug propyphenazone. J Allergy Clin Immunol 2003;111(4):882–8.

66. Bavbek S, Erkekol FO, Dursun B, et al. Meloxicam-associated anaphylactic reaction. J Investig Allergol Clin Immunol 2006;16(5):317–20.

67. Chamberlin KW, Silverman AR. Celecoxib-associated anaphylaxis. Ann Pharmacother 2009;43(4):777–81.

68. Fontaine C, Bousquet PJ, Demoly P. Anaphylactic shock caused by a selective allergy to celecoxib, with no allergy to rofecoxib or sulfamethoxazole. J Allergy Clin Immunol 2005;115(3):633–4.

69. Levy MB, Fink JN. Anaphylaxis to celecoxib. Ann Allergy Asthma Immunol 2001; 87(1):72–3.

70. Brockow K, Romano A, Aberer W, et al. Reactions to iodinated contrast media— a European multicenter study. Allergy 2009;64(2):234–41.

71. Beaudouin E, Kanny G, Morisset M, et al. Immediate hypersensitivity to chlorhexidine: literature review. Eur Ann Allergy Clin Immunol 2004;36(4):123–6.

72. Mertes PM, Malinovsky JM, Mouton-Faivre C, et al. Anaphylaxis to dyes during the perioperative period: reports of 14 clinical cases. J Allergy Clin Immunol 2008;122(2):348–52.

73. Kemp SF, Lockey RF, Simons FE. Epinephrine: the drug of choice for anaphylaxis. A statement of the World Allergy Organization. Allergy 2008;63(8):1061–70.

74. Kemp SF, Lockey RF. Anaphylaxis: a review of causes and mechanisms. J Allergy Clin Immunol 2002;110(3):341–8.

75. Mertes PM, Laxenaire MC, Lienhart A, et al. Reducing the risk of anaphylaxis during anaesthesia: guidelines for clinical practice. J Investig Allergol Clin Immunol 2005;15(2):91–101.

76. Simons FE. Advances in H1-antihistamines. N Engl J Med 2004;351(21):2203–17.

77. Lieberman P. Biphasic anaphylactic reactions. Ann Allergy Asthma Immunol 2005;95(3):217–26 [quiz: 26, 58].

78. Zuberbier T, Ifflander J, Semmler C, et al. Acute urticaria: clinical aspects and therapeutic responsiveness. Acta Derm Venereol 1996;76(4):295–7.

79. Brockow K, Romano A, Blanca M, et al. General considerations for skin test procedures in the diagnosis of drug hypersensitivity. Allergy 2002;57(1):45–51.

80. Romano A, Gaeta F, Valluzzi RL, et al. Diagnosing hypersensitivity reactions to cephalosporins in children. Pediatrics 2008;122(3):521–7.

81. Romano A, Gueant-Rodriguez RM, Viola M, et al. Diagnosing immediate reactions to cephalosporins. Clin Exp Allergy 2005;35(9):1234–42.

82. Aberer W, Bircher A, Romano A, et al. Drug provocation testing in the diagnosis of drug hypersensitivity reactions: general considerations. Allergy 2003;58(9): 854–63.

Delayed Cutaneous Manifestations of Drug Hypersensitivity

Andreas J. Bircher, MD*, Kathrin Scherer, MD

KEYWORDS

- Drug hypersensitivity • Cutaneous manifestation
- Maculopapular exanthem • Urticaria • Vasculitis
- Acute generalized exanthematous pustulosis
- Drug-induced hypersensitivity syndrome/
  drug reaction with eosinophilia and systemic symptoms

Adverse drug reactions (ADRs) affect a considerable number of patients. Between 10% and 15% of treated patients report an unwanted drug reaction, 2% to 5% of them have to be hospitalized, and in 1% to 3% of them mortality may result.[1]

ADRs often involve the skin.[2] Particularly, hypersensitivity reactions may present with cutaneous manifestations only. However, a careful look may often reveal (minor) organ involvement as well, indicating that drug hypersensitivity reactions are systemic immune reactions. On the other hand, in some reactions, the skin involvement may be of minor importance (anaphylaxis or the drug hypersensitivity syndrome [DHS]).[3]

The skin may present a variety of different reaction patterns. The correct identification and diagnosis of the skin lesions are paramount for the diagnosis of drug-induced hypersensitivity. For this reason, as for syphilis, the term "the great imitator" has been attributed to drug-induced hypersensitivity reactions, because they can imitate a variety of other diseases.[4] Therefore, in many clinical situations cutaneous ADRs present a challenge in the differential diagnosis.

INITIAL STEPS OF DIAGNOSIS

The approach to the patient with a presumed drug hypersensitivity is described in another article by B. Schnyder in this issue. In brief, the initial clinical diagnosis requires a detailed description of the morphology, particularly the cutaneous efflorescences and signs. The often-used term "rash" is not specific and clear enough for this

No conflict of interest.
Allergy Unit, Department of Dermatology, University Hospital Basel, Petersgraben 4, CH-4031, Basel, Switzerland
* Corresponding author.
E-mail address: andreas.bircher@unibas.ch

Med Clin N Am 94 (2010) 711–725
doi:10.1016/j.mcna.2010.04.001
0025-7125/10/$ – see front matter © 2010 Elsevier Inc. All rights reserved.

purpose. The clinical investigation comprises a complete examination of the skin and its appendages, including the mucous membranes of the mouth, eyes, and genitals. The type (**Box 1**) and distribution (**Box 2**, **Fig. 1**) of the lesions as well as their evolution (**Fig. 2**) should be noted, for example, predominant affection of the trunk, acral localizations, involvement of face and scalp, or sparing or involvement of light-protected areas. Pruritus of variable severity is typically present. The morphologic presentations of cutaneous hypersensitivity reactions are manifold and variable. Although the skin has only a limited repertoire of inflammatory reaction patterns, a wide spectrum including pruritus, erythema, erythroderma, urticaria, angioedema and macular, papular, vesicular, bullous, vasculitic, hemorrhagic, or necrotic lesions (see **Box 1**) may be observed.[5,6] Some manifestations are rather specific for an ADR, such as fixed drug eruption, whereas others may present a challenge in the differential diagnosis toward other skin disorders, particularly infectious exanthems.[7] A histopathologic examination may be helpful in distinguishing drug eruptions from other dermatoses.[8] Based on the information gathered by clinical investigation and history, a pathogenetic

---

Box 1
Drug induced cutaneous symptoms/signs

Pruritus

    Indirect signs (erosions from scratching)

Urticaria, angioedema

Exanthems

    Macular

    Papular

    Vesicular

    Pustular

    Bullous

    Hemorrhagic

    Necrotic

    Lichenoid

    Psoriasiform

    Pityriasiform

    Exfoliative

    Erythroderma

Mucous membranes

    Erythema

    Erosions

    Aphthous lesions

    Ulcerations

Data from Bircher AJ. Approach to the patient with a drug hypersensitivity reaction–clinical perspectives. In: Pichler W, editor. Drug hypersensitivity. Basel (Switzerland): Karger; 2007. p. 354.

Box 2
Localization and distribution

Localized (central)

    Trunk

    Hand, feet

    Extremities

    Face

Localized (acral)

    Hands, feet

Isolated

Flexural

Disseminated

Generalized

Light (UV)-associated

    Face

    Nose, upper lids, and lip

    Chin shadow

    Back of hand, feet

---

hypothesis of the reaction can be formulated. This facilitates the later selection of allergological test tools, which may help in the identification of the eliciting drug. The suspected drugs should be immediately stopped, particularly if danger signs such as bullous or hemorrhagic widespread lesions or mucosal affections are present.[3]

Etiologic Diagnosis

The next step includes the identification of the potentially eliciting drug or drugs. Information on their dosages, way of administration, and the chronology of the reaction and the identification of cofactors such as underlying disorders (eg, viral infections, hepatopathy, or renal diseases) are required. A standardized approach with a drug questionnaire and consultation of pertinent textbooks is recommended.[9]

Chronology

The time period between the first dose and the occurrence of first symptoms does vary. First, a clear distinction between the situation of an immunologically naive person and a sensitized individual should be made. Sensitization to a drug or its metabolites takes at least 5 to 7 days of exposure but for several reasons it may take up to several weeks or rarely months to be completed. Particularly, intake of a drug at changing intervals and with irregular frequency may facilitate sensitization, whereas the continuous intake typically results more likely in tolerance. This time lag between the initiation of a drug therapy and the beginning of first symptoms represents the induction interval and does not cause any recognizable symptoms. It may be in part influenced by cofactors such as dose, metabolism, dosing intervals, and administration route of the drug among others. Sensitization, however, may also occur through another similar molecule and elicit an allergic reaction on first exposure to a molecule by

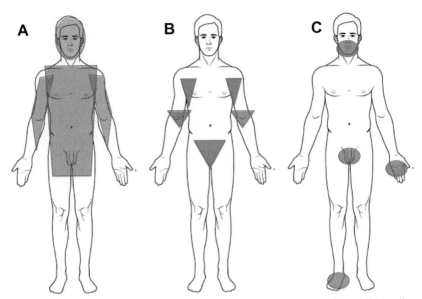

Fig. 1. Patterns of localization and distribution of common drug eruptions. (*A*) Maculopapular exanthem and urticaria: trunk and proximal extremities, rarely head. (*B*) Flexural exanthem (symmetrical drug-related intertriginous and flexural exanthem [SDRIFE]): perigenital and gluteal triangle, large folds (axillae, elbows). (*C*) Fixed drug eruption and angioedema: face and oral cavity, hands and feet, and male genitals. (Image reprinted with permission from Medscape.com, 2009.)

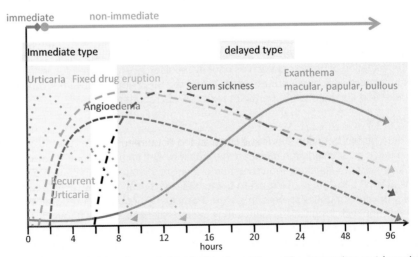

Fig. 2. Characteristic chronology of drug-induced eruptions. The separation at 1 hour into immediate or nonimmediate reactions does not sufficiently reflect the large overlap between the pathophysiologically determined immediate- and delayed-type clinical manifestations.

cross-reactivity. This type of sensitization has been shown not only for the β-lactam ring in penicillins and cephalosporins and quinolones[10] but also for sulfonamides and aromatic antiepileptic drugs. Once an individual is sensitized, the time period between the exposure to the eliciting dose and the first occurrence of symptoms, the so-called reaction interval, varies depending on the pathomechanism and type of eruption (see **Fig. 2**).[4,11] In IgE-mediated reactions, the typical eliciting or reaction period varies between a few minutes and some hours (see the article by Lumsuwan and Demoly elsewhere in this issue for further exploration of this topic). In the so-called pseudoallergic reactions, mainly to nonsteroidal antiinflammatory drugs (NSAIDs) and radio contrast media, the reaction period is also short, although no IgE-mediated mechanism has been definitely proved for NSAIDs, with the exception of reactions from pyrazolones[12] and possibly metabolites from diclofenac.[13] In T cell–mediated (many exanthems) reactions the time delay ranges typically between a few hours and 2 days. Typically, there is also a certain inherent dynamism in the reaction, for example, an exanthema may set out with an erythematous flush or macules within hours, which then turn into papules that peak at 48 to 72 hours, that is, not only the distribution and extent of the eruption but also the single lesions may vary over time. In immediate reactions (eg, urticaria), this aspect is less pronounced; however, also in IgE-mediated reactions, the delay after drug intake (eg, by the oral route) may last up to several hours.[14] Many factors, eg, the route of administration (intravenous > intramuscular > subcutaneous > topical > oral), drug metabolism, and other cofactors (food intake, drug interactions) play a modifying role. For this reason, the somewhat rigid separation between immediate and nonimmediate reactions at 1 hour based on the chronology only[15,16] may be problematic, because there is a considerable overlap of a period of approximately 2 to 6 hours between the reaction period of urticarial and exanthematous eruptions (see **Fig. 2**, **Table 1**). The terms immediate and delayed are also commonly used to depict the pathophysiology (ie, type I [IgE mediated] and type IV [T cell mediated]). This is most important with regard to the selection of appropriate diagnostic tests.

DELAYED OCCURRING CUTANEOUS MANIFESTATIONS OF DRUG HYPERSENSITIVITY

The clinical characteristics of the more common and some more severe drug-related manifestations with a delayed occurrence are reviewed.[7] Also, urticaria and angioedema are briefly mentioned because they may develop with a delay of several hours after exposure to the eliciting drug. Some drug-induced syndromes have been defined to delineate them from other diseases (**Table 2**). However, there is no general agreement on the terminology. More detailed information on the severe bullous reactions such as Stevens-Johnson syndrome (SJS) and toxic epidermal necrolysis (TEN) is presented in other articles of this issue.

General Symptoms

Generally, patients with allergic reactions do not often suffer substantially from the ongoing immune process: many patients may feel surprisingly good considering that a generalized immune reaction takes place. They mainly suffer from pruritus. If, however, nonspecific symptoms, such as general malaise, fatigue, headache, elevated body temperature, and gastrointestinal ailments (vomitus, diarrhea) are present, then they should be considered as an ominous sign of a more severe reaction (in particular acute generalized exanthematous pustulosis [AGEP], SJS/TEN, and DHS/drug reaction with eosinophilia and systemic symptoms [DRESS]).

Table 1
Clinical manifestations, chronology and morphology

Clinical Diagnosis	Chronology of Elicitation	Morphology and Localization
Urticaria, Angioedema	Immediate Typically minutes to 1–2 h, angioedema up to 6 h Rapid change and resolution (Urticaria <24 h) Angioedema 24–72 h	Urticarial wheals, pale swelling surrounded by erythematous border Pruritus No cutaneous sequelae Trunk, face, generalized, mucosae
Anaphylaxis	Immediate Typically few minutes to 1–2 h Rapid change and resolution (<24 h) NB: biphasic anaphylaxis	Flush (face, trunk, folds) Urticaria (disseminated) Angioedema Palmoplantar or inguinal pruritus No cutaneous sequelae
Maculopapular Exanthem	Delayed Typically 6–24 h Peak at 48–72 h Resolution 5–7 d	Macules, papules confluence, desquamation Trunk, proximal extremities, dissemination
Fixed Drug Eruption	Delayed Typically 0.5–8 h Resolution 3–5 d	Erythematous or lilac macule or plaque, central bulla, erosion, permanent hyperpigmentation, burning, pruritus Fixed (identical) Acral localization, mucosa
Pustular Exanthem (AGEP)	Delayed Typically 6–12 h up to 24–48 h Resolution 5–7 d	Confluent erythema, pinpoint nonfollicular pustules, pruritus, massive desquamation Folds, trunk, dissemination generalized
Vesiculobullous exanthems	Delayed Typically 24–48 h Resolution 14–21 d	Macules, bullae, epidermolysis, mucositis Initially painful skin Trunk, face, dissemination generalized

Abbreviation: AGEP, acute generalized exanthematous pustulosis; NB, nota bene.
Data from Bach S, Bircher AJ. Drug hypersensitivity reactions: from clinical manifestations to an allergologic diagnosis. Eur Ann Allergy Clin Immunol 2005;37(6):213–8.

Drug Fever

Fever may be the only manifestation of a drug hypersensitivity reaction; its frequency is estimated at a few percent in all ADRs. Many patients suffer from additional symptoms, such as headaches and myalgias. Physical factors, pyrogens, and immune complexes contributing to the pathogenesis are discussed. Drugs that may elicit an isolated drug fever are antibiotics, cytostatics, sulfonamides, antidepressants, and many others.[17] On the other hand, fever may precede or accompany particularly the more severe drug-induced exanthems, such as DHS or AGEP. In the latter, fever and neutrophilia are the diagnostic criteria.

Pruritus

Itch is a very common symptom of many skin diseases and, in particular, allergic reactions. It may be mediated by histamines in immediate-type symptoms and by proinflammatory cytokines in delayed-type reactions. Pruritus is present in many

Table 2
Major features of some delayed drug-induced syndromes

Drug-Induced Syndromes	Morphology	Localization	Internal Organ Involvement	Systemic Signs	Pertinent Laboratory Findings
SDRIFE (Baboon Syndrome)	Erythema Papules (pustules) Rarely bullae	Flexural/ intertriginous, rarely dissemination	Not affected	Usually none	None
DHS/DRESS	Maculopapular exanthem Erythroderma	Generalized centrofacial edema	Required Lymphadenopathy Hepatitis Pneumonitis Nephritis	Fever Malaise Fatigue	Eosinophilia, atypical lymphocytes Pathologic liver, renal function tests
AGEP	Erythroderma Pustules (small, numerous)	Disseminated generalized, rarely flexural	Possible but rare	High fever (temperature >38°C)	Neutrophilia
SJS/TEN	Macular Bullous lesions Epidermal necrolysis Stomatitis, conjunctivitis	Disseminated generalized	Common Pneumonitis Mucosal lesions (gastrointestinal tract)	Fever Malaise Fatigue	Lymphopenia

Abbreviations: AGEP, acute generalized exanthematous pustulosis; DHS, drug hypersensitivity syndrome; DRESS, drug reaction with eosinophilia and systemic symptoms; SDRIFE, symmetrical drug-related intertriginous and flexural exanthem; SJS, Stevens-Johnson syndrome; TEN, toxic epidermal necrolysis.
Data from Scherer K, Bircher A. Unerwünschte arzneimittelreaktionen an der haut: zwischen trivial und fatal. Internist 2009;50(2):171–8 [in German].

cutaneous drug reactions and may even be the only manifestation of drug hypersensitivity. Drugs associated with isolated pruritus include analgetics and NSAIDs, antibiotics, cardiovascular drugs, opiates, hydroxyethyl starch, radio contrast media, and vitamin A derivates. The pathomechanism is often not elucidated.

Urticaria and Angioedema

Urticaria is a disseminated skin eruption characterized by rapidly emerging, migrating, and itching wheals. A wheal is a rather flat, pale red elevation caused by edema in the upper part of the dermis. Wheals mainly affect trunk and extremities. After clearing they leave the intact skin behind. The lesions typically appear within minutes and usually persist for less than 24 hours at one location. Angioedema is a tense nonpitting edema of the corium layers, affecting mainly the face, lips, oral mucosa, and male genitals. It is usually pale due to vasocompression and causes a tingling and pressure sensation.

Urticaria and angioedema can result not only from a type I (IgE mediated) reaction but also from a nonimmunologic reaction, the so-called pseudoallergic mechanism such as aspirin intolerance. These reactions appear rather rapidly after drug uptake. Eliciting drugs include antibiotics, NSAIDs, radio contrast media, general anesthetic drugs, and many others. According to Coombs and Gell classification, there are also other types of reactions, for example, type III (immune-complex mediated) reactions to antibiotics, which manifest with urticaria only after several hours or even days.[18] This implies that the above-mentioned separation of immediate and nonimmediate reactions at 1 hour is problematic, because particularly urticaria may manifest after several hours or even days. The pathomechanism in such delayed reactions is not elucidated and may involve antibody- or T cell–mediated mechanisms. It is striking that in a study on 20 children with ADR to aminopenicillins with negative skin tests, in more than 50% urticarial manifestations developed after a 5-day oral provocation test. In most children, the symptoms developed 1 to 2 days after completion of the reexposure.[18] This implies that a very schematic approach is problematic.

Maculopapular Exanthems

These are the most common delayed manifestations. They manifest initially with erythematous macules and infiltrated papules, affecting particularly the trunk and the proximal extremities. Classic maculopapular exanthems (eg, seen with amoxicillin) appear after 7 to 10 days, sometimes even after cessation of therapy (eg, after 10 days of aminopenicillin treatment, exanthema appears on day 12). In stronger reactions, exanthems are confluent, resulting in erythrodermia. Typically, a more or less pronounced desquamation occurs after clearing of the inflammatory lesions within 7 to 10 days. The differential diagnosis includes the classic infectious exanthems such as measles and rubella; therefore, these exanthems were also called morbilliform and rubeoliform, respectively. In more severe reactions, elevated eosinophil counts can be observed in approximately 50% of patients, which help to distinguish maculopapular exanthems from viral exanthems. Common elicitors include antibiotics (such as aminopenicillins[15] and quinolones[10]), antiepileptic drugs,[19] and radio contrast media,[20] among many others. According to Coombs and Gell, exanthems normally result from a type IV (T cell mediated) reaction, whereby in maculopapular exanthems cytotoxic $CD4^+$ T cells seem to play the major role (see the article by Pichler W elsewhere in this issue for further exploration of this topic). During initial drug exposure, about 1 week's time is required for expansion of drug-reactive cells and development of symptoms, whereas a sensitized individual may develop symptoms 24 to 48 hours after a renewed drug exposure. First signs such as a discrete erythema may even appear after a few hours.

Flexural Exanthem (Previously Called Baboon Syndrome)

In some instances, a maculopapular exanthem may manifest in a symmetric distribution in the flexural areas. A sharply delineated erythema of the perigenital and perianal area is associated with the affection of the large folds by macules and papules, such as the axilla, the elbows, and the knees (**Fig. 3**). Rarely some pustules or vesicles may be observed. The reaction may later result in a considerable desquamation. Some investigators propose that symmetrical drug-related intertriginous and flexural exanthem (SDRIFE) is a variant of AGEP. However, AGEP requires high fever and neutrophilia, 2 features that are absent in SDRIFE. This particular drug reaction is mainly elicited by aminopenicillins but other drugs have also been implicated. In contrast to most other drug exanthems, men are more often affected by SDRIFE than women. Systemic symptoms and signs are typically absent (see **Table 2**). To delineate this particular drug reaction from systemic contact dermatitis to systemically administered contact allergens, such as mercury or nickel, the neutral acronym SDRIFE has been proposed.[21] The literature on SDRIFE is controversial to the chronology—rather long reaction times from up to 7 days have been reported. However, most cases appear to have a T cell–mediated pathomechanism and follow the above-mentioned chronology patterns.

Drug Hypersensitivity Syndrome

For the so-called DHS, the acronym DRESS has also been proposed.[22] The features of this syndrome have been described in another article in this issue by Kano and Shiohara. Briefly, typical for this syndrome affecting multiple organs is a macular and papular but rarely hemorrhagic or even bullous exanthem. Characteristic of this syndrome is an erythematous, centrofacial swelling. This occasionally fatal hypersensitivity syndrome (lethality 8%)[23] shows the following alarm signs: fever, general malaise, and lymphadenopathy. It may be accompanied by hepatitis (in >50%), nephritis (in circa 10%), and more rarely by pneumonitis or myocarditis. Later, other organs, such as the thyroid gland, may be affected. The symptoms may differ according to the drug used (see the article by Kano and colleagues elsewhere in this issue for further exploration of this topic).

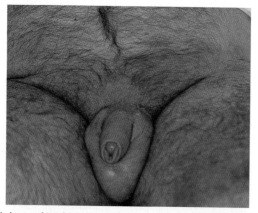

Fig. 3. Symmetrical drug-related intertriginous and flexural exanthem (SDRIFE) to amoxicillin. Characteristic flexural involvement (V-shaped in inguinogenital area).

Fixed Drug Eruption

The clinical manifestation of a fixed drug eruption is virtually pathognomonic for a drug-induced reaction.[24] A livid erythematous and sometimes edematous plaque with often a later-developing bullous center may be observed (**Fig. 4**) Typically, a residual hyperpigmentation persists; rarely there are nonpigmented forms.[25] The reaction always occurs in the same localization upon reexposure to the eliciting drug. The fixed drug eruption is typically singular, but multilocular disseminated forms have been observed. They have to be distinguished from SJS or TEN. Isolated mucosal lesions may be present in the oral cavity or on the male genitals; in women, genital localization is extremely rare. Commonly eliciting agents include sulfonamides, tetracyclines, pyrazolones, NSAIDs, and carbamazepine. In sensitized individuals, the lesions typically occur with a mean time delay of 2 hours (0.5–8 hours). The pathophysiology involves local memory CD8+ T cells, which may be counteracted by regulatory T cells preventing extended or disseminated tissue damage.[24]

Pustular Exanthems

Isolated pustules may be observed in maculopapular exanthems; however, for disseminated forms the acronym AGEP has been proposed.[26] On a generalized erythema, multiple 1- to 3-mm measuring sterile pustules associated with pruritus or burning are observed. The initial lesions may start in the face or in the intertriginous areas after 12 to 24 hours and may disseminate within few days. Fever and leucocytosis are always present. A diagnostic algorithm for this not uncommon drug hypersensitivity reaction has been proposed.[27] The reaction is most often elicited by β-lactam antibiotics, particularly aminopenicillins and cephalosporins, and sometimes by exposure to mercury vapors. The reaction has also been observed to a large number of other drugs.[26,27] (See the article by French and colleagues elsewhere in this issue for further exploration of this topic.) The differential diagnosis includes pustular psoriasis and bacterial infections.

Acute Febrile Neutrophilic Dermatosis (Sweet Syndrome)

Sweet syndrome comprises a symptom complex including fever; neutrophilia; and tender erythematous papules, nodules, and plaques.[28] Three forms of the syndrome are distinguished: classical (idiopathic), malignancy-associated, and drug-induced Sweet syndrome (DISS). For the diagnosis of DISS 5 criteria are required: (1) abrupt onset of painful erythematous plaques or nodules, (2) histopathologic evidence of

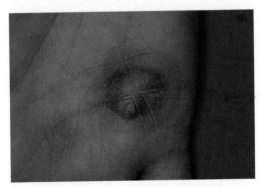

Fig. 4. Fixed drug eruption of the palm due to mefenamic acid.

a dense neutrophilic infiltrate without evidence of leukocytoclastic vasculitis, (3) fever with a temperature greater than 38°C, (4) temporal relationship between drug ingestion and manifestation or temporally related recurrence after oral challenge, and (5) temporally related resolution of lesions after drug withdrawal or treatment with systemic corticosteroids.[28] A large number of drugs have been implicated; however, the best documented evidence exists for granulocyte-macrophage colony-stimulating factor, all-trans retinoic acid, vaccines, and probably for minocycline.[29] Other frequently reported drugs are bortezimib, azathioprine, and sulfonamides.

Pityriasis Rosea–like Drug Eruptions

Pityriasis rosea is a common probably infectious skin disorder; an association with human herpesvirus types 6 and 7[30] and also with human herpesvirus 8[31] has been proposed. Typically, it begins with a solitary, erythematous slightly elevated patch with fine scaling borders called the "herald patch." It occurs usually on the trunk and more rarely on the limbs. After about 2 weeks, a generalized eruption acutely develops. These secondary oval patches are smaller and symmetrically oriented along the cleavage lines (Christmas tree distribution). Many drugs have been incriminated as possible triggers of pityriasis rosea–like eruptions: gold, captopril, tyrosine kinase inhibitors, and NSAIDs among many others. Also, vaccines such as diphtheria, smallpox, pneumococcus, hepatitis B, and BCG have been reported as triggering agents. In drug-induced pityriasis rosea, however, a morphologic atypicality is accompanied by histopathologic features with interface dermatitis and eosinophils. They may be followed by lichen planus–like changes, leaving marked hyperpigmentation, and clear after drug withdrawal.[30]

Lichenoid Drug Reactions

Lichen planus or lichen planus–like reactions have been reported.[32] In terms of location, morphology, and histology, lichen planus and drug-induced lichenoid eruptions may be identical. The skin lesions are small, shiny, polygonal papules with the characteristic Wickham striae. The oral mucosa may also be affected. Most often gold, antimalarials, methyldopa, β-blockers, and lithium salts have been incriminated.[32]

Macular exanthems may proceed into very pruritic infiltrated lesions with the histologic presentation of a pseudolymphoma. They have a slower and more protracted time course, and therefore, the relation to the eliciting drug may be obscure. Cases from carbamazepine, phenytoin,[33] angiotensin-converting enzyme inhibitors, and quinidine have been reported.[22]

Vesicular and Bullous Exanthems

The severe vesicular bullous exanthems are not an entity but include a range of disorders. Among these are the minor and major forms of erythema exsudativum multiforme, SJS, and TEN.[6,34] They are differentiated from each other by the presence or absence of typical target lesions and particularly by the extent of the skin and mucosal manifestations and associated symptoms.[35] In erythema exsudativum multiforme major, SJS, and TEN or Lyell disease, the skin may be initially painful before bullous lesions evolve and affection of the mucosae is always present. This may involve the conjunctival, oral, genital, and perianal mucosa as well as mucosal surfaces of internal organs. Lethal outcome is present in approximately 30% of TEN cases (see the article by French and colleagues elsewhere in this issue for further exploration of this topic).

Serum Sickness–like Disease

Serum sickness classically manifests itself with fever, macular and urticarial exanthems, lymphadenopathy, arthralgia, and sometimes peripheral edemas. Classic serum sickness is an example of an immune complex–mediated type III reaction. The symptoms manifest typically after 6 to 8 hours.[34] Antibiotics such as penicillins,[36] co-trimoxazole, cefaclor, and rifampicin may induce a serum sickness–like disease without measurable immune complexes or complement activation among others. More recently, biologicals such as rituximab have elicited serum sickness–like syndromes based on the development of antirituximab antibodies.[37]

Vasculitis

Drugs may rarely elicit cutaneous or systemic vasculitis.[38] A typical manifestation is the cutaneous small-vessel vasculitis, so-called allergic or hypersensitivity vasculitis. Morphology includes purpura, papules, bullae, and necrotic lesions. Affection of internal organs such as the gastrointestinal tract, the kidneys, the liver, and the central nervous system has to be excluded.[39] Drug-induced vasculitis and drug-induced lupuslike disease are seen in long-term treatments and typically occur with a long delay. Approximately 100 drugs have been reported of inducing vasculitic syndromes. The clinical manifestations vary from isolated cutaneous or organ involvement to severe systemic inflammatory disease dominated by vasculitis. Pathophysiologically, antineutrophil cytoplasmic antibodies with specificity to more than 1 lysosomal antigen have been recently implicated. Combined with presence of antibodies to histones and beta2-glycoprotein 1 they constitute a useful serologic profile for drug-induced vasculitis or drug-induced lupuslike disease.[38]

Erythema nodosum, histologically a septal panniculitis, is a cutaneous reaction pattern presenting with painful nodules on the legs and induced by heterogenous causes.[40] Histology represents a typical panniculitis. Apart from infections (tuberculosis, leprosy) and inflammatory disorders (sarcoidosis, inflammatory bowel disease), some drugs have also been implicated such as sulfonamides, analgesics, antipyretics, oral contraceptives, and some others have been reported.[41]

Other Organs

Particularly the liver and the circulating blood cells may be affected in drug-induced reactions, either as single manifestation or in complex syndromes (see **Table 2**). Also, lymphadenopathy, nephritis, and pneumonitis have been observed, and other organs such as the myocardium, the thyroid gland, and the gastrointestinal tract may be affected. Some of these organs may be involved in the context of drug-induced autoimmune disorders such as lupus[42] and vasculitis.[43] In addition, a variety of drugs elicit exclusive reactions in liver, kidney, or lung, often without skin symptoms; such reactions are difficult to recognize, which often delays the diagnosis. A peripheral eosinophilia may help in the diagnosis and as a hint for a drug allergic process.

Diagnostic Approach

The specific cause-oriented allergy diagnosis should be usually performed the earliest—3 to 4 weeks after complete clearing of all clinical symptoms and signs. On the other hand, after a time interval of more than 6 to 12 months, some drug tests may already have become negative, resulting in false-negative results.

According to the clinical manifestations and the time pattern, a hypothesis of the putative pathogenesis should be generated to select appropriate test procedures.

A histologic analysis of the cutaneous lesions may help to further specify the manifestation and to differentiate it from other skin disorders.[8]

SUMMARY

Drugs and drug allergens may elicit a wide variety of clinical manifestations that are based on various pathogenetic mechanisms. However, there still remain many clinical reactions, in which the pathomechanism is not known, and therefore, no validated diagnostic tools are available. In addition, the preparation of drug allergens for skin tests, the performance of in vitro tests, correctly conducted provocation tests, and the required validation procedures are time consuming and cost intensive. They have been validated only for a minority of drugs and respective forms of clinical reactions. The diagnosis of a drug hypersensitivity reaction is then based on clinical grounds, including a detailed history of previous exposures and reactions, an exact evaluation of the chronology, and a description of the clinical morphology, if necessary supplemented by histology.

REFERENCES

1. Demoly P, Hillaire-Buys D. Classification and epidemiology of hypersensitivity drug reactions. Immunol Allergy Clin North Am 2004;24(3):345–56, v.
2. Bircher AJ. Approach to the patient with a drug hypersensitivity reaction–clinical perspectives. In: Pichler W, editor. Drug hypersensitivity. Basel (Switzerland): Karger; 2007. p. 352–65.
3. Bircher AJ. Symptoms and danger signs in acute drug hypersensitivity. Toxicology 2005;209(2):201–7.
4. Bircher AJ. Arzneimittelallergie und Haut. Stuttgart (Germany): Georg Thieme; 1996. New York.
5. Nigen S, Knowles SR, Shear NH. Drug eruptions: approaching the diagnosis of drug-induced skin diseases. J Drugs Dermatol 2003;2(3):278–99.
6. Roujeau JC. Clinical heterogeneity of drug hypersensitivity. Toxicology 2005; 209(2):123–9.
7. Friedmann PS, Pickard C, Ardern-Jones M, et al. Drug-induced exanthemata: a source of clinical and intellectual confusion. Eur J Dermatol 2010;20(2):1–5.
8. Ramdial PK, Naidoo DK. Drug-induced cutaneous pathology. J Clin Pathol 2009; 62(6):493–504.
9. Demoly P, Kropf R, Bircher A, et al. Drug hypersensitivity: questionnaire. EAACI interest group on drug hypersensitivity. Allergy 1999;54(9):999–1003.
10. Scherer K, Bircher AJ. Hypersensitivity reactions to fluoroquinolones. Curr Allergy Asthma Rep 2005;5(1):15–21.
11. Bircher AJ. Arzneimittelallergie. In: Schultze-Werninghaus G, Fuchs T, Bachert C, et al, editors, Manuale allergologicum, vol. 1. München-Deisenhofen (Germany): Dustri-Verlag; 2004. p. 677–714.
12. Himly M, Jahn-Schmid B, Pittertschatscher K, et al. IgE-mediated immediate-type hypersensitivity to the pyrazolone drug propyphenazone. J Allergy Clin Immunol 2003;111(4):882–8.
13. Scherer K, Ballmer-Weber BK, Bircher AJ. Highlights in nonhymenoptera anaphylaxis. Curr Opin Allergy Clin Immunol 2008;8(4):348–53.
14. Tas E, Pletscher M, Bircher AJ. IgE-mediated urticaria from formaldehyde in a dental root canal compound. J Investig Allergol Clin Immunol 2002;12(2): 130–3.

15. Romano A, Blanca M, Torres MJ, et al. Diagnosis of nonimmediate reactions to beta-lactam antibiotics. Allergy 2004;59(11):1153–60.

16. Torres MJ, Blanca M, Fernandez J, et al. Diagnosis of immediate allergic reactions to beta-lactam antibiotics. Allergy 2003;58(10):961–72.

17. Johnson DH, Cunha BA. Drug fever. Infect Dis Clin North Am 1996;10(1):85–91.

18. Blanca-López N, Zapatero L, Alonso E, et al. Skin testing and drug provocation in the diagnosis of nonimmediate reactions to aminopenicillins in children. Allergy 2009;64(2):229–33.

19. Hyson C, Sadler M. Cross sensitivity of skin rashes with antiepileptic drugs. Can J Neurol Sci 1997;24(3):245–9.

20. Brockow K, Christiansen C, Kanny G, et al. Management of hypersensitivity reactions to iodinated contrast media. Allergy 2005;60(2):150–8.

21. Hausermann P, Harr T, Bircher AJ. Baboon syndrome resulting from systemic drugs: is there strife between SDRIFE and allergic contact dermatitis syndrome? Contact Derm 2004;51(5–6):297–310.

22. Bocquet H, Bagot M, Roujeau JC. Drug-induced pseudolymphoma and drug hypersensitivity syndrome (drug rash with eosinophilia and systemic symptoms: DRESS). Semin Cutan Med Surg 1996;15(4):250–7.

23. Wolkenstein P, Revuz J. Drug-induced severe skin reactions. Incidence, management and prevention. Drug Saf 1995;13(1):56–68.

24. Shiohara T. Fixed drug eruption: pathogenesis and diagnostic tests. Curr Opin Allergy Clin Immunol 2009;9(4):316–21.

25. Lee AY. Fixed drug eruptions. Incidence, recognition, and avoidance. Am J Clin Dermatol 2000;1(5):277–85.

26. Roujeau JC, Bioulac-Sage P, Bourseau C, et al. Acute generalized exanthematous pustulosis. Analysis of 63 cases. Arch Dermatol 1991;127(9):1333–8.

27. Sidoroff A, Halevy S, Bavinck JNB, et al. Acute generalized exanthematous pustulosis (AGEP) – a clinical reaction pattern. J Cutan Pathol 2001;28(3):113–9.

28. Cohen P. Sweet's syndrome - a comprehensive review of an acute febrile neutrophilic dermatosis. Orphanet J Rare Dis 2007;2(1):34.

29. Thompson DF, Montarella KE. Drug-induced Sweet's syndrome. Ann Pharmacother 2007;41:801–11.

30. Drago F, Broccolo F, Rebora A. Pityriasis rosea: an update with a critical appraisal of its possible herpesviral etiology. J Am Acad Dermatol 2009; 61(2):303–18.

31. Prantsidis A, Rigopoulos D, Papatheodorou G, et al. Detection of human herpesvirus 8 in the skin of patients with pityriasis rosea. Acta Derm Venereol 2009; 89(6):604–6.

32. Ellgehausen P, Elsner P, Burg G. Drug-induced lichen planus. Clin Dermatol 1998;16(3):325–32.

33. Van Renterghem D, De Vries EA. Pseudo-lymphoma and anticonvulsant hypersensitivity syndrome during the use of anti-epileptic agents. Tijdschr Geneeskd 1997;53:399–403.

34. Wolf R, Orion E, Marcos B, et al. Life-threatening acute adverse cutaneous drug reactions. Clin Dermatol 2005;23(2):171–81.

35. Auquier-Dunant A, Mockenhaupt M, Naldi L, et al. Correlations between clinical patterns and causes of erythema multiforme majus, Stevens-Johnson syndrome, and toxic epidermal necrolysis: results of an international prospective study. Arch Dermatol 2002;138(8):1019–24.

36. Clark BM, Kotti GH, Shah AD, et al. Severe serum sickness reaction to oral and intramuscular penicillin. Pharmacotherapy 2006;26(5):705–8.

37. Scherer S, Spoerl D, Bircher AJ. Adverse drug reactions to biological response modifiers. J Dtsch Dermatol Ges 2010 [Epub ahead of print].
38. Wiik A. Drug-induced vasculitis. Curr Opin Rheumatol 2008;20(1):35–9.
39. Doyle M, Cuellar M. Drug-induced vasculitis. Expert Opin Drug Saf 2003;2(4): 401–9.
40. Mana J, Marcoval J. Erythema nodosum. Clin Dermatol 2007;25(3):288–94.
41. Bhalla M, Thami GP, Singh N. Ciprofloxacin-induced erythema nodosum. Clin Exp Dermatol 2007;32(1):115–6.
42. Schlienger RG, Bircher AJ, Meier CR. Minocycline-induced lupus. A systematic review. Dermatology 2000;200(3):223–31.
43. Wiik A. Clinical and laboratory characteristics of drug-induced vasculitic syndromes. Arthritis Res Ther 2005;7(5):191–2.

Severe Cutaneous Adverse Reactions: Acute Generalized Exanthematous Pustulosis, Toxic Epidermal Necrolysis and Stevens-Johnson Syndrome

Thomas Harr, MD*, Lars E. French, MD*

KEYWORDS

- Acute generalized exanthematous pustulosis
- Stevens-Johnson syndrome • Toxic epidermal necrolysis
- Intravenous immunoglobulins

Most drug hypersensitivity reactions show skin symptoms. The most severe cutaneous manifestations include pustular and bullous skin eruptions. These 2 manifestations can lead to acute generalized exanthematous pustulosis (AGEP), or Stevens-Johnson syndrome (SJS) and toxic epidermal necrolysis (TEN). These are rare complications, but should be known to any doctor prescribing drugs because they are life threatening, and early stoppage of treatment is mandatory.

ACUTE GENERALIZED EXANTHEMATOUS PUSTULOSIS
Definition

AGEP is an acute febrile, generalized rash, with small uniform noninfective, nonfollicular associated pustules, with a tendency for the skin manifestation to be accentuated in the intertriginous and flexural regions and a predilection for females. In the vast majority of cases, AGEP is induced by drugs, mainly by anti-infectives (antibiotics,

Competing interest: Both authors declare that they have no competing financial interests.
Department of Dermatology, University Hospital Zurich, Gloriastrasse 31, Zurich 8031, Switzerland
* Corresponding author.
E-mail addresses: thomas.harr@usz.ch; lars.french@derm.uzh.ch

Med Clin N Am 94 (2010) 727–742
doi:10.1016/j.mcna.2010.04.004
0025-7125/10/$ – see front matter © 2010 Elsevier Inc. All rights reserved.

medical.theclinics.com

antimalarials, and antifungals). The term AGEP was instituted for the first time in 1980 by Beylot and colleagues,[1] but in the late 1960s a handful of cases atypical for psoriasis had already been described within a large case series of patients with pustular psoriasis.[2]

Clinical Background

AGEP manifests itself within days after the onset of a generalized rash, with nonfollicular associated small uniform pustules on an initially unaffected skin. The intertriginous and flexural parts are particularly affected, leading to discussion with protagonists arguing that AGEP and symmetric drug-related intertriginous and flexural exanthema (systemic drug-related intertriginous and flexural exanthema, Baboon syndrome) might be of the same entity, but with differential manifestation. The manifestation of AGEP very often includes, besides the trunk and extremities, the face in many cases, whereas typically the mucosal membranes (mouth, conjunctivae, genitals) and the palmoplantar surfaces are spared. In almost all cases there are fever and neutrophilia in the peripheral blood, but eosinophilia in the peripheral blood is only seen occasionally. Internal organ involvement is not a typical feature of AGEP. The duration of the rash without therapy is 7 to 21 days (**Fig. 1**).

Differential Diagnoses

The following diseases should be considered: generalized pustular psoriasis (Zumbusch psoriasis), subcorneal pustulosis (Sneddon-Wilkinson disease), subcorneal immunoglobulin A (IgA) dermatosis, infectious folliculitis, viral exanthema with secondary postulation, and Sweet syndrome (neutrophilic dermatosis of the skin).

Generalized pustular psoriasis (Zumbusch psoriasis) is where pustules typically manifest themselves often on lesioned skin, with polyarthritis and palmoplantar involvement. In addition, a positive family history for psoriasis usually exists, and relapses of generalized pustulation occur often.

Subcorneal pustulosis (Sneddon-Wilkinson disease) and subcorneal IgA dermatosis often present with similar clinical features to the aforementioned disease, but sometimes mucosal involvement is seen, and only diagnostic procedures such as a skin biopsy can distinguish the diseases.

Infectious folliculitis is always a major differential diagnosis of AGEP although the typical manifestations are follicular-associated abscesses of bacterial, fungal, or viral pathogens. Unfortunately, a follicular or a nonfollicular association of pustulosis cannot always be made on a macroscopic observation.

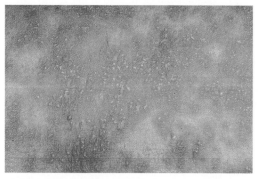

Fig. 1. Acute generalized exanthematous pustulosis.

Viral exanthema with primary vesiculation and secondary pustulation, consisting of pustules that are nonfollicular, has always to be taken into consideration (eg, herpes simplex virus and varicella-zoster virus).

Sweet syndrome (neutrophilic dermatosis of the skin) more often shows firmer vesicles, which are often grouped.

Pustulosis, identical to AGEP, can also be a first manifestation of a drug rash with eosinophilia and systemic symptoms (DRESS) or drug-induced hypersensitivity syndrome (DiHS). In this case the pustules appear after weeks of prior therapy, hepatitis or other internal involvement is present, and the causative drug is a known elicitor of DRESS/DiHS. Eosinophilia (together with neutrophilia) is also present (**Box 1**).

Diagnostics

Besides the clinical picture with aforementioned symptoms, a conventional skin biopsy with direct immunofluorescence should be performed. The typical histologic picture of AGEP is either a subcorneal pustulosis with neutrophils or, to a lesser extent, intraepidermal neutrophilic pustulosis. In certain cases a leukocytic vasculitis can be seen.[3–8] In one study it was shown that the same drug (hydroxychloroquine) can induce AGEP with either a subcorneal or an intraepidermal histologic picture, leading to the conclusion that a singular drug can induce 2 different kinds of pathologic pictures in AGEP.[6]

To distinguish AGEP from other pustoloses, careful examination of the skin histology has to be conducted by the pathologist. Pustular psoriasis typically shows, besides microabscesses, a papillomatosis and acanthosis. Other diseases such as subcorneal pustulosis described by Sneddon and Wilkinson[9] and linear IgA dermatosis additionally need direct immunofluorescence examination for definitive diagnosis; while Sneddon-Wilkinson disease does not show any autoantibodies in the skin or in the peripheral blood, subcorneal variants of linear-IgA dermatosis shows deposits of IgA in the skin. Folliculitis always shows abscesses with a direct link to a follicle, either superficially or in deeper parts of the follicle. Sweet syndrome or neutrophilic dermatosis of the skin reveals typically intradermal accumulation of neutrophils and can therefore be histologically discriminated more easily from AGEP.

In the peripheral blood neutrophilic leukocytosis, sometimes accompanied by mild eosiniphilia can typically be seen. Microbiological evaluation of the pustules should always include bacterial, fungal, and viral cultures, but is usually negative in AGEP.

Experimental studies show on in situ slides and ex vivo besides interleukin-8 expression, chemokine CXCL8 expression and specific T lymphoctyes against the culprit drugs.[10,11] Therefore, diagnostic procedures include in vivo diagnostics with patch testing and ex vivo lymphocyte transformation tests (LTT) or interferon-γ

Box 1
Differential diagnoses of AGEP
Generalized pustular psoriasis (Zumbusch psoriasis)
Subcorneal pustulosis (Sneddon-Wilkinson disease)
Subcorneal IgA dermatosis
Infectious folliculitis
Viral exanthema with secondary pustulation
Sweet syndrome (neutrophilic dermatosis of the skin)

stimulation tests to identify drug-specific T cells, either indirectly with positive delayed-type hypersensitivity by patch tests or by proliferation of T cells or interferon-γ release ex vivo by specific T cells. Patch testing to identify the culprit drug has an intermediate sensitivity, but importantly, besides a readout after 48 and 72 hours, another readout should be performed at either 96 or 120 hours to increase the sensitivity. Not uncommonly, pustule formation, like in acute AGEP, can be seen at the test site. The test should be as early as 1 month after disease resolution. The possibility of induction of AGEP due to patch testing is generally considered to be low. As a further tool besides patch tests, LTT or interferon-γ release tests can be performed in the case of negative or unclear patch tests to increase the sensitivity of diagnostic procedures.[5,12] It has to be kept in mind, however, that these tests should be only performed in specialized laboratories having a strong experience in drug testing, because of the difficulty of reliably performing these tests and interpreting them. After having identified the culprit drug or in case of negative patch tests or ex vivo tests, patients should be always given a document clearly indicating the possible culprit drug or drugs, and potential cross-reactive molecules to reduce risks of a further episode of AGEP.

Demography

Studies including patients in Europe, Israel, and South-East Asia show a tendency of AGEP to be more frequent in females than in males, whereas a single study in Mexico with 12 patients revealed a slight male predominance (7 of 12 patients).[4,7,13,14] The mean age of development of AGEP in the EuroSCAR study (Austria, France, Israel, Italy, the Netherlands, and Germany) was 56 years and in the smaller study from Mexico, 28 years. The overall frequency of AGEP is reported in one article as being up to 5 cases per million inhabitants annually,[8] but is probably higher due to lack of correct workup in patients with pustulosis. Genetic associations are discussed, but clear-cut evidence is missing at the moment.

Etiology

In most AGEP cases, drugs and especially anti-infectives have been identified as the cause of the disease. Some cases make a direct link to systemic mercury exposure days before the onset of AGEP.[15] A case report series of AGEP was reported as a consequence of spider bites.[16]

The EuroSCAR study has identified pristinamycin (macrolide), ampicillin/amoxicillin, quinolones, aromatic sulfonamides, (hydroxy-)chloroquine, terbinafine, and diltiazem.[7] Other less strong associations were made with corticosteroids, macrolides other than pristinamycin, nonsteroidal anti-inflammatory drug (NSAID) of oxicam type, and antiepileptic drugs (with the exception of valproic acid). No association was found with paracetamol (acetaminophen), benzodiazepine, angiotensin-converting inhibitors, β-blockers, calcium channel blockers (with the exception of diltiazem), sartanes, allopurinol, and cephalosporins, which are typical inducers of SJS/TEN. Furthermore, in the EuroSCAR study and in other studies, no pathogenetic link to pustular psoriasis was observed. In addition, human immunodeficiency virus (HIV) drugs such as nevirapine seem not to be associated with an elevated risk of inducing AGEP, contrary to the increased risk for SJS and TEN.

In a Mexican study, similar drugs causing AGEP were identified, as well as 2 cases in which cephalosporin was found to be the cause.[4] The interval between drug intake and the onset of AGEP can be generally divided into groups of 5 days or less of intake and 22 days or less of intake. Typically anti-infectious drugs (pristinamycin, aminopenicillin, quinolones, and anti-infective sulfonamides) lead to development of rash within 5 days, whereas chloroquine, diltiazem, terbinafine, and hydroxychloroquine tend to lead to delayed induction of rash (**Box 2**).[3,4,6,7]

Therapy

There is an absolute necessity to establish a correct diagnosis and to rule out any infectious disease before administering intermediate to high doses of systemic corticosteroids over several days. In addition, local corticosteroids of high potency (class I and class II) can be applied for 5 to 10 days.

STEVENS-JOHNSON SYNDROME AND TOXIC EPIDERMAL NECROLYSIS
Definition and Historical Background

SJS was first described in 1922, as an acute mucocutaneous syndrome in 2 young boys. The condition was characterized by severe purulent conjunctivitis, severe stomatitis with extensive mucosal necrosis, and "erythema multiforme–like" cutaneous lesions. It was later termed Stevens-Johnson syndrome, defined as a severe mucocutaneous disease with a prolonged course and a potentially lethal outcome that is in most cases drug-induced, and should be distinguished from erythema multiforme major (EMM).[17,18]

In 1956, Lyell[18] described 4 patients with an eruption resembling scalding of the skin, which he called toxic epidermal necrolysis. It was only as more patients with TEN were reported in the years after his original publication that it became clear that TEN was drug induced. Nowadays, SJS and TEN are considered to be 2 ends of a spectrum of severe epidermolytic adverse cutaneous drug reactions, differing only by the extent of skin detachment.

Epidemiology

SJS and TEN are rare diseases. The incidence of TEN is 1.89 cases per million inhabitants per year, as reported for Western Germany and Berlin in 1996,[19] with similar frequencies in the United States.[20,21] Regional differences in drug prescription, genetic background (HLA, metabolizing enzymes) of patients, and coexisting diseases including infectious diseases (HIV, tuberculosis), cancer, and radiotherapy[22,23] probably have an impact on the actual incidence of SJS and TEN.

Etiology and Pathogenesis

Genetic susceptibility
To identify genetic factors associated with drug hypersensitivity, populations with various ethnic backgrounds were studied. A unique and strong association among

Box 2
Drugs with high risk for induction of AGEP (EuroSCAR)
Pristinamycin
Ampicillin/amoxicillin
Quinolone
Hydroxychloroquine
Terbinafine
Diltiazem
Anti-infective sulfonamides

HLA, drug hypersensitivity, and ethnic background was described by Chung and colleagues,[24] who showed a strong association between HLA-B*1502, SJS, and carbamazepine in Han Chinese. This strong association with an odds ratio of 2504 led to further studies in a similar ethnic group of Hong Kong Han Chinese with severe adverse reactions to antiepileptic drugs.[25] Severe cutaneous reactions in HLA-B*1502 subjects could be found not only for carbamazepine but also, with a lower odds ratio, for phenytoin and lamotrigine. A second strong association between HLA genotype and severe drug hypersensitivity was found for allopurinol, an antigout drug. Indeed, HLA-B*5801 was found in all Han Chinese patients with a severe adverse drug reaction to allopurinol.[26] In a large European study (Regiscar), HLA-B genotyping was performed in patients with severe cutaneous adverse reactions linked to 5 high-risk drugs (carbamazepine, allopurinol, sulfamethoxazole, lamotrigine, NSAIDs of oxicam type). No HLA association was found for carbamazepine, and this lack of association in patients of European ancestry was confirmed in a smaller study.[27–29] However, the association of HLA-B*1502 with SJS and TEN and carbamazepine use in patients with Asian ancestry was confirmed.[28,29] Moreover, the association of HLA-B*5801 with allopurinol-induced SJS and TEN was confirmed (odds ratio of 80) independent of the ethnic background.[28]

Clinical Features and Background

Acute phase

Initial symptoms of TEN and SJS are usually nonspecific and include fever, stinging eyes, and discomfort on swallowing. These symptoms typically precede cutaneous manifestations by a few days. Early sites of cutaneous involvement are the presternal region of the trunk and the face, palms, and soles. Erythema and erosions of the buccal, genital, and/or ocular mucosa are present in almost all patients, and in some cases the respiratory and the gastrointestinal tract are also affected.[30] The morphology of early skin lesions includes erythematous and livid macules, which may or may not be slightly infiltrated and which have a tendency to rapidly coalescence. It is unlikely that a normal maculopapular exanthema (MPE) is a risk factor for SJS and TEN: for example, amoxicillin, the main cause of MPE, rarely causes TEN, and the massive stimulation of CD8$^+$ T cells and natural killer (NK)-like cells is not found in MPE. However, a painful skin, livid-erythematous macules (and not papular eruptions), malaise, and the use of an SJS/TEN-associated drug should be considered as danger signs and promote an immediate stop to the drug. The development to SJS or TEN from a harmless-looking macular eruption to bullous detachment can occur rapidly, within a few hours. In a second phase, large areas of epidermal detachment develop. In the absence of epidermal detachment, more detailed skin examination should be performed by exerting tangential mechanical pressure on several erythematous zones (Nikolsky sign). The Nikolsky sign is positive if mechanical pressure induces epidermal detachment, but it is not specific for TEN or SJS because it can also be positive, for example, in autoimmune bullous skin diseases (**Fig. 2**).

All aforementioned clinical features are danger signs, and if they are present, immediate histologic workup has to be performed. The extent of skin involvement is a major prognostic factor in SJS and TEN. It should be emphasized that only necrotic skin that is already detached (eg, blisters, erosions) or detachable skin (Nikolsky positive) should be counted for evaluation of extent of the skin involvement. Bastuji-Garin and colleagues[31] proposed to classify patients into 3 groups according to the degree of skin detachment (**Figs. 3** and **4; Table 1**).

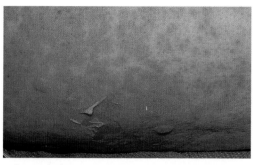

Fig. 2. Toxic epidermal necrolysis.

Late phase and sequelae

Sequelae are common features of late-phase TEN (75% of all cases) with typical manifestations including hyper- and hypopigmentation (62.5%), nail dystrophies (37.5%), conjunctival keratinization (62.5%), and keratoconjunctivitis sicca (50%).[32] Corneal involvement and symblepharon have been observed occasionally. Special attention should be drawn to oral, esophageal, and genital sequelae.[33]

Differential Diagnoses

The major differential diagnoses of SJS/TEN are autoimmune diseases such as linear IgA dermatosis, bullous pemphigoid, and staphylococcal scalded skin syndrome (SSSS). The clinical symptoms often resemble those of SJS/TEN, but histology can distinguish SSSS from SJS/TEN due to typical dermoepidermal detachment and necrosis beneath the stratum corneum in SJS/TEN. Autoimmune bullous diseases histologically show clefts on different layers of the epidermis or subepidermis, with only few necrotic epidermal cells and positive direct immunofixation.

Further differential diagnoses include EMM and AGEP, and in rare cases of TEN without mucosal involvement, disseminated fixed bullous drug eruption should also be considered.

Diagnostics and Pathomechanism of SJS and TEN

The pathogenesis of SJS and TEN is not fully understood but is believed to be immune-mediated. The histopathology of SJS/TEN lesions shows that keratinocyte

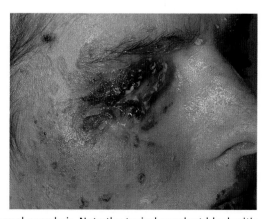

Fig. 3. Toxic epidermal necrolysis. Note the typical purulent blepharitis.

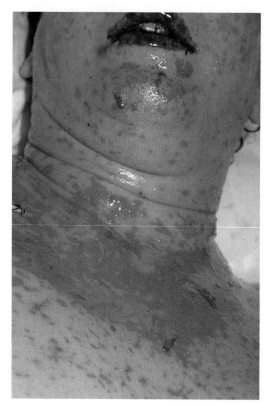

Fig. 4. Toxic epidermal necrolysis.

apoptosis followed by necrosis is the pathogenic basis of the widespread epidermal detachment observed. The clinical, histopathologic, and immunologic findings in SJS and TEN support the currently prevalent concept that SJS and TEN are hypersensitivity reactions to specific drugs. To date, strong evidence suggests a paramount contribution of the cytotoxic molecules FasL and granulysin as key molecules responsible for the disseminated keratinocyte apoptosis in SJS and TEN.[34,35]

The potential role of the apoptosis ligand FasL and the cognate apoptosis receptor Fas in the signaling that triggers keratinocyte apoptosis is supported by the research of several different groups.[35] The functionality of upregulated FasL, or upregulation of FasL on keratinocytes itself in patients with SJS or TEN is still controversial, however.[36] Gene expression analysis of blister fluid cells and analysis of blister fluid from patients with SJS and TEN has also recently identified secretory granulysin as a key molecule responsible for the induction of keratinocyte death in TEN.[34] Blister fluid cells express high levels of granulysin mRNA (a cationic cytolytic protein secreted by cytotoxic T lymphocytes, NK cells, and NK T cells), increased concentrations of the granulysin protein are found in blister fluid, and recombinant granulysin mimics features of SJS/TEN when injected intradermally in mice. In conclusion, and based on our knowledge to date, CD8 T cells as well as the cytolytic molecules FasL and granulysin are key players in the pathogenesis of SJS/TEN.

Table 1
Clinical features that distinguish SJS, SJS-TEN overlap, and TEN

Clinical Entity	SJS	SJS-TEN Overlap	TEN
Primary lesions	Dusky red lesions Flat atypical targets	Dusky red lesions Flat atypical targets	Poorly delineated erythematous plaques Epidermal detachment— spontaneous or by friction Dusky red lesions Flat atypical targets
Distribution	Isolated lesions Confluence (+) on face and trunk	Isolated lesions Confluence (++) on face and trunk	Isolated lesions (rare) Confluence (+++) on face, trunk, and elsewhere
Mucosal involvement	Yes	Yes	Yes
Systemic symptoms	Usually	Always	Always
Detachment (% body surface area)	<10	10–30	>30

Data from Bachot N, Revuz J, Roujeau JC. Intravenous immunoglobulin treatment for Stevens-Johnson syndrome and toxic epidermal necrolysis: a prospective noncomparative study showing no benefit on mortality or progression. Arch Dermatol 2003;139:33.

Drugs

Drug exposure and a resulting hypersensitivity reaction is the cause of the majority of cases of SJS/TEN. In absolute case numbers, allopurinol is the most common cause of SJS and TEN in Europe and Israel,[37] and mostly in patients receiving daily doses of at least 200 mg.

In a case-control study of patients hospitalized for SJS/TEN in selected hospitals in France, Germany, Italy, and Portugal between 1989 and 1993, Roujeau and colleagues[21] reported drugs that are at increased risk of inducing SJS/TEN when used over a short period of time (trimethoprim-sulfamethoxazole and other sulfonamide antibiotics, aminopenicillins, cephalosporins, quinolones, and chlormezanone), and those that are at increased risk when used over months (aromatic antiepileptics [carbamazepine, phenytoin, phenobarbital], valproic acid, NSAIDs of the oxicam type, allopurinol, and corticosteroids). A similar population was studied in the years from 1997 to 2001 by Mockenhaupt and colleagues.[38] However valproic acid might be over estimated as inducer of SJS/TEN as suggested by Rzany and colleagues.[19] In a multinational case-control study in Europe covering more than 100 million inhabitants, the investigators paid special attention to newly marketed drugs and, in addition, identified nevirapine, lamotrigine, and sertraline as drugs with a significantly increased risk of inducing SJS and TEN. A recent survey of TEN in children identified similar drugs as in adults, besides a possibly increased susceptibility to acetaminophen (paracetamol).[39]

An often-addressed issue is the induction of TEN or SJS after vaccination. The vaccine adverse-event reporting system concludes that despite the plausibility of a relationship between vaccination of SJS and TEN, the very small number of reports compared with the large number of vaccinations, and the benefits of vaccinations outweigh the potential risk of SJS/TEN.[40]

Not only the type of drug but also the duration of drug intake is a potential risk factor. Drugs with an intake of less than 8 weeks induce severe drug reactions significantly more often (**Table 2**).[19,41]

Diagnosis and Diagnostic Methods

After an initial clinical judgment and evaluation of the extent of skin and mucosal involvement, a skin biopsy has to be performed as soon as possible. Cryosection stains are available within 1 hour after biopsy and show large numbers of necrotic keratinocytes, skin detachment of the basal epidermal layer, and no intraepidermal clefting.

An additional histologic workup with formaldehyde-fixed paraffin slides, conventional staining, and direct immune fluorescence should be done to definitively confirm the initial cryosection-based histologic diagnosis and to rule out autoimmune blistering diseases.

Management and Therapy

Treatment in the acute stage

Prompt withdrawal of culprit drugs and supportive care Garcia-Doval and colleagues[42] have shown that the earlier the causative drug is withdrawn, the better the prognosis, and that patients exposed to causative drugs with long half-lives have an increased risk of dying.

SJS and TEN are life-threatening conditions, and therefore supportive care is an essential part of the therapeutic approach. A multicenter study conducted in the United States and a smaller study showed a positive correlation of early referral to specialized intensive care units such as burn units, and survival.[33,43]

Wounds should be treated conservatively, with nonadhesive wound dressings being used where required. Topical sulfa-containing medications should be avoided.

Drug therapy To date, specific therapy for SJS and TEN, which has shown efficacy in controlled clinical trials, does not exist.

High-dose intravenous immunoglobulins As a consequence of the discovery of the anti-Fas potential of pooled human intravenous immunoglobulins (IVIG) in vitro,[35] IVIG have been tested for the treatment of TEN, and their effect reported in different noncontrolled studies. To date numerous case reports and 11 noncontrolled clinical studies containing 10 or more patients have analyzed the therapeutic effect of IVIG in TEN. All except 1 study[44] confirm the known excellent tolerability and a low toxic potential of IVIG when used with appropriate precaution in patients with potential risk factors (renal insufficiency, cardiac insufficiency, IgA deficiency, thromboembolic risk).[45]

Taken together, although each study has its potential bias and the 11 studies are not directly comparable, 8 of the 11 studies suggest that there may be a benefit of IVIG used at total doses greater than 2 g/kg over 3 to 4 days on the mortality associated with TEN.[35,44,46–53] Given that in certain studies the early administration of IVIG in

Table 2 Drugs with high risk of inducing SJS/TEN				
Selected Drugs with Increased Risk				
TMP/SMX	Aminopenicillin	Cephalosporin	Quinolone	Carbamazepine
Phenytoin	Phenobarbital	Nevirapine	Oxicam-NSAID	Allopurinol

TEN has shown the potential to reduce mortality, and given the favorable side effect profile of IVIG and the absence of any other clinically proven specific therapeutic alternative, early administration of high-dose immunoglobulin should, in the authors' opinion, be considered in severe forms of TEN.

The concomitant administration of corticosteroids or immunosuppressive agents remains controversial. Only 1 cycle of IVIG treatment administered over a period of 3 to 5 days is usually required in this condition. The dose recommended in TEN differs from that in other autoimmune diseases. A total dose of 3 g/kg body weight is generally recommended. IVIG has also been applied in a few children with SJS/TEN. The incidence of SJS and TEN is lower in children than in adults, but 2 studies point toward a beneficial trend for the use of IVIG.[54,55]

Clinical data are currently insufficient to draw conclusions on the therapeutic efficacy of IVIG in TEN. A multicenter, comparative analysis needs to be performed to determine the role of IVIG in the management of patients with SJS and TEN.

Cyclosporin A (CsA), a calcineurin inhibitor, is an efficient drug in transplantation and autoimmune diseases. Clinical data are currently insufficient to draw conclusions on the therapeutic potential of CsA, also in combination with other drugs, in TEN.[56,57]

Special attention has to be paid to the prevention of ocular complications. Early referral to an ophthalmologist is mandatory for assessment of the extent of eye involvement and prompt treatment with topical steroids. Some of the ocular complications have an inflammatory background, and have to be treated occasionally with ophthalmic steroids and/or extensive lubrication of the eye to prevent progression leading ultimately to the need for corneal transplantation.[58] Visual outcome is reported to be significantly better in patients who receive specific ophthalmologic treatment during the first week of disease.[59]

Systemic steroids were the standard treatment until the early 1990s, although no benefit has been proved in controlled trials, and their use therefore remains controversial. A recent small retrospective monocenter study suggests, however, that a short-course "pulse" of high-dose corticosteroids (dexamethasone) may be of benefit.[60]

Other anti-inflammatory therapies, such as tumor necrosis factor-α inhibitors, were administered in single cases with partial positive effects, but at the moment these medications are not regular therapeutic options. The potential side effect of these drugs with potential enhancement of immunosuppression and consequent increased risk of sepsis should always be taken into consideration.

Allergological Testing

The severity of SJS and TEN does not allow rechallenges or intradermal tests with the culprit drugs because of the risk of inducing a second episode of SJS/TEN. Patch testing is under discussion but is not a regular diagnostic option at the moment. Only one study with patch testing in patients with SJS/TEN has been conducted in recent years . Wolkenstein and colleagues[61] performed patch testing in 22 suspected SJS/TEN patients. Only 2 out of 22 tested patients had a relevant positive test, suggesting a weak sensitivity in SJS and TEN.

The focus currently lies on ex vivo or in vitro tests. The LTT is an ex vivo method established in delayed drug hypersensitivity. The LTT measures the proliferation of T cells to a drug in vitro by generating T-lymphocyte cell lines and clones. Pichler and Tilch[12] report a sensitivity of 60% to 70% for patients allergic to β-lactam antibiotics in classic exanthematic drug rash. Unfortunately, the sensitivity of LTT is still very low in SJS and TEN. To improve the sensitivity in SJS and TEN, LTT should be done within 1 week after onset of the disease to get the highest (but in respect of all cases, still low) sensitivity.[62]

		SCORTEN (Sum of	
SCORTEN Parameter	**Individual Score**	**Individual Scores)**	**Predicted Mortality (%)**
Age >40 years	Yes = 1, No = 0	0–1	3.2
Malignancy	Yes = 1, No = 0	2	12.1
Tachycardia (>120/min)	Yes = 1, No = 0	3	35.8
Initial surface of epidermal detachment >10%	Yes = 1, No = 0	4	58.3
Serum urea >10 mmol/L	Yes = 1, No = 0	≥5	90
Serum glucose >14 mmol/L	Yes = 1, No = 0		
Bicarbonate >20 mmol/L	Yes = 1, No = 0		

Table 3
SCORTEN severity-of-illness score

Novel in vitro methods to identify drug-specific T lymphocytes are a necessity. A new drug-specific cytotoxicity test was recently proposed by Zawodniak and colleagues[63] using a combination method with flow cytometry and enzyme-linked immunospot. Two parameters were evaluated: CD107 (a degranulation marker) expression by flow cytometry, and Granzyme B (a serine protease) synthesis by Elispot. In accordance with the investigators, the authors suggest primarily performing an LTT and, if noncontributive, a cytotoxicity test.

Prognosis

SJS and TEN are severe and life threatening. The average reported mortality rate of SJS is 1% to 5%, and that of TEN 25% to 35%; it can be even higher in elderly patients and those with a large surface area of epidermal detachment. To standardize the evaluation of risk and prognosis in patients with SJS and TEN, different scoring systems have been proposed. The SCORTEN is now the most widely used scoring system and evaluates the following parameters: age, malignancy, tachycardia, initial body surface area of epidermal detachment, serum urea, serum glucose, and bicarbonate (**Table 3**).[64]

REFERENCES

1. Beylot C, Bioulac P, Doutre MS. [Acute generalized exanthematic pustuloses (four cases) (author's transl)]. Ann Dermatol Venereol 1980;107:37 [in French].
2. Baker H, Ryan TJ. Generalized pustular psoriasis. A clinical and epidemiological study of 104 cases. Br J Dermatol 1968;80:771.
3. Beltraminelli HS, Lerch M, Arnold A, et al. Acute generalized exanthematous pustulosis induced by the antifungal terbinafine: case report and review of the literature. Br J Dermatol 2005;152:780.
4. Guevara-Gutierrez E, Uribe-Jimenez E, Diaz-Canchola M, et al. Acute generalized exanthematous pustulosis: report of 12 cases and literature review. Int J Dermatol 2009;48:253.
5. Halevy S, Cohen A, Livni E. Acute generalized exanthematous pustulosis associated with polysensivity to paracetamol and bromhexine: the diagnostic role of in vitro interferon-gamma release test. Clin Exp Dermatol 2000;25:652.

6. Paradisi A, Bugatti L, Sisto T, et al. Acute generalized exanthematous pustulosis induced by hydroxychloroquine: three cases and a review of the literature. Clin Ther 2008;30:930.

7. Sidoroff A, Dunant A, Viboud C, et al. Risk factors for acute generalized exanthematous pustulosis (AGEP)—results of a multinational case-control study (EuroSCAR). Br J Dermatol 2007;157:989.

8. Sidoroff A, Halevy S, Bavinck JN, et al. Acute generalized exanthematous pustulosis (AGEP)—a clinical reaction pattern. J Cutan Pathol 2001;28:113.

9. Sneddon IB, Wilkinson DS. Subcorneal pustular dermatosis. Br J Dermatol 1956; 68:385.

10. Britschgi M, Pichler WJ. Acute generalized exanthematous pustulosis, a clue to neutrophil-mediated inflammatory processes orchestrated by T cells. Curr Opin Allergy Clin Immunol 2002;2:325.

11. Britschgi M, Steiner UC, Schmid S, et al. T-cell involvement in drug-induced acute generalized exanthematous pustulosis. J Clin Invest 2001;107:1433.

12. Pichler WJ, Tilch J. The lymphocyte transformation test in the diagnosis of drug hypersensitivity. Allergy 2004;59:809.

13. Chang SL, Huang YH, Yang CH, et al. Clinical manifestations and characteristics of patients with acute generalized exanthematous pustulosis in Asia. Acta Derm Venereol 2008;88:363.

14. Davidovici B, Dodiuk-Gad R, Rozenman D, et al. Profile of acute generalized exanthematous pustulosis in Israel during 2002–2005: results of the RegiSCAR Study. Isr Med Assoc J 2008;10:410.

15. Lerch M, Bircher AJ. Systemically induced allergic exanthem from mercury. Contact Dermatitis 2004;50:349.

16. Davidovici BB, Pavel D, Cagnano E, et al. Acute generalized exanthematous pustulosis following a spider bite: report of 3 cases. J Am Acad Dermatol 2006;55: 525.

17. Auquier-Dunant A, Mockenhaupt M, Naldi L, et al. Correlations between clinical patterns and causes of erythema multiforme majus, Stevens-Johnson syndrome, and toxic epidermal necrolysis: results of an international prospective study. Arch Dermatol 2002;138:1019.

18. Lyell A. Toxic epidermal necrolysis: an eruption resembling scalding of the skin. Br J Dermatol 1956;68:355.

19. Rzany B, Correia O, Kelly JP, et al. Risk of Stevens-Johnson syndrome and toxic epidermal necrolysis during first weeks of antiepileptic therapy: a case-control study. Study Group of the International Case Control Study on Severe Cutaneous Adverse Reactions. Lancet 1999;353:2190.

20. La Grenade L, Lee L, Weaver J, et al. Comparison of reporting of Stevens-Johnson syndrome and toxic epidermal necrolysis in association with selective COX-2 inhibitors. Drug Saf 2005;28:917.

21. Roujeau JC, Kelly JP, Naldi L, et al. Medication use and the risk of Stevens-Johnson syndrome or toxic epidermal necrolysis. N Engl J Med 1995;333:1600.

22. Aguiar D, Pazo R, Duran I, et al. Toxic epidermal necrolysis in patients receiving anticonvulsants and cranial irradiation: a risk to consider. J Neurooncol 2004;66: 345.

23. Aydin F, Cokluk C, Senturk N, et al. Stevens-Johnson syndrome in two patients treated with cranial irradiation and phenytoin. J Eur Acad Dermatol Venereol 2006;20:588.

24. Chung WH, Hung SI, Hong HS, et al. Medical genetics: a marker for Stevens-Johnson syndrome. Nature 2004;428:486.

25. Man CB, Kwan P, Baum L, et al. Association between HLA-B*1502 allele and anti-epileptic drug-induced cutaneous reactions in Han Chinese. Epilepsia 2007;48: 1015.

26. Hung SI, Chung WH, Liou LB, et al. HLA-B*5801 allele as a genetic marker for severe cutaneous adverse reactions caused by allopurinol. Proc Natl Acad Sci U S A 2005;102:4134.

27. Alfirevic A, Jorgensen AL, Williamson PR, et al. HLA-B locus in Caucasian patients with carbamazepine hypersensitivity. Pharmacogenomics 2006;7:813.

28. Lonjou C, Borot N, Sekula P, et al. A European study of HLA-B in Stevens-Johnson syndrome and toxic epidermal necrolysis related to five high-risk drugs. Pharmacogenet Genomics 2008;18:99.

29. Lonjou C, Thomas L, Borot N, et al. A marker for Stevens-Johnson syndrome: ethnicity matters. Pharmacogenomics J 2006;6:265.

30. Lebargy F, Wolkenstein P, Gisselbrecht M, et al. Pulmonary complications in toxic epidermal necrolysis: a prospective clinical study. Intensive Care Med 1997;23:1237.

31. Bastuji-Garin S, Rzany B, Stern RS, et al. Clinical classification of cases of toxic epidermal necrolysis, Stevens-Johnson syndrome, and erythema multiforme. Arch Dermatol 1993;129:92.

32. Magina S, Lisboa C, Leal V, et al. Dermatological and ophthalmological sequels in toxic epidermal necrolysis. Dermatology 2003;207:33.

33. Oplatek A, Brown K, Sen S, et al. Long-term follow-up of patients treated for toxic epidermal necrolysis. J Burn Care Res 2006;27:26.

34. Chung WH, Hung SI, Yang JY, et al. Granulysin is a key mediator for disseminated keratinocyte death in Stevens-Johnson syndrome and toxic epidermal necrolysis. Nat Med 2008;14:1343.

35. Viard I, Wehrli P, Bullani R, et al. Inhibition of toxic epidermal necrolysis by blockade of CD95 with human intravenous immunoglobulin. Science 1998;282:490.

36. Murata J, Abe R, Shimizu H. Increased soluble Fas ligand levels in patients with Stevens-Johnson syndrome and toxic epidermal necrolysis preceding skin detachment. J Allergy Clin Immunol 2008;122:992.

37. Halevy S, Ghislain PD, Mockenhaupt M, et al. Allopurinol is the most common cause of Stevens-Johnson syndrome and toxic epidermal necrolysis in Europe and Israel. J Am Acad Dermatol 2008;58:25.

38. Mockenhaupt M, Viboud C, Dunant A, et al. Stevens-Johnson syndrome and toxic epidermal necrolysis: assessment of medication risks with emphasis on recently marketed drugs. The EuroSCAR-study. J Invest Dermatol 2008;128:35.

39. Levi N, Bastuji-Garin S, Mockenhaupt M, et al. Medications as risk factors of Stevens-Johnson syndrome and toxic epidermal necrolysis in children: a pooled analysis. Pediatrics 2009;123:e297.

40. Ball R, Ball LK, Wise RP, et al. Stevens-Johnson syndrome and toxic epidermal necrolysis after vaccination: reports to the vaccine adverse event reporting system. Pediatr Infect Dis J 2001;20:219.

41. Tennis P, Stern RS. Risk of serious cutaneous disorders after initiation of use of phenytoin, carbamazepine, or sodium valproate: a record linkage study. Neurology 1997;49:542.

42. Garcia-Doval I, LeCleach L, Bocquet H, et al. Toxic epidermal necrolysis and Stevens-Johnson syndrome: does early withdrawal of causative drugs decrease the risk of death? Arch Dermatol 2000;136:323.

43. Palmieri TL, Greenhalgh DG, Saffle JR, et al. A multicenter review of toxic epidermal necrolysis treated in U.S. burn centers at the end of the twentieth century. J Burn Care Rehabil 2002;23:87.

44. Bachot N, Revuz J, Roujeau JC. Intravenous immunoglobulin treatment for Stevens-Johnson syndrome and toxic epidermal necrolysis: a prospective non-comparative study showing no benefit on mortality or progression. Arch Dermatol 2003;139:33.

45. Prins C, Gelfand EW, French LE. Intravenous immunoglobulin: properties, mode of action and practical use in dermatology. Acta Derm Venereol 2007;87:206.

46. Al-Mutairi N, Arun J, Osama NE, et al. Prospective, noncomparative open study from Kuwait of the role of intravenous immunoglobulin in the treatment of toxic epidermal necrolysis. Int J Dermatol 2004;43:847.

47. Brown KM, Silver GM, Halerz M, et al. Toxic epidermal necrolysis: does immunoglobulin make a difference? J Burn Care Rehabil 2004;25:81.

48. Campione E, Marulli GC, Carrozzo AM, et al. High-dose intravenous immunoglobulin for severe drug reactions: efficacy in toxic epidermal necrolysis. Acta Derm Venereol 2003;83:430.

49. Prins C, Kerdel FA, Padilla RS, et al. Treatment of toxic epidermal necrolysis with high-dose intravenous immunoglobulins: multicenter retrospective analysis of 48 consecutive cases. Arch Dermatol 2003;139:26.

50. Schneck J, Fagot JP, Sekula P, et al. Effects of treatments on the mortality of Stevens-Johnson syndrome and toxic epidermal necrolysis: a retrospective study on patients included in the prospective EuroSCAR Study. J Am Acad Dermatol 2008;58:33.

51. Shortt R, Gomez M, Mittman N, et al. Intravenous immunoglobulin does not improve outcome in toxic epidermal necrolysis. J Burn Care Rehabil 2004;25:246.

52. Tan AW, Thong BY, Yip LW, et al. High-dose intravenous immunoglobulins in the treatment of toxic epidermal necrolysis: an Asian series. J Dermatol 2005;32:1.

53. Trent JT, Kirsner RS, Romanelli P, et al. Analysis of intravenous immunoglobulin for the treatment of toxic epidermal necrolysis using SCORTEN: the University of Miami Experience. Arch Dermatol 2003;139:39.

54. Mangla K, Rastogi S, Goyal P, et al. Efficacy of low dose intravenous immuno-globulins in children with toxic epidermal necrolysis: an open uncontrolled study. Indian J Dermatol Venereol Leprol 2005;71:398.

55. Tristani-Firouzi P, Petersen MJ, Saffle JR, et al. Treatment of toxic epidermal nec-rolysis with intravenous immunoglobulin in children. J Am Acad Dermatol 2002; 47:548.

56. Hashim N, Bandara D, Tan E, et al. Early cyclosporine treatment of incipient toxic epidermal necrolysis induced by concomitant use of lamotrigine and sodium val-proate. Acta Derm Venereol 2004;84:90.

57. Robak E, Robak T, Gora-Tybor J, et al. Toxic epidermal necrolysis in a patient with severe aplastic anemia treated with cyclosporin A and G-CSF. J Med 2001;32:31.

58. Sheridan RL, Schulz JT, Ryan CM, et al. Long-term consequences of toxic epidermal necrolysis in children. Pediatrics 2002;109:74.

59. Sotozono C, Ueta M, Koizumi N, et al. Diagnosis and treatment of Stevens-John-son syndrome and toxic epidermal necrolysis with ocular complications. Ophthalmology 2009;116:685.

60. Kardaun SH, Jonkman MF. Dexamethasone pulse therapy for Stevens-Johnson syndrome/toxic epidermal necrolysis. Acta Derm Venereol 2007;87:144.

61. Wolkenstein P, Chosidow O, Flechet ML, et al. Patch testing in severe cutaneous adverse drug reactions, including Stevens-Johnson syndrome and toxic epidermal necrolysis. Contact Dermatitis 1996;35:234.

62. Kano Y, Hirahara K, Mitsuyama Y, et al. Utility of the lymphocyte transformation test in the diagnosis of drug sensitivity: dependence on its timing and the type of drug eruption. Allergy 2007;62:1439.

63. Zawodniak A, Lochmatter P, Yerly D, et al. In vitro detection of cytotoxic T and NK cells in peripheral blood of patients with various drug-induced skin diseases. Allergy 2010;65:376–84.

64. Bastuji-Garin S, Fouchard N, Bertocchi M, et al. SCORTEN: a severity-of-illness score for toxic epidermal necrolysis. J Invest Dermatol 2000;115:149.

Visceral Involvements and Long-term Sequelae in Drug-induced Hypersensitivity Syndrome

Yoko Kano, MD, PhD*, Tadashi Ishida, MD, Kazuhisa Hirahara, MD, Tetsuo Shiohara, MD, PhD

KEYWORDS

- Drug-induced hypersensitivity syndrome
- Hepatitis • Limbic encephalitis • Renal dysfunction
- Sclerodermoid lesion • Systemic lupus erythematosus
- Type 1 diabetes mellitus • Thyroiditis

Drug-induced hypersensitivity syndrome (DIHS) is a life-threatening adverse systemic reaction characterized by skin rashes, fever, leukocytosis with eosinophilia and/or atypical lymphocytosis, lymph node enlargement, and liver and/or renal dysfunction.[1] The syndrome develops from 2 weeks to more than 6 weeks after initiation of a specific drug therapy. It has been estimated that DIHS occurs in 1 in 1000 to 1 in 10,000 exposures to antiepileptic drugs.[2] Previously, there was no consistent term for this phenomenon. Various terms had been used to refer to this syndrome using the generic names of the culprit drugs, such as phenytoin syndrome, allopurinol hypersensitivity syndrome, and dapson syndrome. Bocquet and colleagues[3] proposed the name drug rash with eosinophilia and systemic symptoms (DRESS) to simplify the nomenclature for drug-hypersensitivity syndromes. Later, Descamps and colleagues[4] and the Japanese Research Committee on Severe Cutaneous Adverse Reaction (J-SCAR) group[5,6] showed a relationship between this drug reaction and human herpesvirus 6 (HHV-6) reactivation. Subsequently, the J-SCAR group coined the

This work was supported by Health and Labor Sciences Research Grants from the Ministry of Health, Labor and Welfare of Japan (to Japanese Research Committee on Severe Cutaneous Adverse Reaction [J-SCAR]).

Department of Dermatology, Kyorin University School of Medicine, 6-20-2 Shinkawa Mitaka, Tokyo 181-8611, Japan

* Corresponding author.

E-mail address: kano@ks.kyorin-u.ac.jp

Med Clin N Am 94 (2010) 743–759

doi:10.1016/j.mcna.2010.03.004

0025-7125/10/$ – see front matter

medical.theclinics.com

term DIHS to reflect its association with HHV-6.[7,8] There is no significant difference in the clinical findings of patients who have been reported to have DRESS versus DIHS, although hypersensitivity reaction includes severe reactions with systemic symptoms without eosinophilia (eg, some hypersensitivity reactions following abacavir or allopurinol). Patients with this illness have a wide variety of complications involving multiple organs during the course of the disease, which persist long after resolution of the cutaneous eruptions, although the explanation for this multiorgan involvement remains unknown.

The severity of DIHS/DRESS is most frequently determined by the degree of visceral involvement. The mortality of DIHS/DRESS approaches 10%, primarily related to systemic involvement, including hepatitis, nephritis, myocarditis, and pneumonitis.[9] This review focuses on the early and late complications observed in patients with DIHS/DRESS.

DIAGNOSIS AND CLINICAL COURSE OF DIHS/DRESS

DIHS/DRESS appears after a 2-week to 3-month exposure to a limited number of drugs, including anticonvulsants, dapsone, allopurinol, and minocycline.[10] The delayed onset in relation to the introduction of the causative drug is 1 of the more important features of DIHS/DRESS. This feature can be used to distinguish DIHS/DRESS from other types of drug eruptions, which typically begin 1 to 2 weeks after initiating therapy.

The criteria for the diagnosis of DRESS proposed by Bocquet and colleagues[3] are as follows: (1) cutaneous drug eruption; (2) hematologic abnormalities including eosinophilia greater than 1.5×10^9/L or the presence of atypical lymphocytes; and (3) systemic involvement including adenopathy greater than 2 cm in diameter, hepatitis (liver transaminase values >2 N), interstitial nephritis, interstitial pneumonia, or carditis. These criteria emphasize 2 important characteristics: multiple organ involvement and eosinophilia.[11]

The criteria for the diagnosis of DIHS established by J-SCAR[8] are as follows: (1) maculopapular rash developing more than 3 weeks after starting a limited number of drugs; (2) prolonged clinical symptoms 2 weeks after discontinuation of the causative drug; (3) fever greater than 38°C; (4) liver abnormalities (eg, alanine aminotransferase [ALT] levels >100 U/L); (5) leukocyte abnormalities such as leukocytosis (>11 $\times 10^9$/L), atypical lymphocytosis (>5%), and/or eosinophilia (>1.5 $\times 10^9$/L); (6) lymphadenopathy; and (7) HHV-6 reactivation. Diagnosis of typical DIHS requires the presence of all 7 criteria. An association between herpesvirus, particularly HHV-6, and DIHS has been increasingly reported; HHV-6 reactivation can be detected 2 to 4 weeks after the onset of this syndrome. Considering that HHV-6 reactivation is rarely detected in patients who develop a milder form of the disease, the detection of this viral reactivation is a useful marker for the diagnosis of DIHS/DRESS.[7,12] The authors have recently shown that various herpesvirus reactivations, such as Epstein-Barr virus (EBV), cytomegalovirus (CMV), and HHV-7, in addition to HHV-6, contribute to the internal organ involvement and the relapse of symptoms observed long after discontinuation of the causative drugs.[13] In some patients with DIHS, sequential herpesvirus reactivations can be detected during the acute phase of DIHS, coincident with the various clinical symptoms. However, it is still a matter of debate to what extent herpesvirus reactivations are responsible for clinical symptoms and particularly exacerbations of symptoms like hepatitis.

Clinical features of this disease include the stepwise development of multiorgan failure and the frequent deterioration of clinical signs such as fever, skin rashes, and liver or renal dysfunction, occurring even after discontinuation of the causative drug (**Fig. 1**). Fever usually precedes the skin rash by several days and is followed by a pruritic diffuse macular, sometimes reddish to lilac exanthema; some patients have a pustular eruption; occasionally the rash is maculopapular or erythema multiformelike. The patient's temperature ranges from 38 to 40°C, with temperature spikes that generate a concern for an underlying upper respiratory infection. The fever often persists for weeks. The maculopapular rash initially develops on the upper trunk and face, followed by involvement of lower extremities. Marked periorbital edema, a characteristic cutaneous manifestation of this syndrome, is frequently observed. The skin rash progresses to an exfoliative dermatitis or erythrodermic condition. Bilateral cervical, axillary, and inguinal lymphadenopathy, with tenderness, are commonly present. In many cases, these clinical features can be seen for weeks or months after cessation of the causative drug.[14]

Differentiation of DIHS from viral eruptions is the most challenging aspect of the diagnosis and care of patients afflicted with this disorder. Because the clinical presentation of DIHS/DRESS can resemble viral infections as well as autoimmune conditions, a careful drug history and physical examination are critical for making the correct diagnosis. Many of the patients are initially misdiagnosed with a viral illness, such as EBV or CMV-induced infectious mononucleosis or measles. However, these viral infections can be distinguished by the lack of eosinophilia and/or hypogammaglobulinemia. Kawasaki disease is more easily excluded by established diagnostic criteria and laboratory testing. Serum sicknesslike reaction can be distinguished by the presence of urticarial lesions and lack of internal organ involvement.[15] Clinical manifestations of DIHS/DRESS can be indistinguishable from atopic erythroderma with a bacterial infection; however, hepatitis and/or nephritis are not commonly observed in an atopic condition. Pseudolymphomas have also been reported to develop in association with causative drugs such as phenytoin and carbamazepine.[16] A diagnosis of

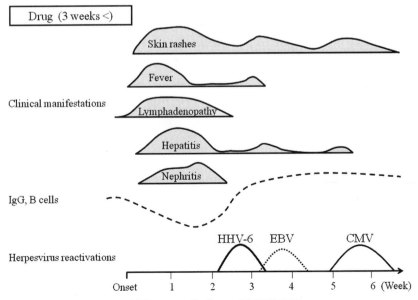

Fig. 1. Clinical symptoms and laboratory findings of DIHS/DRESS.

drug-induced pseudolymphoma is usually based on histologic findings or clinical presentation, ranging from solitary nodules to multiple infiltrative papules or plaques, without evidence of extracutaneous lymphoma, or resolution of the eruption with cessation of the drug.[17]

To identify the drug responsible for the eruption, in vivo and in vitro tests, such as patch tests and lymphocyte transformation tests (LTTs), are often performed. In particular, positive LTT reactions are only observed more than 4 weeks after disease onset and strong positive reactions can be observed at more than 1 year after discontinuation of the causative drug.[18]

VISCERAL ORGAN FAILURES OBSERVED DURING THE COURSE OF DIHS/DRESS

A variety of visceral involvements are observed at various time points after onset despite withdrawal of the causative drug. **Box 1** lists visceral involvements that appear from the onset of the symptoms to clinical resolution of the disease. Some of them are strongly related to herpesvirus reactivation.

Hematologic Abnormalities

Hematologic alterations occur in most patients. Leukocytosis with atypical lymphocytes and/or varying degrees of eosinophilia is a prominent feature of this syndrome. Nevertheless, leukopenia or lymphopenia often precedes leukocytosis, although this is not usually recognized because it occurs several days before the initial presentation. More than 1.5×10^9 eosinophils/L is recognized as eosinophilia in this syndrome. The eosinophilia may often be delayed for 1 to 2 weeks and can occur even after an increase in liver enzymes returns to baseline.

HPS is rarely observed during the course of DIHS/DRESS. HPS is associated with and triggered by various conditions such as viral infections, and particularly EBV-related disorders, malignant tumors, or autoimmune diseases. HPS associated with DIHS/DRESS occurs approximately 2 weeks after onset of the disease. A decrease in leukocyte and platelet counts is commonly detected along with an increase in serum lactate dehydrogenase. Bone marrow aspirates in hemophagocytosis usually show an increased number of macrophages. Descamps and colleagues[4] have described a patient with severe phenobarbital-induced DIHS/DRESS in whom a fulminant HPS associated with HHV-6 reactivation was noted. Another report details how HPS associated with reactivation of EBV can occur as part of DIHS/DRESS in a patient treated

---

Box 1
Visceral organ involvements in acute stage

Enterocolitis/intestinal bleeding

Hemophagocytic syndrome (HPS)

Hepatitis

Limbic encephalitis

Myocarditis

Nephritis

Parotitis

Pneumonitis/pleuritis

Syndrome of inappropriate secretion of antidiuretic hormone (SIADH)

for rheumatoid arthritis with sulfasalazine. EBV DNA in this patient was detected in the serum during the course of DIHS/DRESS. It is therefore likely that herpesvirus reactivation may contribute to the appearance of HPS in patients with DIHS/DRESS.[19]

Hepatic Involvement

As reported, hepatitis is the most common organ dysfunction in DIHS/DRESS. Hepatomegaly accompanied by splenomegaly is frequently observed (**Fig. 2**). Liver abnormalities occur in up to 70% of patients and are characterized by a marked increase in serum ALT.[20,21] The finding of an ALT level greater than 100 U/L is 1 of the criteria for DIHS established by J-SCAR.[8] Increases in liver enzymes usually persist for several days after discontinuation of the offending drug. Prolonged prothrombin times and/or partial thromboplastin times are observed in severe cases.[22] Severe hepatitis portends a prolonged course characterized by multiple exacerbations and remissions of the skin rash and the liver disease.[23] Among causative drugs, hepatitis is often observed in phenytoin-, minocycline-, or dapson-induced DIHS/DRESS.[10] Although most patients recover spontaneously, hepatic necrosis in the setting of coagulopathy and sepsis can cause death. The hepatitis is usually anicteric, but if it is icteric, it tends to have a poorer prognosis. Icterus is often observed in patients who have leprosy with dapson-induced DIHS/DRESS. Cholangitis is rarely observed as a part of dapson-induced DIHS/DRESS.[24] Liver involvement displays a mixed hepatocellular and cholestatic pattern. Results of hepatitis A, hepatitis B, and hepatitis C viral analyses are usually negative; however, underlying persistent viral infection, such as hepatitis B and hepatitis C virus infection, often causes a deterioration in liver function and prolongs liver dysfunction. According to the analysis of 62 cases by Tohyama and colleagues,[25] the flaring of symptoms such as fever and hepatitis was closely related to HHV-6 reactivation in patients with DIHS/DRESS. A patient reported by Eshki and colleagues[26] required a liver transplantation in an emergency setting; in this patient, a significant increase in anti-HHV-6 IgG antibody titers was detected in a serum sample collected several months before the transplantation. This case is important in that it confirmed that HHV-6 reactivation is a pretransplantation episode.

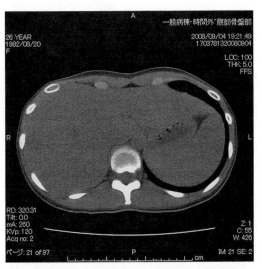

Fig. 2. Hepatomegaly in a patient with phenytoin-induced hypersensitivity syndrome showed by CT.

Fulminant hepatitis associated with DIHS/DRESS was reported in a patient who underwent intravenous intensive corticosteroid therapy, with a beneficial outcome.[27] A recent article has reported that fulminant liver failure after additional vancomycin treatment was observed in a patient with sulfasalazine-induced DIHS/DRESS.[28] Liver histology in this patient revealed infiltration of granzyme B[+]CD3[+] lymphocytes close to apoptotic hepatocytes. This patient developed recurrent skin rashes, eosinophilia and moderate hepatitis after liver transplantation; HHV-6 DNA was not detected in the affected liver.

There are no strict guidelines for corticosteroid therapy in patients with hepatitis: In Europe, 1 mg/kg body weight/d of prednisolone is recommended, if ALT or aspartate aminotransferase values are more than 500 IU. Tapering is performed according to clinical course, whereby too early CS reduction tends to go along with transient exacerbations (liver enzymes, eosinophilia, and additional drug intolerance).

Renal Involvement

Renal involvement occurs in 11% of patients with DIHS/DRESS.[29] In the criteria for DIHS/DRESS, renal dysfunction can be substituted for liver abnormalities. Regarding multiple visceral involvement, renal involvement is particularly evident in allopurinol-induced DIHS/DRESS.[10] In more than 80% of cases of allopurinol-induced DIHS/DRESS, patients showed evidence of renal impairment before commencing allopurinol. Because renal function declines steadily with age, elderly people are most vulnerable to developing this particular complication.[30] In many cases, laboratory studies show worsening renal insufficiency, ranging from a mild increase in serum creatinine levels to severe interstitial nephritis. In severe renal dysfunction, laboratory findings show high serum urea nitrogen and creatinine levels and low creatinine clearance. Urine analysis may reveal a substantial content of eosinophils. Kidney ultrasound examination is commonly normal and clinical symptoms are usually absent. A case of a patient with sulfasalazine-induced DIHS/DRESS who developed renal failure after corticosteroids withdrawal has been reported. Hemodialysis was shown to be effective in this patient.[31] A kidney biopsy showed acute interstitial nephritis with an intense lymphocytic infiltrate and tubular necrosis.[32] No specific deposits were detected by the immunofluorescence study. Accumulated case reports have shown that severe renal insufficiency increases the risk of mortality.

Pulmonary Involvement

Although pulmonary involvement is rarely reported in DIHS/DRESS, interstitial pneumonia with eosinophilia is often observed in patients who have minocycline-induced DIHS/DRESS.[10] It is possible that the cases with less severe pulmonary involvement are not reported, leading to a reporting bias with regard to the severity of the published cases.

Pulmonary complications include abnormal pulmonary function, acute interstitial pneumonitis, lymphocytic interstitial pneumonia, and acute respiratory distress syndrome (ARDS). Clinical symptoms such as a nonproductive cough and breathlessness are highly suggestive of pulmonary involvement. Pleuritis can also be observed during the course of DIHS/DRESS. Most patients with pulmonary involvement survive with no permanent sequelae; however, it may be life threatening in patients who show the characteristic findings of ARDS.[33]

Lazoglu and colleagues[34] have reported a patient who developed Loeffler syndrome during the course of anticonvulsant hypersensitivity syndrome. Physical examination of this patient revealed marked rhonchi and increased fremitus in the lung fields. Chest radiographs showed bilateral infiltrates and contrast-enhanced computed tomography (CT) of the chest revealed fluffy bilateral infiltrates. Abacavir-induced severe hypersensitivity reaction, occurring exclusively in genetically susceptible individuals (HLA-B5701*), also often shows some pulmonary involvement.[35,36] Eosinophilia is often not present in these reactions, and the term DRESS therefore not used for abacavir-induced hypersensitivity reactions.

According to our and J-SCAR members' cases, it is likely that infectious pneumonia induced by *Pneumocystis jiroveci* or *Cryptococcus neoformans* could develop following the clinical resolution in patients with DIHS/DRESS.

Cardiac Involvement

Cardiac involvement is rarely observed during the course of the disease in patients with DIHS/DRESS. According to reports, myocarditis associated with DIHS/DRESS can develop at the onset of the disease or approximately 40 days after onset (**Fig. 3**).[37,38] Clinically, symptoms suggestive of myocarditis include heart failure symptoms such as chest pain, unexpected tachycardia, breathlessness, and low blood pressure during the early course of DIHS/DRESS, although some patients are completely asymptomatic. Chest radiographs show cardiomegaly and pleural effusions and the electrocardiogram usually shows nonspecific ST-T changes, sinus tachycardia, or arrhythmias. The echocardiogram shows significant reduction in ejection fraction. Increases of serum cardiac enzymes, such as creatinine kinase and creatinine kinase MB-fraction, are detected but increased troponin-I levels are not seen.[39] Cardiac findings like these, especially if they are of recent onset in the presence of signs and symptoms of DIHS/DRESS, should be considered strongly suggestive of drug-induced myocarditis as part of DIHS/DRESS. Although endomyocardial biopsy remains the gold standard for the diagnosis of myocarditis, this is a highly invasive procedure that is not routinely performed.[38] Therefore, the diagnosis of myocarditis is still largely dependent on clinical suspicion rather than definitive diagnosis. In this setting, the final diagnosis of myocarditis is based on the presence of signs and symptoms of DIHS/DRESS, associated with recent onset of electrocardiogram changes, increased serum cardiac enzymes and a structurally normal heart and coronary arteries.[38,40] Regardless of the cause, in patients with myocarditis and symptoms of heart failure, initial therapy should include besides corticosteroids (1 mg

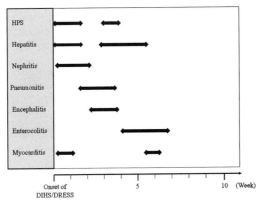

Fig. 3. Time interval between onset and visceral involvements during the course of DIHS/DRESS.

prednisolone/kg body weight/d), diuretics, an angiotensin-converting enzyme inhibitor and a β-blocker.[40]

Recently, complete atrioventricular block-associated dapson-induced DIHS/DRESS has been reported. In this case, the atrioventricular block, as confirmed by electrocardiogram, was considered 1 of the multiple internal organ dysfunctions related to DIHS/DRESS, primarily because dyspnea, numbness of the limbs for several minutes, and sudden onset syncope were observed in conjunction with the onset of clinical signs and symptoms of DIHS/DRESS.[41]

Neurologic Involvement

Neurologic complications observed in DIHS/DRESS include meningitis and encephalitis. Meningoencephalitis develops approximately 2 to 4 weeks after the onset of this syndrome (see **Fig. 3**). The clinical features of this disease include coma, seizure, headache, and speech disturbance. Neurologic symptoms such as arm weakness and cranial nerve palsies are also observed. An electroencephalogram shows diffuse slow waves, with an occasional solitary spike, in the frontal and temporal leads without periodic patterns. A magnetic resonance imaging (MRI) scan of the brain shows bilateral lesions involving the amygdala, mesial temporal lobes, insula, and cingulate gyrus.[42] The predilection for the hippocampal region in encephalitis is suggestive of limbic encephalitis. In accordance with the apparent fixed latency of HHV-6 reactivation after onset of DIHS/DRESS, the limbic encephalitis may be caused by reactivation of HHV-6 during the course of the disease. Masaki and colleagues[43] have reported a patient with allopurinol-induced DIHS/DRESS who developed encephalitis after reduction of systemic corticosteroids. Laboratory analysis showed an increase in anti-HHV-6 IgG titers and detection of HHV-6 DNA by means of polymerase chain reaction (PCR) assay in the cerebrospinal fluid (CSF). However, viral DNA cannot necessarily be detected in CSF samples obtained from patients with DIHS/DRESS after the onset of encephalitis.[44] These results may indicate secondary encephalitis or inappropriate timings of sampling. The progression of meningoencephalitis observed in DIHS/DRESS is similar to that observed in patients who have received a bone marrow transplant.

The authors have reported a case of SIADH, coincident with the clinical symptoms of limbic encephalitis, in a patient with DHS/DRESS.[44] A similar unusual presentation of limbic encephalitis caused by HHV-6, associated with hyponatremia, has been previously described in several hematopoietic cell transplant recipients who developed graft-versus-host disease (GVHD). These 2 cases suggest that DIHS/DRESS and GVHD may have a common underlying condition, specifically reactivation of latent herpesvirus.[45,46] Recent reports offer evidence that HHV-6 reactivation may underlie a characteristic limbic encephalitis syndrome following hematopoietic cell transplant; the cardinal features of this syndrome include memory loss, insomnia, electroencephalographic evidence of temporal lobe seizure activity, MRI signal intensity abnormalities of the temporal lobe, and SIADH.[47]

Gastrointestinal Involvement

Abrupt gastrointestinal bleeding can be observed during the course of DIHS/DRESS. This is a life-threatening manifestation of the syndrome and is caused by CMV ulcers. CMV disease is a serious viral infection that occurs primarily in immunocompromised patients and rarely in immunocompetent patients. The gastrointestinal ulcers can be misdiagnosed as steroid-induced gastric ulcers in these patients unless special attention is given to the possibility of CMV disease. Endoscopic examination reveals arterial bleeding from punched-out gastric ulcerations.[48] Because of the high mortality associated with these ulcerations, early intervention with emergency endoscopic clipping and blood transfusion is usually required.

The gastrointestinal manifestation often appears concomitantly with cutaneous CMV ulcers on the shoulders and trunk. Biopsy specimens obtained from the gastric mucosa and the skin show cytomegalic cells with the characteristic owl's eye intranuclear inclusions in the infiltrating cells. The CMV infection is usually confirmed by immunohistochemical analysis using anti-CMV monoclonal antibody.[48] Autopsy results obtained from a patient with severe DIHS/DRESS revealed disseminated CMV infection involving the lung, myocardium, kidney, adrenal gland, liver, pancreas, spleen, and skin.[49]

Although it is uncommon to suspect CMV reactivation during the disease, the presence of scratch dermatitis and erythematous rashes, unexplained slight fever, and lumbar pain are considered as symptoms suggestive of the development of gastrointestinal CMV disease. In addition, a reduction in platelet and white blood cell counts and a decreased serum globulin level are also useful markers predictive of CMV reactivation. To detect CMV reactivation, examination of CMV antigenemia in the peripheral blood is the most useful diagnostic tool because this is not a time-consuming technique.

CMV reactivation occurs in a predictable time course during the course of DIHS/DRESS. In most patients, CMV DNA is detected during a 4- to 5-week period after the onset of disease (see **Fig. 3**), regardless of the administration of systemic corticosteroids, at approximately 10 days to 3 weeks after HHV-6 reactivation.[48,50] Although comprehensive explanations are unavailable, several preexisting factors that contribute to CMV reactivation are reported in retrospective studies. The results indicate that elderly patients, particularly those older than 60 years, and male patients with antecedent high HHV-6 DNA loads are at risk for overt CMV disease.[48]

If CMV antigenemia is positive in patients with DIHS/DRESS, treatment with the antiviral agent ganciclovir is recommended until CMV antigenemia becomes negative.

Involvement of Other Organ Systems

A patient with anticonvulsant hypersensitivity syndrome developed enlargement of the parotid glands with cervical lymphadenopathy in the acute stage.[34] Descamps and colleagues documented a patient with DIHS/DRESS who showed pancreatitis and increased serum amylase and lipase levels. Herpes labialis and herpes zoster are also observed in patients with DIHS/DRESS.[13,20] The former is often recognized as an epiphenomenon of the disease, whereas the latter may precede the onset of this disease. These herpetic cutaneous lesions should be considered as a reactivation event in the sequential reactivations of herpesviruses occurring in patients with DIHS/DRESS.

LONG-TERM SEQUELAE OBSERVED AFTER SYMPTOM-FREE INTERVAL IN DIHS

Several articles, including the authors', have shown the occurrence of autoimmune diseases and/or production of autoantibodies after resolution of DIHS/DRESS (**Box 2**). These autoimmune diseases include type 1 diabetes mellitus (DM),[51–56] autoimmune thyroid disease,[38,56] sclerodermoid GVHD-like lesions,[57] and lupus erythematosus[58,59] (**Fig. 4**). Some of these autoimmune diseases are similar to those seen after bone marrow transplantation. According to the reports, autoimmune diseases have developed from several months to years after the apparent clinical resolution of DIHS/DRESS. Because of the long symptom-free interval, it is difficult to establish an association between DIHS/DRESS and autoimmune diseases. The association

> **Box 2**
> **Visceral organ involvements in late stage**
>
> Bullous pemphigoid (BP)
>
> Enteropathy
>
> Sclerodermoid lesions
>
> Systemic lupus erythematosus
>
> Type 1 DM
>
> Thyroiditis

between DIHS/DRESS and these autoimmune diseases is overlooked unless physicians pay special attention to the previous history of DIHS/DRESS and the presence of viral reactivations that trigger the development of autoimmune diseases.

Type 1 DM

In rare cases, fulminant type 1 DM may develop in association with DIHS/DRESS. Type 1 DM is classified into classic autoimmune type 1A DM and idiopathic type 1B DM. Diagnosis of type 1 DM is confirmed by low levels of serum C-peptide. Fulminant type 1 DM has been recently characterized by its rapid onset with an absence of diabetes-related autoantibodies. In type 1 DM diabetes-related autoantibodies, such as antiglutamic acid decarboxylase (GAD) and islet cell antibodies, are usually not detected, indicating that β-cell failure is not of autoimmune origin.[51,52,60] Initial clinical manifestations of fulminant type 1 DM reveal vomiting and dull epigastric pain. Laboratory findings show hyperglycemia, hyperosmolarity, and metabolic acidosis. These findings are compatible with diabetic ketoacidosis. Increases of pancreatic exocrine enzyme levels such as lipase and amylase are observed during the course of the disease, consistent with acute pancreatitis.[53] De novo onset type 1 DM appears around 3 weeks and 10 months after the onset of the clinical symptoms of DIHS/DRESS[51–54,60] (see **Fig. 4**); type 1 DM develops during corticosteroid treatment of DIHS/DRESS in most patients. Early detection and intervention for this serious complication should be given to patients with DIHS/DRESS. The cause of this particular appearance of type 1 DM remains unknown. Based on previous reports implicating viral agents such as enteroviruses, rubella, mumps, and CMV in the potential triggers,[61] it seems likely that herpesvirus reactivation could contribute to the development of the type 1 DM in patients with DIHS/DRESS. In addition,

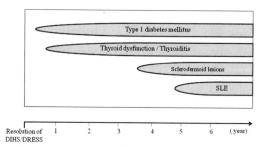

Fig. 4. Autoimmune diseases after clinical resolution of DIHS/DRESS. SLE, systemic lupus erythematosus.

because analyses of HLA antigens showed that DQA1*0303 and DQB1*0401 are associated with fulminant type 1 DM, DIHS/DRESS may have triggered the fulminant type 1 DM in this particular group.[62]

On the other hand, in autoimmune type 1 DM, various autoantibodies including IA_2, anti-GAD, are detected. Autoimmune type 1 DM is not common in patients with DIHS/ DRESS. The coexistence of autoimmune type 1 DM and Graves disease has been observed in relation to DIHS/DRESS. In a reported case, 4 months after the diagnosis of DIHS/DRESS, manifestations of type 1 DM developed; low anti-GAD antibody titers are detected.[55] In addition, Brown and colleagues[56] have recently reported a case of a patient with minocycline-induced DIHS/DRESS who developed autoimmune hyper-thyroidism, type 1 DM, and additional serologic findings suggestive of evolving systemic autoimmunity. In this case, clinical manifestations of autoimmune type 1 DM developed 7 months after discontinuation of the causative drug (see **Fig. 4**); various autoantibodies including IA_2, anti-GAD, -thyroid peroxidase (TPO), -thyroglob-ulin, -nuclear, and -SSA antibodies were also detected during this period; HLA antigen typing revealed DQA1*0303. Such findings arouse suspicion of the development of autoimmune diseases like polyglandular autoimmune syndrome in patients with DIHS/DRESS.[63]

After the diagnosis of type 1 DM, prompt insulin injection therapy should be commenced. When the diagnosis is overlooked, consequences can be life threatening.

Thyroid Dysfunction/Thyroiditis

In some patients with DIHS/DRESS, endocrinologic evaluation reveals various thyroid gland abnormalities, such as increased free thyroxine (T4), low thyroid-stimulating hormone (TSH), and increased TSH levels. These abnormal findings may escape detection if thyroid markers are not evaluated. Levothyroxine replacement therapy may be required for hypothyroidism. Of those patients who show thyroid dysfunction, some may later develop autoimmune thyroid disease.

Graves disease could also develop after the resolution of DIHS/DRESS. The interval between the discontinuation of the causative drug and the onset of Graves disease is approximately 2 to 4 months. According to Brown and colleagues,[56] at first low TSH and high free thyroxine (FT_4) levels and markedly increased antithyroglobulin and anti-TPO antibody titers are detected without any symptoms; anti-TSH receptor antibodies are negative. Markers of Graves disease are also negative, and a diagnosis of autoim-mune thyroiditis in the thyrotoxic phase is usually made.[56] Approximately 5 months after cessation of the causative drug, the patient develops clinical symptoms such as palpitation, irritability, and difficulty sleeping with laboratory findings compatible with Graves disease (see **Fig. 4**). Thyrotoxicosis was also observed as the presenting symptom in a patient with dapson-induced DIHS/DRESS.[38]

On the other hand, Hashimoto disease, revealing anti-TPO and antithyroglobulin antibodies, is also observed after the resolution of clinical symptoms of DIHS/DRESS. The authors have experienced a patient with increased anti-TPO antibodies and antithyroglobulin antibodies during the course of DIHS/DRESS with multiple herpes-virus reactivations such as HHV-6, EBV, HHV-7, and CMV. The patient developed Hashimoto disease 3 years after resolution of the clinical symptoms of the disease with a significant increase in anti-TPO and antithyroglobulin, and goiter.

According to our analyses, approximately 3 months to 1 year after resolution of DIHS/DRESS, antithyroid antibodies are detected in our patients with DIHS/ DRESS without any clinical manifestations. Therefore, we examined several autoanti-body titers, including antinuclear antibody (ANA) titer, anti-TPO antibodies, and antithyroglobulin antibodies at the acute stage as well as up to 1 year after resolution of DIHS/DRESS. Our analyses showed that anti-TPO and antithyroglobulin antibodies increased in some patients without any clinical symptoms or functional alterations of the thyroid gland (T. Ishida, unpublished data, 2010).

Sclerodermoid Lesions

The authors have reported a patient who developed systemic sclerosis-like lesions 3 to 4 years after zonisamide-induced DIHS/DRESS[57] (see **Fig. 4**). The patient presented with multiple brownish, indurated plaques with xerosis on the extremities. In this patient, a wide variety of manifestations were observed, including pancytopenia, diffuse alopecia, thyroid dysfunction, and sclereodermoid lesions, with an increase in various autoantibody titers. The patient's past history revealed that fever, liver dysfunction, and skin rashes had occurred along with HHV-6 reactivation, which fulfilled the criteria for DIHS/DRESS. ANA and rheumatoid factor were negative during the course of DIHS/DRESS but became detectable with the appearance of diffuse alopecia. A dramatic increase in ANA was found at the initial presentation to our department because of sclerodermoid GVHD-like lesions, indicating that the disease process of DIHS/DRESS may act as a trigger for the development of autoimmune disease.[57,58] Autoimmune-like lesions resembling scleroderma or lupus erythematosus often develop as manifestations of chronic GVHD after organ transplantation. Generalized sclerodermatous lesions appeared between days 332 and 876 in a group of patients, after donor leukocyte infusion, in this setting.[64] Autoimmune reactions ranging from thyroid dysfunction to sclerodermoid GVHD-like lesions appeared 1 to 4 years after the onset of DIHS/DRESS in this patient, a time frame similar to that of chronic GVHD.

Systemic Lupus Erythematosus

A patient who developed systemic lupus erythematosus after resolution of carbamazepine-induced DIHS/DRESS with reactivation of HHV-6 and EBV has been reported.[58,59] After resolution of DIHS/DRESS, the patient remained asymptomatic for 4 years until he presented with cervical lymphadenopathy and erythematous lesions on the face and chest. Clinical manifestations and histology of his lymphadenopathy were consistent with a diagnosis of Kikuchi-Fujimoto disease. One week later, his erythematous lesions deteriorated, evolving into the typical lesions of lupus erythematosus on the face, chest, and back (**Fig. 5**). Laboratory findings showed leukopenia, positive ANA, and decreased serum C3 and C4 levels. Histologic examination of the erythematous lesion showed vacuolar changes of basal cell layer with a moderate lymphocytic infiltration around follicles and sweat glands. The lupus band test of the skin lesion was positive and lupus nephritis was confirmed by renal biopsy. Expression of EBV-encoded RNA was detected in the lymph node by in situ hybridization. The presence of EBV DNA was also confirmed by PCR in the lymph node.[59] EBV reactivations in this patient may have been involved in the pathogenesis of systemic lupus erythematosus after Kikuchi-Fujimoto disease. These findings could be interpreted as an indication that herpesvirus reactivation and/or the immune response to them can occur during the disease process of DIHS/DRESS and may render refractory individuals susceptible to autoimmune disease.

Autoimmune Bullous Diseases

Autoimmune bullous disease and autoantibodies rarely appear after the onset of DIHS/DRESS. Kijima and colleagues[65] have reported a case of a patient who developed recalcitrant bullous lesions on the trunk and extremities 77 days after the onset of symptoms,

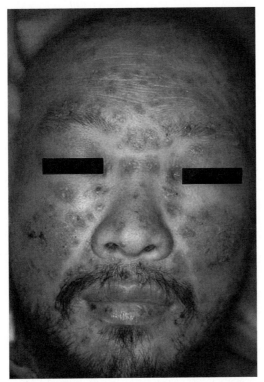

Fig. 5. Typical lesions of lupus erythematosus developed after DIHS/DRESS.

with an increase in peripheral eosinophil counts during treatment with systemic cortico-steroids for DIHS/DRESS. In this case, the final diagnosis of BP was made from lesional and circulating IgG autoantibodies at the basement membrane shown by direct and indirect immunofluorescence, and the detection of a high index of anti-BP 180 anti-bodies by enzyme-linked immunosorbent assay.[65] In a separate case, vesicular lesions on the lower leg developed after aggravation of symptoms caused by addition of val-proate to the regimen in a patient with carbamazepine-induced DIHS/DRESS. Circu-lating autoantibodies against 190-kDa antigen, which are usually found in patients with pemphigus foliaceus and paraneoplastic pemphigus, were detected in the serum by indirect immunofluorescence and immunoblot analyses.[66]

Other Late Complications

Newell and colleagues[22] have reported a pediatric patient with aniticonvulsant-induced DIHS/DRESS who developed chronic protein-losing enteropathy.

SUMMARY

DIHS/DRESS is a severe drug-induced systemic reaction with several herpesvirus reactivations. Multiple visceral organ failure such as hepatitis, nephritis, myocarditis, and pneumonitis can appear during the course of disease. The severity of DIHS/DRESS is most frequently determined by the presence of visceral involvement and mortality is related to the degree of systemic involvement. On the other hand, autoim-mune diseases such as thyroid disease, sclerodermoid lesions, and lupus erythematosus develop after a disease-free interval of several years. The immune dysfunction in DIHS/DRESS may serve as an excellent tool for investigating the pathogenesis of autoimmune diseases occurring after viral infections. To identify patients at risk for developing autoimmune diseases, thereby improving overall patient management, patients with DIHS/DRESS, in particular those with symptoms suggestive of viral reactivation, should be carefully followed up even after resolution of clinical symptoms. Studies of DIHS/DRESS may provide further insight into the pathogenesis of visceral organ diseases.

REFERENCES

1. Sullivan JR, Shear NH. The drug hypersensitivity syndrome: what is the pathogenesis? Arch Dermatol 2001;137(3):357–64.
2. Gennis MA, Vemuri R, Burns EA, et al. Familial occurrence of hypersensitivity to phenytoin. Am J Med 1991;91(6):631–4.
3. Bocquet H, Martine B, Roujeau JC. Drug-induced pseudolymphoma and drug hypersensitivity syndrome (drug rash with eosinophilia and systemic symptoms: DRESS). Semin Cutan Med Surg 1996;15(4):250–7.
4. Descamps V, Bouscarat F, Laglenne S, et al. Human herpesvirus 6 infection associated with anticonvulsant hypersensitivity syndrome and reactive haemophagocytic syndrome. Br J Dermatol 1997;137(4):605–8.
5. Suzuki Y, Inagi R, Aono T, et al. Human herpesvirus 6 infection as a risk factor of the development of severe drug-induced hypersensitivity. Arch Dermatol 1998; 134(9):1108–12.
6. Tohyama M, Yahata Y, Yasukawa M, et al. Severe hypersensitivity syndrome due to sulfasalazine associated with reactivation of human herpesvirus 6. Arch Dermatol 1998;134(9):1113–7.
7. Hashimoto K, Yasukawa M, Tohyama M. Human herpesvirus 6 and drug allergy. Curr Opin Allergy Clin Immunol 2003;3(4):255–60.
8. Shiohara T, Iijima M, Ikezawa Z, et al. The diagnosis of a DRESS syndrome has been sufficiently established on the basis of typical clinical features and viral reactivations. Br J Dermatol 2007;156(5):1083–4.
9. Ghislain PD, Roujeau JC. Treatment of severe drug reactions: Stevens-Johnson syndrome, toxic epidermal necrolysis and hypersensitivity syndrome. Dermatol online J 2002;8(1):5.
10. Kano Y, Shiohara T. The variable clinical picture of drug-induced hypersensitivity syndrome (DIHS)/drug rash with eosinophilia and systemic symptoms (DRESS) in relation to the eliciting drug. Immunol Allergy Clin North Am 2009;29(3): 481–501.
11. Roujeau JC. Clinical heterogeneity of drug hypersensitivity. Toxicology 2005; 209(2):123–9.
12. Shiohara T, Kano Y. Complex interaction between drug allergy and viral infection. Clin Rev Allergy Immunol 2007;33(1–2):124–33.
13. Kano Y, Hirahara K, Sakuma K, et al. Several herpesviruses can reactivate in a severe drug-induced multiorgan reaction in the same sequential order as in graft-versus-host disease. Br J Dermatol 2006;155(2):301–6.
14. Kano Y, Inaoka M, Shiohara T. Association between anticonvulsant hypersensitivity syndrome and human herpesvirus 6 reactivation and hypogammaglobulinemia. Arch Dermatol 2004;140(2):183–8.
15. Carroll MC, Yueng-Yue KA, Esterly NB, et al. Drug-induced hypersensitivity syndrome in pediatric patients. Pediatrics 2001;108(2):485–92.

16. Callot V, Roujeau JC, Bagot M, et al. Drug-induced pseudolymphoma and hypersensitivity syndrome. Two different clinical entities. Arch Dermatol 1996;132(11): 1315–21.

17. Rijlaarsdam JU, Scheffer E, Meijer CJ, et al. Cutaneous pseudo-T cell lymphomas. A clinicopathologic study of 20 patients. Cancer 1992;69(3): 717–24.

18. Kano Y, Hirahara K, Mitsuyama Y, et al. Utility of the lymphocyte transformation test in the diagnosis of drug sensitivity: dependence on its timing and type of drug eruption. Allergy 2007;62(12):1439–44.

19. Komatsuda A, Okamoto Y, Hatakeyama T, et al. Sulfasalazine-induced hypersensitivity syndrome and haemophagocytic syndrome associated with reactivation of Epstein-Barr virus. Clin Rheumatol 2008;27(3):395–7.

20. Shiohara T, Takahashi R, Kano Y. Drug-induced hypersensitivity syndrome and viral reactivation. In: Pichler WJ, editor. Drug hypersensitivity. Basel: Karger; 2007. p. 251–66.

21. Hari Y, Frutig-Schnyder K, Hurni M, et al. T cell involvement in cutaneous drug eruptions. Clin Exp Allergy 2001;31(9):1398–408.

22. Newell BD, Moinfar M, Mancini AJ, et al. Retrospective analysis of 32 pediatric patients with anticonvulsant hypersensitivity syndrome (ACHSS). Pediatr Dermatol 2009;26(5):536–46.

23. Shiohara T, Inaoka M, Kano Y. Drug-induced hypersensitivity syndrome (DIHS): a reaction induced by a complex interplay among herpesviruses and antiviral and antidrug immune responses. Allergol Int 2006;55(1):1–8.

24. Itha S, Kumar A, Dhingra S, et al. Dapsone induced cholangitis as a part of dapsone syndrome: a case report. BMC Gastroenterol 2003;3:21.

25. Tohyama M, Hashimoto K, Yasukawa M, et al. Association of human herpesvirus 6 reactivation with the flaring and severity of drug-induced hypersensitivity syndrome. Br J Dermatol 2007;157(5):934–40.

26. Eshki M, Allanore L, Musset P, et al. Twelve-year analysis of severe cases of drug reaction with eosinophilia and systemic symptoms. Arch Dermatol 2009;145(1): 67–72.

27. Descloux E, Argaud L, Dumortier J, et al. Favourable issue of a fulminant hepatitis associated with sulfasalazine DRESS syndrome without liver transplantation. Intensive Care Med 2005;31(12):1727–8.

28. Mennicke M, Zawodniak A, Keller M, et al. Fulminant liver failure after vancomycin in a sulfasalazine-induced DRESS syndrome: fatal recurrence after liver transplantation. Am J Transplant 2009;9(9):2197–202.

29. Roujeau JC, Stren RS. Severe adverse cutaneous reactions to drugs. N Engl J Med 1994;331(19):1272–85.

30. Kumar A, Edward N, White MI, et al. Allopurinol, erythema multiforme, and renal insufficiency. BMJ 1996;312(7024):173–4.

31. Higuchi M, Agatsuma T, Iizima M, et al. A case of drug-induced hypersensitivity syndrome with multiple organ involvement treated with plasma exchange. Ther Apher Dial 2005;9(5):412–6.

32. Augusto J-F, Sayegh J, Simon A, et al. A case of sulphasalazine-induced DRESS syndrome with delayed acute interstitial nephritis. Nephrol Dial Transplant 2009; 24(9):2940–2.

33. Roca B, Calvo B, Ferrer D. Minocycline hypersensitivity reaction with acute respiratory distress syndrome. Intensive Care Med 2003;29(2):338.

34. Lazoglu AH, Boglioli LR, Dorsett B, et al. Phenytoin-related immunodeficiency associated with Loeffler's syndrome. Ann Allergy Asthma Immunol 1995;74(6):479–82.

35. Hetherrington S, McGuirk S, Powell G, et al. Hypersensitivity reactions during therapy with the nucleoside reverse transcriptase inhibitor abacavir. Clin Ther 2001;23(10):1603–14.

36. Mallal S, Nolan D, Witt C, et al. Association between presence of HLA-B*5701, HLA-DR7, and HLA-DQ3 and hypersensitivity to HIV-1 reverse-transcriptase inhibitor abacavir. Lancet 2002;359(9308):727–32.

37. Sekiguchi A, Kashiwagi T, Ishida-Yamamoto A, et al. Drug-induced hypersensitivity syndrome due to mexiletine associated with human herpesvirus 6 and cytomegalovirus reactivation. J Dermatol 2005;32(4):278–81.

38. Teo RY, Tay YK, Tan CH, et al. Presumed dapson-induced drug hypersensitivity syndrome causing reversible hypersensitivity myocarditis and thyrotoxicosis. Ann Acad Med Singap 2006;35(11):833–6.

39. Ben m'rad M, Lecler-Mercier S, Blanche P, et al. Drug-induced hypersensitivity syndrome clinical and biologic patterns in 24 patients. Medicine 2009;88(3): 131–40.

40. Zaldi AN. Anticonvulsant hypersensitivity syndrome leading to reversible myocarditis. Can J Clin Pharmacol 2005;12(1):e33–40.

41. Zhu KJ, He FT, Jin N, et al. Complete atrioventricular block associated with dapson therapy: a rare complication of dapson-induced hypersensitivity syndrome. J Clin Pharm Ther 2009;34(4):489–92.

42. Fujino Y, Nakajima M, Inoue H, et al. Human herpesvirus 6 encephalitis associated with hypersensitivity syndrome. Ann Neurol 2002;51(6):771–4.

43. Masaki T, Fukunaga A, Tohyama M, et al. Human herpes virus 6 encephalitis in allopurinol-induced hypersensitivity syndrome. Acta Derm Venereol 2003;83(2): 128–31.

44. Sakuma K, Kano Y, Fukuhara M, et al. Syndrome of inappropriate secretion of antidiretic hormone associated with limbic encephalitis in a patient with drug-induced hypersensitivity syndrome. Clin Exp Dermatol 2008;33(3):287–90.

45. Chik KW, Chan PK, Li CK, et al. Human herpesvirus-6 encephalitis after unrelated umbilical cord blood transplant in children. Bone Marrow Transplant 2002;29(12): 991–4.

46. Wainwright MS, Martin PL, Morse RP, et al. Human herpesvirus 6 limbic encephalitis after stem cell transplantation. Ann Neurol 2001;50(5):612–9.

47. Gewurtz BE, Marty FM, Baden LR, et al. Human herpesvirus 6 encephalitis. Curr Infect Dis Rep 2008;10(4):292–9.

48. Asano Y, Kagawa H, Kano Y, et al. Cytomegalovirus disease during severe drug eruptions: report of 2 cases and retrospective study of 18 patients with drug-induced hypersensitivity syndrome. Arch Dermatol 2009;145(9):1030–6.

49. Arakawa M, Kakuto Y, Ichikawa K, et al. Allopurinol hypersensitivity syndrome associated with systemic cytomegalovirus infection and systemic bacteremia. Intern Med 2001;40(4):331–5.

50. Seishima M, Yamanaka S, Fujisawa T, et al. Reactivation of human herpesvirus (HHV) family members other than HHV-6 in drug-induced hypersensitivity syndrome. Br J Dermatol 2006;155(2):344–9.

51. Seino Y, Yamauchi M, Hirai C, et al. A case of fulminant Type 1 diabetes associated with mexiletine hypersensitivity syndrome. Diabet Med 2004;21(10):1156–7.

52. Chiou CC, Chung WH, Hung SI, et al. Fulmimant type 1 diabetes mellitus caused by drug hypersensitivity syndrome with human herpesvirus 6. J Am Acad Dermatol 2006;54(Suppl 2):S14–7.

53. Sommers LM, Schoene RB. Allopurinol hypersensitivity syndrome associated with pancreatic exocrine abnormalities and new-onset diabetes mellitus. Arch Intern Med 2002;162(10):1190–2.

54. Chiou CC, Yang LC, Hung SI, et al. Clinicopathological features and prognosis of drug rash with eosinophilia and systemic symptoms: a study of 30 cases in Taiwan. J Eur Acad Dermatol Venereol 2008;22(9):1044–9.

55. Ozaki N, Miura Y, Sakakibara A, et al. A case of hypersensitivity syndrome induced by methimazole for Graves' disease. Thyroid 2005;15(12):1333–6.

56. Brown RJ, Rother KI, Artman H, et al. Minocycline-induced drug hypersensitivity syndrome followed by multiple autoimmune sequelae. Arch Dermatol 2009; 145(1):63–6.

57. Kano Y, Sakuma K, Shiohara T. Sclerodermoid graft-versus-host disease-like lesions occurring after drug-induced hypersensitivity syndrome. Br J Dermatol 2007;156(5):1061–3.

58. Aota N, Shiohara T. Viral connection between drug rashes and autoimmune diseases: how autoimmune responses are generated after resolution of drug rashes. Autoimmun Rev 2009;8(6):488–94.

59. Aota N, Hirahara K, Kano Y, et al. Systemic lupus erythematosus presenting with Kikuchi-Fujimoto's disease as a long-term sequela of drug-induced hypersensitivity syndrome: a possible role of Epstein-Barr virus reactivation. Dermatology 2009;218(3):275–7.

60. Sekine N, Motokura T, Oki T, et al. Rapid loss of insulin secretion in a patient with fulminant type 1 diabetes mellitus and carbamazepine hypersensitivity syndrome. JAMA 2001;285(9):1153–4.

61. Van der Welf N, Kroese FGM, Rozing J, et al. Viral infections as potential triggers of type 1 diabetes. Diabetes Metab Res Rev 2007;23(3):169–83.

62. Tanaka S, Kobayashi T, Nakanishi K, et al. Association of HLA-DQ genotype in autoantibody-negative and rapid-onset type 1 diabetes. Diabetes Care 2002; 25(12):2302–7.

63. Van den Driessche A, Eenkhoom V, Van Gaal L, et al. Type 1 diabetes and auto-immune polyglandular syndrome: a clinical review. Neth J Med 2009;67(11): 376–87.

64. Jones-Caballero M, Fernandez-Herrera J, Cordoba-Guijarro S, et al. Sclerodermatous graft-versus-host disease after donor leukocyte infusion. Br J Dermatol 1998;139(5):889–92.

65. Kijima A, Inui S, Nakamura T, et al. Does drug-induced hypersensitivity syndrome elicit bullous pemphigoid? Allergol Int 2008;57(2):181–2.

66. Yun SJ, Lee JB, Kim EJ, et al. Drug rash with eosinophilia and systemic symptoms induced by valproate and carbamazepine: formation of circulating autoantibody against 190-kDa antigen. Acta Derm Venereol 2006;86(3):241–4.

Perioperative Anaphylaxis

P.M. Mertes, MD, PhD[a,b,*], K. Tajima, MD[a,b],
M.A. Regnier-Kimmoun, MD[a,b], M. Lambert, MD[a,c],
G. Iohom, MD, PhD[d], R.M. Guéant-Rodriguez, MD, PhD[e,f],
J.M. Malinovsky, MD, PhD[g]

KEYWORDS

- Anesthesia • Anaphylaxis • Tryptase • Skin test
- Neuromuscular blocking agent • Latex
- Antibiotics • Epinephrine

The practice of anesthesiology has become increasingly safe throughout the years. Practicing clinicians and researchers have the opportunity to examine more closely those rare and serious adverse events that may threaten patient well-being. Immediate hypersensitivity reactions, the most severe appearing as anaphylaxis, which sometimes occur during anesthesia, are 1 such example. The effective anticipation, prevention, and treatment of these reactions is largely based on the knowledge and vigilance of the attending clinicians. Immediate hypersensitivity reactions occur, however, only once in every 5000 to 10,000 anesthetics. Therefore, individual anesthetists are likely to encounter only a few cases in their working lifetimes, hence the rapidity with which the diagnosis is made and appropriate management instituted varies considerably. For this reason, a structured approach to preventing, diagnosing, and managing perioperative anaphylaxis is justified.

[a] Service d'Anesthésie-Réanimation Chirurgicale, CHU de Nancy, Hôpital Central, 29 Avenue de Lattre de Tassigny, 54035 Nancy Cedex, France
[b] Unité Inserm U911, Faculté de Médecine, 9 Avenue de la Forêt de Haye, 54505 Vandoeuvre les Nancy, France
[c] Unité Inserm U684, Faculté de Médecine, 9 Avenue de la Forêt de Haye, 54505 Vandoeuvre les Nancy, France
[d] Department of Anaesthesia and Intensive Care Medicine, Cork University Hospital, University College Cork, Cork, Ireland
[e] Laboratoire de Biochimie Biologie Moléculaire Nutrition Métabolisme, CHU de Brabois, Avenue du Morvan, 54511 Vandoeuvre les Nancy, France
[f] Unité de Pathologie Cellulaire et Moléculaire en Nutrition, Inserm U724, Faculté de Médecine, 9 Avenue de la Forêt de Haye, 54505 Vandoeuvre les Nancy, France
[g] Service d'Anesthésie et Réanimation, CHU de Reims, Pôle URAD, Hôpital Maison Blanche, 45 rue Cognacq-Jay, 51092 Reims, France
* Corresponding author. Service d'Anesthésie-Réanimation Chirurgicale, CHU de Nancy, Hôpital Central, 29 Avenue de Lattre de Tassigny, 54035 Nancy Cedex.
E-mail address: pm.mertes@chu-nancy.fr

Med Clin N Am 94 (2010) 761–789
doi:10.1016/j.mcna.2010.04.002
0025-7125/10/$ – see front matter © 2010 Elsevier Inc. All rights reserved.

medical.theclinics.com

EPIDEMIOLOGY

General anesthesia is a unique situation described as a reversible state of unconsciousness, amnesia, analgesia, and immobility as a result of administering several drugs in a short period.[1] Many of these drugs can elicit adverse reactions either related to their pharmacologic properties and usually dose dependent, or unrelated to the pharmacologic properties and less dose dependent. The latter reactions comprise drug intolerance, idiosyncratic reactions, and anaphylactic reactions, which can be either immune mediated (allergic) or nonimmune mediated (pseudoallergic or anaphylactoid reactions). In an attempt to counteract unclear and heterogeneous use of terms, the nomenclature task force of the European Academy of Allergy and Immunology, and the World Allergy Organization, have proposed that anaphylactic-type reactions should be reclassified into allergic anaphylaxis and nonallergic anaphylaxis.[2,3] This proposal has not been universally accepted.[4]

The true incidence of anaphylactic reactions with their associated morbidity and mortality remains poorly defined as a result of uncertainties about reporting accuracy and exhaustiveness. Despite reported variations, probably reflecting differences in clinical practice and reporting systems, overall incidences seem to be similar between countries. The estimated incidence of all immune- and nonimmune-mediated immediate hypersensitivity reactions is 1 in 5000 to 1 in 13,000 anesthetics in Australia, 1 in 5000 in Thailand, 1 in 4600 in France, 1 in 1 250 to 1 in 5000 in New Zealand, and 1 in 3500 in England.[5–9] The estimated incidence of allergic anaphylaxis is 1 in 10,000 to 1 in 20,000 in Australia,[10] 1 in 13,000 in France,[11] 1 in 10,263 in Spain,[12] 1 in 5500 in Thailand,[9] and 1 in 1700 to 1 in 20,000 in Norway.[13] In most series, allergic reactions represent at least 60% of all hypersensitivity reactions observed within the perioperative period.[12,14–17] Reported expected mortality ranges from 3% to 9%.[18,19] The overall morbidity remains unknown.

MECHANISM

Allergic anaphylaxis is most commonly caused by the interaction of an allergen with specific immunoglobulin E (IgE) antibodies. These antibodies, in sensitized individuals, bind to high-affinity FcɛRI receptors located in the plasma membrane of tissue mast cells and blood basophils, and to low-affinity FcɛRII receptors on lymphocytes, eosinophils, and platelets. This interaction stimulates the cells to release preformed and newly synthesized inflammatory mediators, such as histamine, tryptase, phospholipid-derived mediators (eg, prostaglandin D_2, leukotrienes, thromboxane A_2, and platelet-activating factor) as well as several chemokines and cytokines, which account for the clinical features. Target organs commonly include the skin, mucous membranes, cardiovascular and respiratory systems, and the gastrointestinal tract. Allergic anaphylaxis for some substances (eg, dextrans) may be caused by IgG antibodies that produce immune complexes with the antigen (dextran macromolecules), and thereby activate the complement system.[20]

The precise mechanisms of nonimmune-mediated reactions remain difficult to establish. They are usually considered to result from a direct pharmacologic stimulation of mast cells and basophils, causing release of inflammatory mediators.[21] However, other mechanisms may be involved.[22,23] Nonallergic anaphylaxis does not entail an immunologic mechanism and, therefore, previous contact with the culprit substance is not necessary. However, in allergic anaphylaxis, involving drug-specific IgE, previous contact is not obligatory, and sensitization may have occurred via cross-reactive substances (see later discussion).

INVESTIGATION OF AN ALLERGIC REACTION

Any suspected hypersensitivity reaction during anesthesia must be extensively investigated using combined peri- and postoperative testing. It is important to confirm the nature of the reaction, to identify the responsible drug, to detect possible cross-reactivity in cases of anaphylaxis to a neuromuscular blocking agent (NMBA), and to provide recommendations for future anesthetic procedures.[24,25] Serious attempts have been made to standardize and validate in vitro and in vivo techniques for the diagnosis of drug allergy.[24–28] However, none of the available diagnostic tests is absolutely accurate. False-positive test results may merely cause an inconvenience (unnecessary avoidance of a safe drug), whereas false-negative or equivocal results may be extremely dangerous and severely undermine correct secondary prevention. Whenever possible, confirmation of the incriminated allergen should be based on immunologic assessment using more than 1 test. In the event of discrepancies between different tests, an alternative compound that tested completely negative is advocated.

The diagnostic strategy is based on a detailed history including concurrent morbidity, previous anesthetic history, and any known allergies, and on a series of investigations performed immediately and days to weeks later. Biologic investigations include mediator release assays at the time of the reaction,[29] quantification of specific IgE, immediately or best during the first 6 months after the event took place,[29,30] skin tests,[26] and other biologic assays such as histamine release tests or basophil activation assays.[28,31] Early tests are essentially designed to determine whether or not an immunologic mechanism is involved, or at least whether mast cells were activated (tryptase determinations). Skin tests are performed later, but best in the first year after the event, and attempt to identify the drug responsible.

Clinical Picture of Anesthesia-related Anaphylaxis

Anaphylaxis is generally an unanticipated reaction. The initial diagnosis is presumptive, although essential, because anaphylaxis may progress within minutes to become life threatening. The first line of evidence for the diagnosis of anaphylaxis includes the features and severity of clinical signs and the timing between the introduction of a suspected allergen and the onset of symptoms, whereas the required dosage of resuscitative medications gives insight as to the severity of the reaction.

The signs and symptoms of anaphylaxis occurring during anesthesia differ to some extent from those of anaphylaxis not associated with anesthesia. All early symptoms usually observed in the awake patient such as malaise, pruritus, dizziness, and dyspnea are absent in the anaesthetized patient. The most commonly reported initial features are pulselessness, difficulty to ventilate, and desaturation.[10] In our experience, a decreased end-tidal CO_2 is also of diagnostic value.[32] Cutaneous signs may be difficult to notice in a completely draped patient. In addition, many signs such as tachycardia, hypotension, or increased airway resistance may be the result of an interaction between the clinical status of the patient and the drugs administered during the procedure, dose-related side effect of the drugs, or inadequate depth of anesthesia. The differential diagnosis of anesthesia-related anaphylaxis is shown in **Table 1**.

Clinical manifestations show striking variations of intensity in different patients, ranging from mild hypersensitivity reactions to severe anaphylactic shock and death.[7,14] However, when a classification based on symptom severity is applied, allergic reactions are usually more severe than nonimmune-mediated reactions (**Table 2**).[16,17] The absence of cutaneous symptoms does not exclude the diagnosis

Table 1
Differential diagnosis of anaphylaxis during anesthesia
Drug overdose and interactions
Cardiac/vascular drug effects
Asthma
Arrhythmia
Myocardial infarction
Pericardial tamponade
Pulmonary edema
Pulmonary embolism
Tension pneumothorax
Hemorrhagic shock
Venous embolism
Sepsis
C1 esterase inhibitor deficiency
Mastocytosis
Malignant hyperthermia (succinylcholine)
Myotonias and masseter spasm (succinylcholine)
Hyperkalemia (succinylcholine)

of anaphylaxis. In addition, clinical features may occur in isolation such as a sudden cardiac arrest without any other clinical signs.[17] As a result, an anaphylactic reaction restricted to a single clinical symptom (eg, bronchospasm, tachycardia with hypotension) can easily be misdiagnosed because many other pathologic conditions may have an identical clinical presentation. In mild cases restricted to a single symptom, spontaneous recovery may be observed even in the absence of any specific treatment. Under such circumstances, the lack of a proper diagnosis and appropriate allergy assessment may lead to fatal reexposure.

Anaphylaxis may occur at any time during anesthesia, and may progress slowly or rapidly. Ninety percent of reactions appear at anesthesia induction, within minutes or seconds after the intravenous injection of the offending agent such as an NMBA or an antibiotic.[7,33] If the signs appear later, during the maintenance of anesthesia, they suggest an allergy to latex, volume expanders, or dyes. Latex allergy should also be considered when gynecologic procedures are performed. Particles from obstetricians' gloves, which accumulate in the uterus during obstetric maneuvers, could suddenly be released into the systemic blood flow following oxytocin injection.[11] Anaphylactic reactions to antibiotics have also been reported following removal of tourniquet during orthopedic surgery.[34]

Table 2	
Grade of severity: classification of immediate hypersensitivity reactions	
Grade	**Symptoms**
I	Generalized cutaneous signs: erythema, urticaria, with or without angioedema
II	Moderate multiorgan involvement with cutaneous signs, hypotension and tachycardia, bronchial hyperreactivity: cough, difficulty to ventilate
III	Severe life-threatening multiorgan involvement: collapse, tachycardia or bradycardia, arrhythmias, bronchospasm. Cutaneous signs may be present or may occur only after arterial blood pressure is restored
IV	Cardiac and/or respiratory arrest

Histamine and Tryptase

During an IgE-mediated reaction, basophils and mast cells are activated, then degranulate and release mediators into the extracellular fluid compartment. These mediators can be measured in the patient's serum and have proved to be useful for the diagnosis of anaphylaxis during anesthesia.[16,29,35–37] Histamine concentrations are maximal almost immediately and decrease thereafter, with a half-life of about 20 minutes. Therefore, circulating levels should be assayed within the first hour of a reaction. In mild cases, only early serum levels may be increased.[35] Histamine assays should be avoided during pregnancy (particularly near term) and in patients receiving high doses of heparin because of a high rate of false negativity caused by accelerated histamine degradation. When increased, circulating histamine levels confirm basophil cell degranulation, which can result from direct or IgE-mediated activation. In our most recent study, the sensitivity of this test for the diagnosis of anaphylaxis was estimated at 75%, its specificity at 51%, the positive predictive value at 75%, and the negative predictive value at 51%. Urinary methylhistamine assays are no longer recommended in view of their low sensitivity compared with tryptase and histamine assays.

Tryptase reaches a peak in the patient's serum 30 minutes after the first clinical manifestations. Its half-life is 90 minutes, and the levels usually decrease with time but in some cases increased levels can still be detected for up to 6 hours or more after the onset of anaphylaxis.[29] Basophils and mast cells differ in the amount of tryptase contained in their granules. Mast cells contain high tryptase levels (12–35 pg/cell) and basophils low levels (<0.05 pg/cell). Thus, although increased tryptase levels can be observed in different situations, an increased tryptase concentration of more than 25 µg/L is usually regarded as specific for mast cell activation, independent of its cause.[29,31] The absence of an increased serum tryptase level, however, does not rule out an allergic reaction.[31] In our most recent series, the sensitivity of tryptase measurement for the diagnosis of anaphylaxis was estimated at 64%, its specificity at 89.3%, positive predictive value at 92.6%, and negative predictive value at 54.3%.[16] To rule out an underlying mastocytosis with constitutive increased tryptase levels and higher tendency to anaphylaxis, tryptase levels should be determined again after 2 to 3 days.

Specific IgE Assay

In vitro tests are available to detect the presence of serum-specific IgE antibodies. Baldo and Fisher[38] were the first to show that drug-reactive IgEs were involved in anaphylactic reactions, using NMBAs coupled to epoxy Sepharose in a radioimmunoassay (RIA). The detection of antidrug-specific IgEs in serum is performed by a sandwich-type immunoassay in which the serum IgE is first adsorbed to a reactive phase and subsequently quantified via the binding of an anti-IgE tracer. The reactive phase is prepared by covalently coupling a drug derivative to a solid-phase such as nitrocellulose membrane or a polymer.

IgE binding on different NMBA solid phases and competitive inhibition assays with several muscle relaxants and other drugs and chemicals including morphine showed a cross-reactivity of specific IgE.[38–40] However, some patients do not react with all NMBA, showing that the substituted ammonium ion is at least not always the only part of the epitope. Gueant and colleagues[41] improved an RIA method for detecting NMBA IgE in serum using a quaternary ammonium compound coupled to Sepharose (QAS-RIA). The sensitivity of this test was estimated at 88%. An inhibition step in the presence of 130 nmol of soluble drug is performed and the highest percentage is observed with the incriminated drug in most cases (83.3%). Guilloux and colleagues[42] have developed an RIA test by coupling a *p*-aminophenylphosphorylcholine on agarose (PAPPC RIA). PAPPC contains a larger choline derivative (quaternary ammonium ion), including a secondary ammonium group, an aromatic ring, and a phosphate group. Both methods were found to have similar sensitivity and specificity. Recently, Fisher and Baldo[40] suggested the use of a morphine-based immunoassay for the detection of specific IgE to ammonium ions in the sera of sensitized subjects. More recently, Ebo and colleagues[43] investigated the diagnostic value of quantification of IgE by ImmunoCAP (Phadia AB, Uppsala, Sweden) in the diagnosis of rocuronium allergy. They also studied whether IgE inhibition tests can predict clinical cross-reactivity between NMBAs. They concluded that the rocuronium ImmunoCAP constitutes a reliable technique to diagnose rocuronium allergy, provided an assay-specific decision threshold is applied, because these assays reach a sensitivity of more than 85% and absolute specificity.

Specific IgE against thiopental, morphine, phenoperidine, and propofol have also been detected in serum of sensitized patients, using IgE-RIA.[44,45] The presence of hydrophobic IgE reacting nonspecifically with propofol has been reported.[46] With respect to latex, a radioallergosorbent test is available. Although considered less sensitive than the skin-prick test (SPT), 92.8% sensitivity has been reported.[47] In vitro assays to quantify specific IgEs for several penicillin determinants (Phadia penicilloyl G [c1], penicilloyl V [c2], amoxycilloyl [c6], ampicilloyl [c5], and cefaclor [c7]) are available but are generally considered less sensitive than skin tests.[48]

These factors have recently led to limiting the recommended indications for specific IgE assays to the diagnosis of anaphylaxis to NMBAs, thiopental, and latex.[24] These tests are usually performed several weeks after the reaction but can already be performed at the time of the reaction.[24,29,30]

Skin Testing

Skin tests coupled with history remain the mainstay of the diagnosis of an IgE-mediated reaction. Intradermal or SPTs are usually performed 4 to 6 weeks after a reaction. Up to 4 weeks following an allergic reaction, the intracellular stocks of histamine and other mediators are still lower than normal.[49] Skin tests to NMBAs may remain positive for years, whereas positivity to β-lactams declines with time. Ideally, testing should be performed by a professional experienced in performing and interpreting tests with anesthetic agents.[24]

SPTs and intradermal tests (IDTs) with dilutions of commercially available drug preparations are advised. Although highly reliable, skin tests are not infallible.[50] Standardized procedures and dilutions must be precisely defined for each agent tested to avoid false-positive results. Control tests using saline (negative control) and codeine (positive control) must accompany skin tests, to determine whether or not the skin is apt to release histamine and react to it. Skin tests are interpreted after 15 to 20 minutes. An SPT is considered positive when the diameter of the wheal is at least equal to half of that produced by the positive control test and at least 3 mm greater than the negative control. IDTs are considered positive when the diameter of the wheal is twice or more the diameter of the injection wheal.

A certain degree of controversy remains as to the maximal concentrations to be used when sensitization to NMBAs is investigated.[51,52] Detailed recommendations for skin and intradermal test dilutions of anesthetic drugs including NMBAs have been proposed by the Société Française d'Anesthésie et de Réanimation (SFAR; French Society of Anesthesia and Intensive Care Medicine) and the Société Française d'Allergologie (SFA; French Society of Allergology) (**Table 3**).[24] The accuracy of these recommended maximal concentrations has been further confirmed in a prospective

Table 3
Maximal concentrations normally nonreactive for SPT and IDT

Available Agents	Concentration (mg/mL)	SPT Dilution	SPT C_{max} (mg/mL)	IDT Dilution	IDT C_{max} (mg/mL)
NMBAs					
Atracurium	10	1/10	1	1/1000	10
Cisatracurium	2	Undiluted	2	1/100	20
Mivacurium	2	1/10	0.2	1/1000	2
Pancuronium	2	Undiluted	2	1/10	200
Rocuronium	10	Undiluted	10	1/200	50
Suxamethonium	50	1/5	10	1/500	100
Vecuronium	4	Undiluted	4	1/10	400
Hypnotics					
Etomidate	2	Undiluted	2	1/10	200
Midazolam	5	Undiluted	5	1/10	500
Propofol	10	Undiluted	10	1/10	1000
Thiopental	25	Undiluted	25	1/10	2500
Ketamine	100	1/10	10	1/100	1000
Opioids					
Alfentanil	0.5	Undiluted	0.5	1/10	50
Fentanyl	0.05	Undiluted	0.05	1/10	5
Morphine	10	1/10	1	1/1000	10
Remifentanil	0.05	Undiluted	0.05	1/10	5
Sufentanil	0.005	Undiluted	0.005	1/10	0.5
Local anesthetics					
Bupivacaine	2.5	Undiluted	2,5	1/10	250
Lidocaine	10	Undiluted	10	1/10	1000
Mepivacaine	10	Undiluted	10	1/10	1000
Ropivacaine	2	Undiluted	2	1/10	200
Antibiotics					
PPL		Undiluted	0.035	Undiluted	35
MDM (penicillin)		Undiluted	1	Undiluted	1000
Penicillin G		Undiluted	$20–25 \times 10^{3,a}$	Undiluted	$20–25 \times 10^{3,a}$
AX, AMP		Undiluted	20–25	Undiluted	$20–25 \times 10^3$
Other penicillins					
Cephalosporins		Undiluted	1–2	Undiluted	$1–2 \times 10^3$
Vancomycin	500			$1/5 \times 10^6$	0.1
Gentamycin	40	Undiluted		$1/10^2$	400
Miscellaneous					
Chlorhexidine	0.5	Undiluted	0.5	1/10	50
Patent blue	25	Undiluted	25	1/10	2500
Methylene blue	10	Undiluted	10	1/100	100

Abbreviation: C_{max}, maximal concentration.
[a] For penicillin G, concentrations are expressed in IU/ml (not mg/ml).

study conducted in 120 healthy volunteers tested with all available NMBAs at increasing concentrations on the anterior part of the forearm and on the back. Results were similar at both injection sites.[26] Because of the frequent but not systematic cross-reactivity observed with muscle relaxants, all available NMBAs should be tested.[14,24,31,53] This practice may help avoid future adverse reactions and provide documented advice for the future administration of anesthesia.[14,24] However, no diagnostic procedure is devoid of false-positive or -negative results. Although rare, some cases of renewed allergic reactions following exposure to an NMBA considered to be safe have been reported in the literature.[50,54] Therefore when administering an NMBA to a sensitized patient with a negative skin test, one should bear in mind the risk/ benefit ratio. In addition, any new muscle relaxant should be routinely tested in patients known to be allergic to NMBAs to detect possible cross-reactivity.[24]

The estimated sensitivity of skin tests for muscle relaxants is approximately 94% to 97%.[55] There has been some controversy concerning the advantages of prick versus intradermal testing. Studies comparing both techniques show little difference between them.[56,57] However, reliability of prick testing over time has not been assessed, and the reliability of prick tests alone in the individual patient has been questioned by some investigators.[58] Consequently, prick testing is advised for the diagnosis of the muscle relaxant responsible for an anaphylactic reaction, but intradermal testing should be preferred when investigating cross-reaction.

The diagnostic approach to β-lactam antibiotic-related allergic reactions has recently been standardized under the aegis of the European Network for Drug Allergy, the European Academy of Allergy and Clinical Immunology (EAACI) interest group on drug hypersensitivity.[59,60] Skin tests start with SPT, which are, if negative, followed by IDT. Skin testing should not be limited to the classic and commercial reagents benzyl-penicilloyl poly-L-lysine (PPL) and so-called minor determinants mixture (MDM), but should include amoxicillin (AX) and ampicillin (AMP), as well as the culprit compound(s). Maximum concentrations for SPT and IDT for PPL, MDM, AX, AMP and other penicillins, and for most cephalosporins are summarized in **Table 3**. The specificity of skin testing with β-lactams is between 97% and 99%, whereas the sensitivity is only around 50% to 70%. Therefore, oral provocation tests in patients with suggestive clinical history and negative skin test is recommended.

Skin test sensitivity for other substances varies. It is optimal for synthetic gelatins, but poor for barbiturates, opioids, and benzodiazepines.[14] Latex sensitization must be investigated by SPTs.[61] SPTs and IDTs have been proposed in the literature for the diagnosis of sensitization to blue dyes. However, false-negative SPTs have been occasionally reported. These reports strongly suggest favoring IDTs using up to a 1:100 dilution for the diagnosis of sensitization to blue dyes in patients with a history of a possible immediate hypersensitivity reaction to dyes.[62]

Mediator Release Tests

Basophil activation assays

Allergen-induced mediator release tests quantify mediators released during effector cell degranulation, mainly peripheral blood basophils, following stimulation with specific antigen. There are 2 categories of mediator release tests: histamine release tests and sulphidoleukotriene release tests (cellular allergen stimulation test [CAST]). Mata and colleagues[63] have evaluated the in vitro leukocyte histamine release (LHR) tests for the diagnosis of allergy to muscle relaxant drugs in 40 patients and a control group of 44 subjects with negative LHR. LHR tests were positive in 65% of the allergic patients, for a threshold corresponding to specificity at 100%. The concordance between LHR test and QAS-RIA was 64%.[63,64] Despite a good specificity, their diagnostic application remains limited because of the labor-intense experimental conditions and insufficient sensitivity. Therefore they are not used as routine diagnostic tests.[24] They could be useful when cross-reactivity among muscle relaxants is investigated with a view to future anesthesia in sensitized patients. Similarly, monitoring of serotonin,[65] eosinophil cationic protein,[66] or leukotriene C4 (LTC4)[67] release have also been published; however, these assays cannot be recommended for routine clinical use at the present time.

Flow cytometry

Flow-assisted allergy diagnosis relies on quantification of shifts in expression of basophilic activation markers after challenge with a specific allergen using specific antibodies conjugated with a fluorochrome or a dye. Activated basophils not only secrete quantifiable bioactive mediators but also upregulate the expression of different markers, which can be detected efficiently by flow cytometry using specific monoclonal antibodies.[28,68–71] Currently, the most commonly used antibody in allergy diagnosis is anti-CD63 and, to a lesser extent anti-CD203c. This technique has been clinically validated for several classic IgE-mediated allergies including indoor and outdoor inhalational allergies, primary and secondary food allergies, natural rubber latex allergy, hymenoptera venom allergy, and some drug allergies.[28] Although it does not allow differentiating between IgE-dependent and IgE-independent basophil activation, it is anticipated that it might constitute a unique tool in the diagnosis of IgE-independent hypersensitivity reactions as well as for the diagnosis of IgE-mediated anaphylaxis when a specific IgE assay is unavailable.[28,72] However, several methodological issues remain to be addressed. These issues include applying the test to whole blood or isolated basophils, the need for preactivation with interleukin 3 (IL-3), the choice of appropriate dose for different allergens, positive and negative controls, characterization and activation markers, and the appropriate diagnostic threshold for different allergens.[28] Nevertheless, once fully validated, the basophil activation test using flow cytometry will probably represent an interesting diagnostic tool for NMBA anaphylaxis and for cross-sensitization studies.

Challenge Tests

Indications for these tests are limited. They are restricted to local anesthetics, β-lactams, and latex.[73–75] They should be performed only if there is a negative skin test. Local anesthetics can be tested by subcutaneously injecting 0.5 to 2 mL of undiluted anesthetic solution (without epinephrine). The test is considered negative if no adverse reaction occurs within 30 minutes after injection.[76] Oral provocation tests are useful for the diagnosis of β-lactam hypersensitivity.[74,75]

Advice to Patients

Because the purpose of investigations is to identify the drug or substance responsible and the mechanism behind the reaction, to make subsequent anesthesia as safe as possible, a close collaboration between allergologist and anesthesiologist is highly desirable. In view of the constantly evolving anesthesiology practices, and of the complexity of allergy investigation, establishing specialized allergoanesthesia centers should be promoted. At the end of the allergic work-up, the patient should be warned against any substance that has tested positive, and a warning card or bracelet should be issued. A detailed letter containing information on the reaction, on the drugs given, on the results of follow-up investigations, and advice for future anesthetics should be issued to the patient, the referring anesthesiologist, and the patient's general practitioner.

CAUSAL AGENTS

The overall distribution of the various causal agents incriminated in allergic anaphylaxis during anesthesia is similar in most reported series. Every agent used during the perioperative period may be involved. NMBAs represent the most frequently incriminated substances ranging from 50% to 70%, followed by latex (12%–16.7%) and antibiotics (15%) (**Table 4**). Dyes, hypnotic agents, local anesthetics, opioids, colloids, aprotinin, protamine, chlorhexidine, or nonsteroidal antiinflammatory drugs (NSAIDs) are less frequently involved. Mechanisms and available diagnostic tools are summarized in **Table 5**.

NMBAs

Hypersensitivity reactions to NMBAs are mainly acute IgE-dependent allergic reactions. However, striking differences can be observed between countries. In France, the incidence of IgE-mediated hypersensitivity reactions to NMBAs in 1996 was estimated at 1 in 6500 anesthetics involving a muscle relaxant,[11] representing around 60% of all IgE-mediated reactions. It was estimated at 1 per 3000 to 1 per 110,000 exposures in Norway, representing 93.2% of IgE-mediated reactions.[13] However, IgE-mediated reactions involving NMBAs seem to be less frequent in Denmark and Sweden.[33,77,78] Allergic reactions to NMBAs have also been reported for smaller series in the United States.[79]

Differences regarding the relative risk of allergic reactions between NMBAs have been recognized in large epidemiologic surveys.[11,13–16,80] In most reports, suxamethonium seems to be more frequently involved.[13–16,19] In contrast, pancuronium and cisatracurium are the NMBAs associated with the lowest incidence of anaphylaxis during anesthesia.[14–17] Some controversy has arisen concerning a potential increased prevalence of allergic reactions to rocuronium. A trend toward increased frequency of allergic anaphylaxis to rocuronium was initially reported in Norway and France,[81,82] but not in Australia,[83] the United Kingdom,[84] and the United States.[79] Because of statistical limitations, analysis of epidemiologic data from Norway was unable to confirm whether or not rocuronium represented an increased risk.[13] At the same time, surveys conducted in France by the GERAP (Groupe d'Etudes des Réactions

Table 4
Substances responsible for IgE-mediated perioperative hypersensitivity reactions in France (results in percent from 7 consecutive surveys)

	1984–1989	1990–1991	1992–1994	1994–1996	1997–1998	1999–2000	2001–2002
	n = 821	n = 813	n = 1030	n = 734	n = 486	n = 518	n = 502
NMBAs	81	70.2	59.2	61.6	69.2	58.2	54
Latex	0.5	12.5	19	16.6	12.1	16.7	22.3
Hypnotics	11	5.6	8	5.1	3.7	3.4	0.8
Opioids	3	1.7	3.5	2.7	1.4	1.3	2.4
Colloids	0.5	4.6	5	3.1	2.7	4	2.8
Antibiotics	2	2.6	3.1	8.3	8	15.1	14.7
Other	2	2.8	2.2	2.6	2.9	1.3	3
Total	100%	100%	100%	100%	100%	100%	100%

Abbreviation: n = number of cases.
Data from Mertes PM, Laxenaire MC. [Anaphylactic and anaphylactoid reactions occurring during anesthesia in France. Seventh epidemiologic survey (January 2001–December 2002)]. Ann Fr Anesth Reanim 2004;23(12):1133–43.

Table 5
Usual mechanisms and diagnostic procedures for the most frequently involved substances in immediate hypersensitivity reactions during the perioperative period

		NMBAs	Latex	β-Lactam Antibiotics	Hypnotics	Opioids	Gelatines	LA	NSAIDs	Dyes
Mechanism		IgE	IgE	IgE	IgE	NSHR	IgE	Non-IgE	COX-1	IgE ?
History		S	S	S	S	S	S	S	S	S
In vitro tests[a]	Tryptase (and histamine)	S	S	S	S	S	S	S	S	S
	Specific IgE	Succinylcholine Rocuronium Morphine-based QAS PAPPC	S	S	NA	NR	S	NA	NR	NA
	BAT	S	S	S	NR	NR	S	NR	S	S
In vivo tests[b]	SPT	S	S	S	S	S	S	S	NR	S
	IDT	S	NR	S	S	S	S	S	NR	S
	Challenge test	NR	S	S	NR	NR	NR	S	S	NR

Abbreviations: LA, local anesthetic; NA, not available; NR, not relevant; NSHR, nonspecific histamine release; S, standard.
[a] Tryptase (and histamine) measurement during the acute event can be helpful in discriminating anaphylaxis from other types of reaction; tryptase determination should be repeated 2–4 days or later after the incidence to rule out a mastocytosis. In vitro tests have rarely been validated. Prudence is called on their interpretation. BAT is not considered a standard technique yet by all laboratories in all situations.
[b] Skin and challenge tests have to be performed according to existing guidelines.

Anaphylactoïdes Peranesthésiques), a network of 40 French allergoanesthesia outpatient clinics whose aim is to promote the survey of allergic and nonimmune-mediated reactions occurring during anesthesia, still seem to indicate a trend toward an increased risk when the respective market shares of the different NMBAs are taken into account.[15–17] This apparent increased incidence of anaphylaxis to rocuronium might be a result of biased reporting of adverse effects of new drugs,[85] statistical issues,[86] differences in the influence of environmental factors[87] or genotypic differences.[88] Further large epidemiologic studies are necessary to elucidate this problem.

Structure-activity studies designed to explore the molecular basis of specific IgE binding have established that quaternary and tertiary ammonium ions were the main component of the allergenic sites on the reactive drugs.[39] To explain the possible differences observed regarding the risk of allergic reactions with the different NMBAs, it has been suggested that the flexibility of the chain between the ammonium ions as well as the distance between the substituted ammonium ions might be of importance during the elicitation phase of IgE-mediated reactions.[89] Flexible molecules, such as succinylcholine, were considered more potent in stimulating sensitized cells than rigid molecules, such as pancuronium. This hypothesis would be contradicted if a higher risk of sensitization associated with rocuronium were to be confirmed. Similarly, in the past, alcuronium has been claimed to be a high risk for anaphylaxis. If an increased risk with rocuronium is further confirmed by epidemiologic surveys, propenyl ammonium groups present in rocuronium and alcuronium might be involved in this apparent increased allergenicity. These considerations represent an important issue in the design of an ideal NMBA with a reduced risk of allergic reactions.

Cross-sensitization among the different agents has been reported to be frequent, varying between 60% and 70% of patients allergic to NMBAs, but it is not constant.[11,16,17] The patterns of cross-reactivity vary considerably between patients. Cross-reactivity to all NMBAs is unusual, but seems to be more frequent with amino-steroid NMBAs than with benzylisoquinoline-derived NMBAs.[23]

Quaternary and tertiary ammonium ions are the main component of the allergenic sites on the reactive drugs.[39] However, the IgE recognition site of the molecule depends also on the molecular environment of the ammonium ion, a function of the hydrophobicity and distance with polar groups such as hydroxyls. This finding may explain the heterogeneity of the cross-reactivity among patients. Another possible hypothesis is that the antigenic determinant may extend to the adjacent part of the molecule. IgE antibodies could also be complementary to structures other than the ammonium group.[82]

Another intriguing aspect of allergic reactions to NMBAs concerns the dogma of previous exposure. In 15% to 50% of cases, these reactions are reported at the first known contact with an NMBA.[7,14,16,80] This finding suggests a possible cross-reaction with IgE antibodies generated by previous contact with apparently unrelated chemicals. This is a particularly attractive hypothesis in patients who react to small and ubiquitous epitopes such as a substituted ammonium group. These structures occur widely in many drugs but also in foods, cosmetics, disinfectants, and industrial materials. Hence, there seems to be ample opportunity for sensitive individuals to come into contact with and synthesize IgE antibodies to these unusual, and previously unsuspected, antigenic determinants. Recently, Florvaag and colleagues[77] hypothesized that the striking difference in the rate of allergic reactions to NMBAs, which is more than 6 times as common in Norway as in Sweden, could be caused by differences in preoperative sensitization. They reported a higher prevalence of IgE antibodies to quaternary and/or tertiary ammonium ion among blood donors and atopic patients from Norway when compared with Sweden. This study also pointed out that amongst the common quaternary ammonium ion-containing household chemicals and drugs present in the environment of both populations, the only difference was cough mixtures containing pholcodine, which were present in Norway but not in Sweden. The later report that pholcodine exposure in patients having experienced an allergic reaction to an NMBA[90] was responsible for a significant increase in specific IgEs to NMBAs led to the hypothesis that pholcodine exposure could lead to IgE-sensitization to pholcodine and other quaternary ammonium ions and thereby increase the risk of allergic reaction to NMBAs. This hypothesis is further supported by the results of an international prevalence study involving several countries across Europe and the United States, showing a statistically significant association between pholcodine consumption and prevalence of IgE-sensitization to pholcodine and succinylcholine in several countries.[91] However, the results also indicate that other, yet unknown, substances may be involved in IgE-sensitization toward NMBAs.

Nonallergic anaphylaxis may represent 20% to 50% of adverse reactions to NMBAs.[13,15–17,19] Although the precise mechanisms of these reactions remain difficult to establish, they usually result from direct nonspecific mast cell and basophil activation.[21] Reactions resulting from direct histamine release are usually less severe than IgE-mediated reactions,[16,17] with the exception of a subset of patients who have been considered as superresponders to the histamine-releasing effect of NMBAs. Histamine release is predominantly found with the use of the benzylisoquinolines d-tubocurarine, atracurium, and mivacurium, and the aminosteroid rapacuronium.[92] Recently, severe bronchospasm following administration of rapacuronium was reported in children. Increased airway resistance related to rapacuronium administration has been reported in children and adults. It has been suggested that the higher affinity of rapacuronium for M_2 versus M_3 muscarinic receptors could account for the high incidence of bronchospasm observed in clinical practice.[93] As a result of these adverse reactions, rapacuronium has been withdrawn from the market in the United States.

Latex

IgE-mediated latex allergy is a well-defined condition with recognized risk groups, established diagnostic tools, and adequate prevention strategies. It is the second most common cause of anaphylaxis during anesthesia in the general population.[17] The prevalence of latex sensitization varies depending on the population studied. As with all allergy-causing substances, it increases with increased exposure. Genetic factors may also be involved.[94] In children subjected to numerous operations, particularly those suffering from spina bifida, it is the primary cause of anaphylaxis.[95–97] Adults requiring multiple surgical procedures or health care workers are also at increased risk,[7] as well as patients allergic to several plant allergens (especially avocado, banana, kiwi, chestnut, *Ficus benjamina*) because of cross-allergy with latex (latex fruit syndrome).[98]

Primary prevention by providing a latex-free environment during surgery and anesthesia and on pediatric wards has been shown to significantly reduce the prevalence of latex sensitization.[99,100] In addition, a low incidence of allergic reactions caused by latex has been reported in countries where a strategy aimed to reduce latex exposure has been implemented.[13] Therefore, attempts to ban latex from use in clinical products should be encouraged.

In Europe, investigation of sensitization to latex is performed by SPTs using commercial extracts with an excellent sensitivity (75%–90%). If commercial latex extracts are not available, latex gloves extracts can be used, although their amount of latex proteins is not standardized. Sensitization can also be confirmed by quantification of specific IgEs. The use of latex recombinant proteins seems promising and may help to discriminate between sensitizations to anaphylaxis-related latex proteins (eg, Hev b1, 2, 5, 6, 13) or sensitization to less relevant proteins (eg, the profilin Hev b8).[101–103] Although these tests are reliable, in case of equivocal results some patients might need additional tests such as basophil activation or challenge tests (wearing latex gloves for 15 minutes) to establish diagnosis.

Antibiotics

Penicillins and cephalosporins elicit approximately 70% of perioperative anaphylactic reactions to antibiotics. They represent 12% to 15% of the perioperative reactions observed in France.[16,17] Cross-reactivity between penicillins and cephalosporins is attributed to the common β-lactam ring or the side chains attached to it. A recent meta-analysis suggested that patients allergic to penicillin or AX have a higher incidence of allergic reactions to first-generation cephalosporins and cefamandole but not to later-generation cephalosporins.[104,105] In Europe, the diagnostic approach for allergic reactions to β-lactam antibiotics has been standardized using algorithms combining skin tests, quantification of specific IgEs, and in selected cases drug provocation tests.[60]

Vancomycin, which is increasingly used for prophylaxis, has also been incriminated in some cases. However, in most cases, the adverse reactions observed are related to the chemically mediated basophil degranulation causing the red-man syndrome, which is associated with rapid vancomycin administration.[106] Allergic reactions with vancomycin remain rare. Sensitization can be confirmed using skin tests at a concentration less than 10 μg/mL.

Quinolones constitute the third most important group of antibiotics involved in perioperative anaphylaxis. The positive diagnosis of sensitization is hampered by the lack of validated skin test and specific IgE assays. Antibiotics such as bacitracin and rifamycin, applied locally to irrigate wounds, can also elicit potentially life-threatening anaphylaxis.

Hypnotics

Hypnotics commonly used in anesthesia are thiopental, propofol, midazolam, etomidate, ketamine, and inhaled anesthetics. Allergic reactions incriminating these drugs seem to be rare. The incidence of hypersensitivity reactions with thiopental was estimated to be 1:30,000.[107] It has been suggested that most of the generalized reactions were related to its ability to elicit direct LHR. However, there is evidence for IgE-mediated anaphylactic reactions based on skin tests and specific IgE assay.[108,109] Recently, thiopental was involved in less than 1% of allergic reactions in France,[17] probably as a result of its decreased use. Since Cremophor EL, used as a solvent for some nonbarbiturate hypnotics, has been avoided, many previously reported hypersensitivity reactions have disappeared. In the last French surveys, reactions to propofol accounted for less than 2.5% of allergic reactions. It has been suggested that propofol should be omitted in patients with allergy to eggs or soy, because of the presence of lecithins in the propofol vehicle,[110] but this has not been confirmed in daily practice.[24,48] Allergic reactions to midazolam, etomidate, or ketamine seem to be rare.[16,17] No immune-mediated immediate hypersensitivity reaction involving isoflurane, desflurane, or sevoflurane has been reported despite their wide use. Allergic reactions to hypnotics can be investigated using the concentration limits provided in **Table 3**.

Opioids

Life-threatening reactions to opioids are uncommon. Because of the capacity of morphine, codeine phosphate, or pethidine to induce direct nonspecific skin mast cell activation, but not heart or lung mast cell and basophil activation, these reactions are usually limited to pruritus, urticaria, and mild hypotension. They are frequently misinterpreted as drug allergy. Fentanyl and its derivatives do not induce nonspecific mediator release from mast cells. Only 12 cases were recorded in the last 2 years' epidemiologic survey in France, 9 of them being related to morphine administration.[17]

There is no evidence of cross-reactivity between the different opioid subclasses phenanthrenes (eg, morphine, codeine), phenylpiperedines (alfentanyl, fentanyl, remifentanyl, sufentanyl, and meperidine) and diphenylheptanes (methadone and propoxyphene) in the literature.[48] Cross-reactivity between morphine and codeine is frequent, whereas cross-reactivity between phenylpiperedines is uncommon. Morphine cross-reacts strongly with IgE antibodies from patients allergic to NMBAs via the tertiary methylamino group they both contain.[111] However, as narcotics are only monovalent compounds, they are not able to cross-link 2 IgE molecules on the surface of mastocytes and therefore are not able to elicit a clinical reaction. Recently, it has been suggested that exposure to pholcodine may have a role in events leading to allergic sensitization to NMBAs.[87]

The diagnosis of opiate allergy remains a clinical challenge. Skin tests may be helpful; however, because histamine may induce direct histamine release, the maximal concentration recommended for skin testing should not be exceeded (see **Table 3**). As discussed earlier, the clinical relevance of specific IgEs to morphine is questionable.

Local Anesthetics

Local anesthetics include amine (lidocaine, mepivacaine, prilocaine, bupivacaine, levobupivacaine, ropivacaine), and ester derivatives of benzoic acid (chloroprocaine, procaine, tetracaine). Allergic reactions to local anesthetics are rare despite their frequent use. It is estimated that less than 1% of all reactions to local anesthetics have an allergic mechanism.[15,76] Inadvertent intravascular injection leading to excessive blood concentrations of local anesthetics, systemic absorption of epinephrine added to the local anesthetic, or vasovagal near-syncope are by far the most common causes of adverse reactions associated with these drugs. Although severe anaphylactic reactions have been reported with both types of local anesthetics, ester local anesthetics, having the capability of producing metabolites related to para-aminobenzoic acid, are more likely to provoke an allergic reaction. Amide local anesthetics have been involved in less than 0.6% of the perioperative reactions.[17] Allergy to local anesthetics may also be caused by methylparaben, paraben, or metabisulfite used as a preservative in commercial preparations. Challenge tests following negative skin tests remain the gold standard to diagnose anaphylaxis from local anesthetics.[24] These tests should be applied liberally, not only to confirm the lack of sensitization following negative skin tests but also to reassure patients of the safe future administration of local anesthetics.

Colloids

All synthetic colloids used to restore intravascular volume have been shown to produce clinical anaphylaxis. The overall incidence of reactions has been estimated to range between 0.033%[112] and 0.22%.[113] Gelatins and dextrans are more frequently incriminated than albumin or hetastarch. Direct release of histamine has been reported with urea-linked gelatin, antihistamines being efficient for the prevention of these reactions.[114] Evidence for IgE-mediated adverse reactions to gelatin has also been reported.[113] In addition, adverse reactions to urea-linked gelatin (0.852%) seem to be more frequent than with modified fluid gelatin (0.338%),[113] whereas IgG-mediated adverse reactions to hydroxyethyl starch are less frequent. Adverse reactions to dextrans were estimated at 0.275%, to albumine 0.099%, and to hydroxyethyl starch solutions 0.058%.[113] Allergic reactions to dextrans are related to the presence of dextran-reactive antibodies of the IgG class. They can be prevented by hapten dextran (1 kDa) administration before starting the first administration of dextran. Although rare, several allergic reactions have been reported following application of this prevention protocol.[115–117]

Diagnosis of IgE-mediated gelatin allergy is generally established using skin tests. Specific IgE assays or basophil activation tests may also be used. Anaphylaxis to hydroxyethyl starch can be confirmed by skin tests. The clinical relevance of IgG, IgM, and IgA antibodies against hydroxyethyl starch remains unknown (159).[118] The diagnostic value of skin tests with dextrans is not established.

Dyes

Vital dyes have been used for many years in a variety of clinical situations and have long been considered a rare cause of anaphylaxis. This situation may in part be a result of misleading nomenclature.[119] Patent blue V (also called E131, acid blue 3, disulfine blue) and isosulfan blue (also called patent blue violet or lymphazurine), which belong to the group of triarylmethan dyes and share the same formula, are the most commonly used. A recent literature review that includes various names of these dyes reveals an impressive number of case reports of hypersensitivity reactions,[120] and it has been suggested that sensitization occurs using everyday products containing blue dyes. In view of the increasing use of blue dyes for lymphatic mapping for sentinel lymph node biopsy, the incidence of anaphylaxis to these drugs can be expected to increase. The mechanism underlying the allergic reaction to patent blue remains unclear. Direct mast cell and/or basophil activation and cross-linking of specific IgE antibodies are possible causative factors. Evidence supporting an IgE-mediated mechanism at least in some patients comes from 2 clinical reports: 1 showing an immune-mediated mechanism by a passive transfer test,[121] the second showing the presence of specific IgE detected by an enzyme-linked immunosorbent assay test.[122]

Methylene blue has also been shown to be an effective dye for sentinel lymph node localization, with only a limited number of complications reported. Anaphylactic reactions involving methylene blue seem to be rare, perhaps because this small molecule does not bind to plasma proteins, thus reducing the risk of sensitization to a hapten-protein complex. This dye differs structurally from isosulfan blue and patent blue V. Therefore, cross-reactivity was not expected. However, several reports of sensitization to patent blue and methylene blue have previously been reported.[62,123] These reports support the systematic investigation of a possible cross-reactivity before the use of an alternate dye.

The clinical diagnosis of reactions elicited by dyes is difficult. Reactions are usually delayed (ie, 30 minutes following injection), long lasting, and justify prolonged monitoring in intensive care if prolonged epinephrine administration is necessary.[62] Anaphylaxis can be confirmed by skin and basophil activation tests. Because several false-negative prick tests have been reported in the literature, the use of IDT in case of negative prick test is recommended.[62] Intradermal and basophil activation tests can also contribute to the identification of potential cross-reactive and safe alternative dyes.

ASPIRIN AND OTHER NSAIDS

With the increase in consumption of NSAIDs used in multimodal postoperative analgesia,[124] these are likely to be among the most common drugs inducing hypersensitivity reactions. Bronchospasms, urticaria, angioedema, and anaphylaxis from these drugs are most often of a nonimmunologic nature, and result from inhibition of the cyclooxygenase 1 (COX-1) isoenzyme with subsequent depletion of prostaglandin E_2 and unrestrained synthesis of cysteinyl leukotrienes, and release of mediators from mast cells and eosinophils (see the article by Mario Sánchez-Borges elsewhere in this issue for further exploration of this topic). Several potential genetic polymorphisms have been suggested to play a causative role in aspirin-induced asthma or urticaria.[125–127] Weak COX-1 inhibitors, such as paracetamol (acetaminophen), and partial inhibitors of COX-1 and COX-2, such as nimesulide and meloxicam, elicit symptoms more rarely and only at high drug doses. Selective COX-2 inhibitors rarely precipitate immediate hypersensitivity reactions and are generally (but not always) well tolerated.[128,129] Nevertheless, NSAIDs, in particular diclofenac and pyrazolone derivatives, can induce an IgE-mediated hypersensitivity reaction as well. Thus, a history of cross-reactivities between multiple NSAIDs implies a non-IgE-mediated process, whereas a history of monosensitivity to 1 NSAID implies an IgE-mediated process, although specific antibodies are often elusive.[130]

There are no reliable cutaneous tests allowing identification of NSAID hypersensitivity in patients with multiple NSAID intolerance. It has been assumed that there were no reliable in vitro tests for this condition and diagnostic confirmation can be ascertained only by provocation challenge. Several recent studies using a leukotriene release test (CAST) or a basophil activation test (BAT) on blood basophils, or a combination of both tests, yields some positive results (70%–75%) in a sizeable number of clinically validated cases, with high specificity (more than 85%).[131,132] These studies need to be confirmed. A challenge test is still considered by many investigators the gold standard for establishing or excluding a diagnosis of NSAID hypersensitivity and identifying safe alternatives.[48,133] In specific cases, drug desensitization can also be performed.[134]

Aprotinin

Aprotinin, a naturally occurring serine protease inhibitor, may be administered either by the intravenous route or as a component of biologic sealants. Its widespread clinical use is based on its ability to decrease blood loss, and, as a consequence, transfusion requirements. Anaphylactic reactions are mediated by IgG and IgE antibodies. The risk of anaphylactic reactions has been estimated between 0.5% and 5.8% when used intravenously during cardiac surgery, and at 5 in 100,000 applications when used as a biologic sealant.[135,136] Patients previously treated with this drug present an increased risk and any new administration should be avoided for at least 6 months following an initial exposure.[137] Aprotinin used to reduce blood loss has recently been withdrawn from the market. The diagnosis is confirmed by prick tests (pure solution) followed by IDTs (up to 1:10 dilution) in case of negativity.

Other Agents

Several cases of allergic reactions to antiseptics have been reported in the literature. They mainly entail allergic reactions to chlorhexidine following insertion of central catheters impregnated with this antiseptic, after intraurethral use or topical application.[138] Only rare cases of anaphylaxis following topical use of povidone-iodine have been reported.[17]

Protamine has also been incriminated. Its use to reverse heparin anticoagulation has increased over the last 2 decades. Reactions may involve several mechanisms, including IgE, IgG, and complement activation. In a recent systematic literature review analyzing 9 retrospective studies and 16 prospective studies, the incidence of anaphylactic reactions was estimated at 0.19% (retrospective studies) and 0.69% (prospective studies), respectively.[139]

Many clinical cases involving many other substances have been published in the literature. This situation underlines the importance of a careful and systematic investigation of all substances used during the procedure in case of perioperative anaphylaxis.

RISK FACTORS FOR PERIOPERATIVE ANAPHYLAXIS

Allergy to anesthetic agents is the first factor to consider. Any unexplained life-threatening reaction during a previous anesthesia might be an allergic reaction and is a major risk factor for a renewed reaction if the responsible drug is readministered.[16] Ideally, all patients having experienced an episode of perioperative anaphylaxis would have undergone complete allergoanesthetic follow-up before further anesthetics. The practical reality is different. In addition, in many countries, the allergologic assessment is not routinely performed.

Sometimes patients require anesthesia for emergency surgery, at times when little or no information about a previous reaction is available. In this case, regional anesthesia is preferred whenever possible, and a latex-free environment should be provided.[24,25] If general anesthesia is necessary, volatile anesthetics should be used if possible, as allergy to these has never been described. If a reaction to an NMBA is suspected, it is important to try to avoid other NMBAs, because cross-reactions are not uncommon within this group.[24,25] If the anesthetic chart from the reaction is available, all drugs and substances administered to the patient before the reaction should be avoided if possible.

A latex-free environment should be made available to patients having experienced clinical manifestations of allergy when exposed to latex, to patients subjected to many surgical or urologic cannulation procedures (because of the high incidence of sensitization to latex), to children who have undergone repeated operations (particularly those with spina bifida), and to patients with clinical manifestations of allergy to tropical fruits (eg, avocado, kiwi, banana, fig, chestnut, sweet pepper, melon, pineapple, papaya) because of a high rate of cross-reactivity with latex.

In contrast, patients who are atopic (except for latex) or those who are allergic to a drug (except for antibiotics that may be injected as perioperative antibiotic prophylaxis because of the risk of cross-reactivity between β-lactams) unlikely to be used during the perioperative period are not considered to be at risk for perioperative anaphylaxis.[24]

TREATMENT

There is a wide array of reaction severity and responsiveness to treatment. In addition, no controlled trials of treatment in human beings are available. As a result, the ultimate judgment with regards to a particular clinical procedure or treatment scheme must be made by the clinician in light of the clinical presentation and available diagnostic and treatment options.[140] During anesthesia, the patient is usually monitored and has intravenous access, which gives the optimum conditions for prompt and successful treatment, provided that the diagnosis is made early by the attending anesthetist. Treatment is aimed at interrupting contact with the responsible antigen, modulating the effects of the released mediators and inhibiting mediator production and release. Because the identification of the exact offending agent at the time of reaction is virtually impossible, all drugs as well as surgery should be interrupted unless otherwise impossible. Maintenance of airway patency is imperative and oxygen 100% should be administered. The cornerstones of treatment are epinephrine and fluid therapy (**Table 6**).[4,24,25,141–143]

Epinephrine is a highly potent and efficient treatment agent in most cases of anaphylaxis. It opposes the deleterious systemic adverse effects of the released mediators, through its vasoconstricting (α-mediated), positive inotropic (β1-mediated), bronchodilatating (β2-mediated) properties, and by reducing mast-cell and basophil mediator release.[144] There is no absolute contraindication during anaphylaxis for the use of epinephrine. It should be administered as early as possible and titrated carefully to clinical response. Poor outcomes during anaphylaxis, including deaths, are associated with either late or no administration of epinephrine, as well as with inadequate or excessive dosing.[24,145]

Epinephrine administration should be tailored to the severity of symptoms (see **Table 5**). It should not be injected during grade I reactions. Administration should be rapid and goal-oriented, using titrated boluses starting at an initial dose of 10 to 20 μg in grade II reactions, and 100 to 200 μg in case of grade III reactions, repeated every 1 to 2 minutes as necessary. Prolonged inotropic support may also be required in some patients (starting dose: 0.05 to 0.1 μg/kg/min, titrated to effect). Grade IV reactions (cardiac arrest) require cardiopulmonary resuscitation and high doses of epinephrine (1 mg every 2 minutes, repeated and/or increased as needed). Epinephrine doses should be goal oriented and adapted to body weight and age in children (see **Table 6**).

In some cases, epinephrine may fail to restore cardiovascular homeostasis. In cases resistant to epinephrine, the use of vasoactive drugs such as noradrenaline, metaraminol, glucagon, vasopressin, vasopressin analogs, or even methylene blue has been advocated. Previous treatment with β-blockers is a potential risk factor explaining an absence of tachycardia, as well as resistance of arterial hypotension to epinephrine.[53] Glucagon (initial dose 1–5 mg, followed by 1–2.5 mg/h infusion) is recommended in this clinical setting. Several case reports suggest that arginine vasopressin (AVP) might be considered as a potential rescue therapy during anaphylaxis. [146–152] Experimental work provides support for the possible use of AVP during anaphylaxis.[153,154] However, AVP was detrimental when injected alone in the early course of anaphylaxis or when higher doses were used. Methylene blue, which interferes with nitric oxide-mediated vascular smooth muscle relaxation, was also recently successfully used in catecholamine- and vasopressin-resistant anaphylaxis.[155] More clinical information is needed to better evaluate the value of these rescue therapies.

Fluid therapy is important to counteract the large fluid shifts associated with vasodilatation and capillary leakage. Similar to epinephrine administration, fluid therapy should be goal oriented. A commonly used sequence is to rapidly restore the vascular volume either with isotonic saline (10–25 mL/kg for 20 minutes repeated if necessary), or with colloid (10 mL/kg). Colloids should replace saline when the volume of this exceeds 30 mL/kg, avoiding the administration of the substance or substances that are suspected to be the cause of the reaction.

Bronchospasm is usually reversible with epinephrine. However, in case of persistent bronchospasm, inhaled β_2-agonists (salbutamol or albuterol) are indicated. Intravenous administration (5–25 μg/min) should be considered if necessary.

Corticosteroids and antihistamines are often recommended as secondary treatment of anaphylaxis. They could be useful for angioedema, and cutaneous symptoms. Relapse of the anaphylactic reaction can occur up to 24 hours after the initial reaction, therefore careful consideration must be given to the level of monitoring/observation of the patient following successful treatment of an anaphylactic reaction.

Table 6
Emergency management of anaphylactic reactions during anesthesia

Primary treatment

General measures

Inform the surgeon

Request immediate assistance

Cease all drugs, colloids, blood products
(and latex if suspected)

Maintain airway with 100% oxygen

Elevate the legs, if practical

Epinephrine	**Adults**
Titrate dose according to symptoms severity and clinical response	Grade 2: 10–20 µg Grade 3: 100–200 µg Grade 4: 1 mg IV infusion starting dose: 0.05–0.1 µg/kg/min
Repeat dose every 1 to 2 min as necessary	
If large doses are needed, use IV infusion	**Children**
	Grade 2 to 3: 1–5 µg/kg Grade 4: 10 µg/kg

Fluid therapy	
NaCl 9 mg/L or colloids according to clinical response	**Crystalloid** : 10–25 mL/kg for 20 min, more may be needed **Colloid**: 10 mL/kg for 20 min, more may be needed

Anaphylaxis resistant to epinephrine	
Glucagon (failure of large doses of epinephrine in patients on β-blockers)	Initial dose 1–5 mg, followed by 1–2.5 mg/h infusion
Norepinephrine	Initial dose 0.05–0.1 mg/kg/min
Vasopressin	Increments of 2–10 IU IV until response

Secondary treatment

Bronchospasm

β₂-agonist may be used for symptomatic treatment of bronchospasm, but is not first-line treatment. IV administration may be considered if necessary, following hemodynamic recovery	Inhaled β$_2$-agonists (salbutamol or albuterol) IV: 5–25 µg/min
Antihistamines	H$_1$ antagonist: diphenhydramine 0.5–1 mg/kg IV) H$_2$ antagonist: ranitidine 50 mg IV
Corticosteroids	**Adults**: Hydrocortisone 250 mg IV or methylprednisolone 80 mg IV **Children**: Hydrocortisone 50–100 mg IV or methylprednisolone 2 mg/kg IV

Further care

Patient may relapse, admit to intensive care
unit in grade 3 or 4 reactions

Take bloods for testing as soon as possible

Arrange for allergy testing at 1 month

Abbreviation: IV, intravenous.

SUMMARY

Perioperative anaphylaxis is a significant adverse event during anesthesia. It remains underestimated because it is underreported. NMBAs, latex, and antibiotics are the most frequently incriminated drugs, although other drugs used during the perioperative period might be involved. Because no premedication can effectively prevent an allergic reaction, any suspected hypersensitivity reaction must be extensively investigated using combined peri- and postoperative testing. Patients must be fully informed of the results of investigations, and advised to provide a detailed report before future anesthesia. Wearing a warning bracelet or possession of a warning card is strongly indicated.

With the exception of high-risk patients, systematic preoperative screening for sensitization against anesthetic drugs is not justified at this time. Particular attention must be paid to patients who have already experienced an anaphylactic reaction during anesthesia, those alleging an allergy to muscle relaxants, or those at risk of latex sensitization. In these cases, the choice of the safest possible anesthetic agents should be based on the result of a rigorously performed allergologic assessment.

In view of the relative complexity of allergy investigation, allergoanesthesia centers should be promoted to provide all necessary expert support coupled with an active policy to identify patients at risk.

REFERENCES

1. Ishizawa Y. Mechanisms of anesthetic actions and the brain. J Anesth 2007; 21(2):187–99.
2. Johansson SG, Bieber T, Dahl R, et al. Revised nomenclature for allergy for global use: report of the Nomenclature Review Committee of the World Allergy Organization, October 2003. J Allergy Clin Immunol 2004;113(5):832–6.
3. Johansson SG, Hourihane JO, Bousquet J, et al. A revised nomenclature for allergy. An EAACI position statement from the EAACI nomenclature task force. Allergy 2001;56(9):813–24.
4. Sampson HA, Munoz-Furlong A, Campbell RL, et al. Second symposium on the definition and management of anaphylaxis: summary report–Second National Institute of Allergy and Infectious Disease/Food Allergy and Anaphylaxis Network symposium. J Allergy Clin Immunol 2006;117(2):391–7.
5. Fisher MM, More DG. The epidemiology and clinical features of anaphylactic reactions in anaesthesia. Anaesth Intensive Care 1981;9(3):226–34.
6. Laxenaire MC. Quelle est la réalité du risqué allergique en anesthésie. Incidence. Morbidité-Mortalité. Substances responsable. Tableaux cliniques [What is the real risk of drug hypersensitivity in anesthesia? Incidence. Clinical aspects. Morbidity-mortality. Substances responsible]. Ann Fr Anesth Reanim 2002;21(Suppl 1):38s–54s [in French].
7. Mertes PM, Laxenaire MC. Allergic reactions occurring during anaesthesia. Eur J Anaesthesiol 2002;19:240–62.
8. Watkins J. Adverse anaesthetic reactions. An update from a proposed national reporting and advisory service. Anaesthesia 1985;40(8):797–800.
9. Thienthong S, Hintong T, Pulnitiporn A. The Thai Anesthesia Incidents Study (THAI Study) of perioperative allergic reactions. J Med Assoc Thai 2005; 88(Suppl 7):S128–33.
10. Whittington T, Fisher MM. Anaphylactic and anaphylactoid reactions. Clin Anaesthesiol B Clin Anaesthesiol 1998;12:301–23.

11. Laxenaire MC. Epidémiologie des réactions anaphylactoïdes peranesthésiques. Quatrième enquête multicentrique (juillet 1994–décembre 1996). Ann Fr Anesth Reanim 1999;18:796–809.

12. Escolano F, Valero A, Huguet J, et al. Estudio epidemiológico prospectivo de perioperatorio reacciones anafilácticas se producen en Cataluña (1996–7) [Prospective epidemiologic study of perioperative anaphylactoid reactions occurring in Catalonia (1996–7)]. Rev Esp Anestesiol Reanim 2002;49(6): 286–93 [in Spanish].

13. Harboe T, Guttormsen AB, Irgens A, et al. Anaphylaxis during anesthesia in Norway: a 6-year single-center follow-up study. Anesthesiology 2005;102(5):897–903.

14. Fisher M, Baldo BA. Anaphylaxis during anaesthesia: current aspects of diagnosis and prevention. Eur J Anaesthesiol 1994;11(4):263–84.

15. Laxenaire M, Mertes PM, GERAP. Anaphylaxis during anaesthesia. Results of a 2 year survey in France. Br J Anaesth 2001;21(1):549–58.

16. Mertes PM, Laxenaire MC, Alla F. Anaphylactic and anaphylactoid reactions occurring during anesthesia in France in 1999–2000. Anesthesiology 2003; 99(3):536–45.

17. Mertes PM, Laxenaire MC. Les réactions anaphylactiques et anaphylactoides peranesthésiques en France. Septiéme enquête épidémiologique (Janvier 2001–Décembre 2002) [Anaphylactic and anaphylactoid reactions occurring during anaesthesia in France. Seventh epidemiologic survey (January 2001–December 2002)]. Ann Fr Anesth Reanim 2004;23(12):1133–43 [in French].

18. Mitsuhata H, Matsumoto S, Hasegawa J. The epidemiology and clinical features of anaphylactic and anaphylactoid reactions in the perioperative period in Japan. Masui 1992;41:1664–9.

19. Light KP, Lovell AT, Butt H, et al. Adverse effects of neuromuscular blocking agents based on yellow card reporting in the U.K.: are there differences between males and females? Pharmacoepidemiol Drug Saf 2006;15(3):151–60.

20. Hedin H, Richter W. Pathomechanisms of dextran-induced anaphylactoid/anaphylactic reactions in man. Int Arch Allergy Appl Immunol 1982;68(2):122–6.

21. Moss J. Muscle relaxants and histamine release. Acta Anaesthesiol Scand Suppl 1995;106:7–12.

22. Jooste EH, Sharma A, Zhang Y, et al. Rapacuronium augments acetylcholine-induced bronchoconstriction via positive allosteric interactions at the M3 muscarinic receptor. Anesthesiology 2005;103(6):1195–203.

23. Mertes PM, Aimone-Gastin I, Gueant-Rodriguez RM, et al. Hypersensitivity reactions to neuromuscular blocking agents. Curr Pharm Des 2008;14(27):2809–25.

24. Mertes PM, Laxenaire MC, Lienhart A, et al. Reducing the risk of anaphylaxis during anaesthesia: guidelines for clinical practice. J Investig Allergol Clin Immunol 2005;15(2):91–101.

25. Kroigaard M, Garvey LH, Gillberg L, et al. Scandinavian Clinical Practice Guidelines on the diagnosis, management and follow-up of anaphylaxis during anaesthesia. Acta Anaesthesiol Scand 2007;51(6):655–70.

26. Mertes PM, Moneret-Vautrin DA, Leynadier F, et al. Skin reactions to intradermal neuromuscular blocking agent injections: a randomized multicenter trial in healthy volunteers. Anesthesiology 2007;107(2):245–52.

27. Fisher MM. The preoperative detection of risk of anaphylaxis during anaesthesia. Anaesth Intensive Care 2007;35(6):899–902.

28. Ebo DG, Bridts CH, Hagendorens MM, et al. Basophil activation test by flow cytometry: present and future applications in allergology. Cytometry B Clin Cytom 2008;74(4):201–10.

29. Laroche D, Lefrancois C, Gerard JL, et al. Early diagnosis of anaphylactic reactions to neuromuscular blocking drugs. Br J Anaesth 1992;69(6):611–4.

30. Guttormsen AB, Johansson SG, Oman H, et al. No consumption of IgE antibody in serum during allergic drug anaphylaxis. Allergy 2007;62(11):1326–30.

31. Mertes PM, Laxenaire MC. Allergy and anaphylaxis in anaesthesia. Minerva Anestesiol 2004;70(5):285–91.

32. Baumann A, Studnicska D, Audibert G, et al. Refractory anaphylactic cardiac arrest after succinylcholine administration. Anesth Analg 2009;109(1):137–40.

33. Kroigaard M, Garvey LH, Menne T, et al. Allergic reactions in anaesthesia: are suspected causes confirmed on subsequent testing? Br J Anaesth 2005; 95(4):468–71.

34. Laxenaire MC, Mouton C, Frederic A, et al. Anaphylactic shock after tourniquet removal in orthopedic surgery. Ann Fr Anesth Reanim 1996;15(2):179–84.

35. Laroche D, Dubois F, Gérard J, et al. Radioimmunoassy for plasma histamine: a study of false positive and false negative values. Br J Anaesth 1995;74:430–7.

36. Fisher MM, Baldo BA. Mast cell tryptase in anaesthetic anaphylactoid reactions. Br J Anaesth 1998;80(1):26–9.

37. Malinovsky JM, Decagny S, Wessel F, et al. Systematic follow-up increases incidence of anaphylaxis during adverse reactions in anesthetized patients. Acta Anaesthesiol Scand 2008;52(2):175–81.

38. Baldo BA, Fisher MM. Anaphylaxis to muscle relaxant drugs: cross-reactivity and molecular basis of binding of IgE antibodies detected by radioimmunoassay. Mol Immunol 1983;20(12):1393–400.

39. Baldo BA, Fisher MM. Substituted ammonium ions as allergenic determinants in drug allergy. Nature 1983;306(5940):262–4.

40. Fisher MM, Baldo BA. Immunoassays in the diagnosis of anaphylaxis to neuromuscular blocking drugs: the value of morphine for the detection of IgE antibodies in allergic subjects. Anaesth Intensive Care 2000;28:167–70.

41. Gueant JL, Mata E, Monin B, et al. Evaluation of a new reactive solid phase for radioimmunoassay of serum specific IgE against muscle relaxant drugs. Allergy 1991;46(6):452–8.

42. Guilloux L, Ricard-Blum S, Ville G, et al. A new radioimmunoassay using a commercially available solid support for the detection of IgE antibodies against muscle relaxants. J Allergy Clin Immunol 1992;90(2):153–9.

43. Ebo DG, Venemalm L, Bridts CH, et al. Immunoglobulin E antibodies to rocuronium: a new diagnostic tool. Anesthesiology 2007;107(2):253–9.

44. Baldo BA, Fisher MM, Harle DG. Allergy to thiopentone. Clin Rev Allergy 1991; 9(3–4):295–308.

45. Fisher MM, Harle DG, Baldo BA. Anaphylactoid reactions to narcotic analgesics. Clin Rev Allergy 1991;9(3–4):309–18.

46. Gueant JL, Mata E, Masson C, et al. Non-specific cross-reactivity of hydrophobic serum IgE to hydrophobic drugs. Mol Immunol 1995;32(4):259–66.

47. Hemery ML, Arnoux B, Rongier M, et al. Correlation between former and new assays of latex IgE-specific determination using the K82 and K82 recombinant allergens from the Pharmacia Diagnostics laboratory. Allergy 2005;60(1): 131–2.

48. Ebo DG, Fisher MM, Hagendorens MM, et al. Anaphylaxis during anaesthesia: diagnostic approach. Allergy 2007;62(5):471–87.

49. Soetens FM. Anaphylaxis during anaesthesia: diagnosis and treatment. Acta Anaesthesiol Belg 2004;55(3):229–37.

50. Fisher MM, Merefield D, Baldo B. Failure to prevent an anaphylactic reaction to a second neuromuscular blocking drug during anaesthesia. Br J Anaesth 1999; 82(5):770–3.

51. Levy JH, Gottge M, Szlam F, et al. Weal and flare responses to intradermal rocuronium and cisatracurium in humans. Br J Anaesth 2000;85:844–9.

52. Berg CM, Heier T, Wilhelmsen V, et al. Rocuronium and cisatracurium-positive skin tests in non-allergic volunteers: determination of drug concentration thresholds using a dilution titration technique. Acta Anaesthesiol Scand 2003;47(5): 576–82.

53. Mertes PM, Laxenaire M. Anaphylaxis during general anaesthesia. Prevention and management. CNS Drugs 2000;14(2):115–33.

54. Thacker MA, Davis FM. Subsequent general anaesthesia in patients with a history of previous anaphylactoid/anaphylactic reaction to muscle relaxant. Anaesth Intensive Care 1999;27(2):190–3.

55. Laxenaire MC, Moneret-Vautrin DA. Allergy and anaesthesia. Curr Opin Anaesthesiol 1992;5:436–41.

56. Leynadier F, Sansarricq M, Didier JM, et al. Prick tests in the diagnosis of anaphylaxis to general anaesthetics. Br J Anaesth 1987;59(6):683–9.

57. Fisher MM, Bowey CJ. Intradermal compared with prick testing in the diagnosis of anaesthetic allergy. Br J Anaesth 1997;79(1):59–63.

58. McKinnon RP. Allergic reactions during anaesthesia. Curr Opin Anaesthesiol 1996;9:267–70.

59. Blanca M, Romano A, Torres MJ, et al. Update on the evaluation of hypersensitivity reactions to betalactams. Allergy 2009;64(2):183–93.

60. Torres MJ, Blanca M, Fernandez J, et al. Diagnosis of immediate allergic reactions to beta-lactam antibiotics. Allergy 2003;58(10):961–72.

61. Turjanmaa K, Palosuo T, Alenius H, et al. Latex allergy diagnosis: in vivo and in vitro standardization of a natural rubber latex extract. Allergy 1997;52(1): 41–50.

62. Mertes PM, Malinovsky JM, Mouton-Faivre C, et al. Anaphylaxis to dyes during the perioperative period: reports of 14 clinical cases. J Allergy Clin Immunol 2008;122(2):348–52.

63. Mata E, Gueant JL, Moneret-Vautrin DA, et al. Clinical evaluation of in vitro leukocyte histamine release in allergy to muscle relaxant drugs. Allergy 1992;47(5):471–6.

64. Gueant JL, Masson C, Laxenaire MC. Biological tests for diagnosing the IgE-mediate allergy to anaesthetic drugs. In: Assem K, editor. Monographs in allergy. Basel: Karger; 1992. p. 94–107.

65. Bermejo N, Guéant J, Mata E, et al. Platelet serotonin is a mediator potentially involved in anaphylactic reaction to neuromuscular blocking drugs. Br J Anaesth 1993;70(3):322–5.

66. Assem E. Release of eosinophil cationic protein (ECP) in anaphylactoid anaesthetic reactions in vivo and in vitro. Agents Actions 1994;41:C11–3.

67. Assem E. Leukotriene C4 release from blood cells in vitro in patients with anaphylactoid reactions to neuromuscular blockers. Agents Actions 1993;38: C242–4.

68. Abuaf N, Rajoely B, Ghazouani E, et al. Validation of a flow cytometric assay detecting in vitro basophil activation for the diagnosis of muscle relaxant allergy. J Allergy Clin Immunol 1999;104(2 Pt 1):411–8.

69. Sabbah A, Drouet M, Sainte-Laudry J, et al. Apport diagnostique de la cytométrie en flux en allergologie [Contribution of flow cytometry to allergologic diagnosis]. Allerg Immunol (Paris) 1997;29(1):15–21 [in French].

70. Sainte-Laudy J, Vallon C, Guerin JC. Analysis of membrane expression of the CD63 human basophil activation marker. Applications to allergologic diagnosis. Allerg Immunol (Paris) 1994;26(6):211–4.

71. Monneret G, Benoit Y, Gutowski M, et al. Detection of basophil activation by flow cytométrie in patients with allergy to muscle-relaxant drugs. Anesthesiology 2000;92(1):275–7.

72. De Weck AL, Sanz ML, Gamboa PM, et al. Diagnostic tests based on human basophils: more potentials and perspectives than pitfalls. II. Technical issues. J Investig Allergol Clin Immunol 2008;18(3):143–55.

73. Prévention du risque allergique peranesthésique. Recommandations pour la pratique clinique. 2001. Available at: http://wwwsfar.org. Accessed April 15, 2001.

74. Bousquet PJ, Pipet A, Bousquet-Rouanet L, et al. Oral challenges are needed in the diagnosis of beta-lactam hypersensitivity. Clin Exp Allergy 2008;38(1):185–90.

75. Demoly P, Romano A, Botelho C, et al. Determining the negative predictive value of provocation tests with beta-lactams. Allergy 2009;65(3):327–32.

76. Fisher MM, Bowey CJ. Alleged allergy to local anaesthetics. Anaesth Intensive Care 1997;25(6):611–4.

77. Florvaag E, Johansson SG, Oman H, et al. Prevalence of IgE antibodies to morphine. Relation to the high and low incidences of NMBA anaphylaxis in Norway and Sweden, respectively. Acta Anaesthesiol Scand 2005;49(4):437–44.

78. Garvey LH, Roed-Petersen J, Menne T, et al. Danish Anaesthesia Allergy Centre – preliminary results. Acta Anaesthesiol Scand 2001;45(10):1204–9.

79. Bhananker SM, O'Donnell JT, Salemi JR, et al. The risk of anaphylactic reactions to rocuronium in the United States is comparable to that of vecuronium: an analysis of food and drug administration reporting of adverse events. Anesth Analg 2005;101(3):819–22.

80. Galletly DC, Treuren BC. Anaphylactoid reactions during anaesthesia. Seven years' experience of intradermal testing. Anaesthesia 1985;40(4):329–33.

81. Heier T, Guttormsen AB. Anaphylactic reactions during induction of anaesthesia using rocuronium for muscle relaxation: a report including 3 cases. Acta Anaesthesiol Scand 2000;44(7):775–81.

82. Laxenaire MC, Gastin I, Moneret-Vautrin DA, et al. Cross-reactivity of rocuronium with other neuromuscular blocking agents. Eur J Anaesthesiol Suppl 1995;11:55–64.

83. Rose M, Fisher M. Rocuronium: high risk for anaphylaxis? Br J Anaesth 2001;86(5):678–82.

84. Watkins J. Incidence of UK reactions involving rocuronium may simply reflect market use. Br J Anaesth 2001;87(3):522.

85. Mertes PM, Guttormsen AB, Harboe T, et al. Can spontaneous adverse event reporting systems really be used to compare rates of adverse events between drugs? Anesth Analg 2007;104(2):471–2.

86. Laake JH, Rottingen JA. Rocuronium and anaphylaxis–a statistical challenge. Acta Anaesthesiol Scand 2001;45(10):1196–203.

87. Florvaag E, Johansson SG. The pholcodine story. Immunol Allergy Clin North Am 2009;29(3):419–27.

88. Gueant JL, Gueant-Rodriguez RM, Cornejo-Garcia JA, et al. Gene variants of IL13, IL4, and IL4RA are predictors of beta-lactam allergy. J Allergy Clin Immunol 2009;123(2):509–10.

89. Birnbaum J, Vervloet D. Allergy to muscle relaxants. Clin Rev Allergy 1991;9(3–4):281–93.

90. Harboe T, Johansson SG, Florvaag E, et al. Pholcodine exposure raises serum IgE in patients with previous anaphylaxis to neuromuscular blocking agents. Allergy 2007;62(12):1445–50.

91. Johansson SG, Florvaag E, Oman H, et al. National pholcodine consumption and prevalence of IgE-sensitization: a multicentre study. Allergy 2009;65(4): 498–502.

92. Doenicke AW, Czeslick E, Moss J, et al. Onset time, endotracheal intubating conditions, and plasma histamine after cisatracurium and vecuronium administration. Anesth Analg 1998;87(2):434–8.

93. Jooste E, Klafter F, Hirshman CA, et al. A mechanism for rapacuronium-induced bronchospasm: M2 muscarinic receptor antagonism. Anesthesiology 2003; 98(4):906–11.

94. Brown RH, Hamilton RG, Mintz M, et al. Genetic predisposition to latex allergy: role of interleukin 13 and interleukin 18. Anesthesiology 2005;102(3):496–502.

95. Karila C, Brunet-Langot D, Labbez F, et al. Anaphylaxis during anesthesia: results of a 12-year survey at a French pediatric center. Allergy 2005;60(6): 828–34.

96. Niggemann B, Breiteneder H. Latex allergy in children. Int Arch Allergy Immunol 2000;121(2):98–107.

97. Hourihane JO, Allard JM, Wade AM, et al. Impact of repeated surgical procedures on the incidence and prevalence of latex allergy: a prospective study of 1263 children. J Pediatr 2002;140(4):479–82.

98. Rolland JM, O'Hehir RE. Latex allergy: a model for therapy. Clin Exp Allergy 2008;38(6):898–912.

99. Cremer R, Kleine-Diepenbruck U, Hering F, et al. Reduction of latex sensitisation in spina bifida patients by a primary prophylaxis programme (five years experience). Eur J Pediatr Surg 2002;12(Suppl 1):S19–21.

100. Cremer R, Lorbacher M, Hering F, et al. Natural rubber latex sensitisation and allergy in patients with spina bifida, urogenital disorders and oesophageal atresia compared with a normal paediatric population. Eur J Pediatr Surg 2007;17(3):194–8.

101. Antonicelli L, Micucci C, Mistrello G, et al. Improving latex-allergy diagnosis: the clinical role of Hev b8-specific IgE. Allergy 2008;63(5):620–1.

102. Lee MF, Tsai JJ, Hwang GY, et al. Identification of immunoglobulin E (IgE)-binding epitopes and recombinant IgE reactivities of a latex cross-reacting Indian jujube Ziz m 1 allergen. Clin Exp Immunol 2008;152(3):464–71.

103. Quercia O, Stefanini GF, Scardovi A, et al. Patients monosensitised to Hev b 8 (Hevea brasiliensis latex profilin) may safely undergo major surgery in a normal (non-latex safe) environment. Eur Ann Allergy Clin Immunol 2009;41(4):112–6.

104. Harper NJ, Dixon T, Dugue P, et al. Suspected anaphylactic reactions associated with anaesthesia. Anaesthesia 2009;64(2):199–211.

105. Pichichero ME, Casey JR. Safe use of selected cephalosporins in penicillin-allergic patients: a meta-analysis. Otolaryngol Head Neck Surg 2007;136(3): 340–7.

106. Renz CL, Thurn JD, Finn HA, et al. Antihistamine prophylaxis permits rapid vancomycin infusion. Crit Care Med 1999;27(9):1732–7.

107. Clarke RS. Epidemiology of adverse reactions in anaesthesia in the United Kingdom. Klin Wochenschr 1982;60(17):1003–5.

108. Harle D, Baldo B, Fisher M. The molecular basis of IgE antibody binding to thiopentone. Binding of IgE from thiopentone-allergic and non-allergic subjects. Mol Immunol 1990;27:853–8.

109. Fisher M, Ross J, Harle D, et al. Anaphylaxis to thiopentone: an unusual outbreak in a single hospital. Anaesth Intensive Care 1989;17(3):361–5.
110. Hofer KN, McCarthy MW, Buck ML, et al. Possible anaphylaxis after propofol in a child with food allergy. Ann Pharmacother 2003;37(3):398–401.
111. Baldo BA, Fisher MM, Pham NH. On the origin and specificity of antibodies to neuromuscular blocking (muscle relaxant) drugs: an immunochemical perspective. Clin Exp Allergy 2009;39(3):325–44.
112. Ring J, Messmer K. Incidence and severity of anaphylactoid reactions to colloid volume substitutes. Lancet 1977;1(8009):466–9.
113. Laxenaire MC, Charpentier C, Feldman L. Anaphylactoid reactions to colloid plasma substitutes: incidence, risk factors, mechanisms. A French multicenter prospective study. Ann Fr Anesth Reanim 1994;13(3):301–10.
114. Lorenz W, Duda D, Dick W, et al. Incidence and clinical importance of perioperative histamine release: randomised study of volume loading and antihistamines after induction of anaesthesia. Trial Group Mainz/Marburg. Lancet 1994; 343(8903):933–40.
115. Ljungstrom KG, Willman B, Hedin H. Hapten inhibition of dextran anaphylaxis. Nine years of post-marketing surveillance of dextran 1. Ann Fr Anesth Reanim 1993;12(2):219–22.
116. Berg EM, Fasting S, Sellevold OF. Serious complications with dextran-70 despite hapten prophylaxis. Is it best avoided prior to delivery? Anaesthesia 1991;46(12):1033–5.
117. Ljungstrom KG. Dextran 40 therapy made safer by pretreatment with dextran 1. Plast Reconstr Surg 2007;120(1):337–40.
118. Dieterich HJ, Kraft D, Sirtl C, et al. Hydroxyethyl starch antibodies in humans: incidence and clinical relevance. Anesth Analg 1998;86(5):1123–6.
119. Scherer K, Bircher AJ, Figueiredo V. Blue dyes in medicine–a confusing terminology. Contact Dermatitis 2006;54(4):231–2.
120. Cimmino VM, Brown AC, Szocik JF, et al. Allergic reactions to isosulfan blue during sentinel node biopsy–a common event. Surgery 2001;130(3):439–42.
121. Pevny I, Bohndorf W. Allergie wegen Patent-blau Sensibilisierung [Group allergy due to patent blue sensitization]. Med Klin 1972;67(20):698–702 [in German].
122. Wohrl S, Focke M, Hinterhuber G, et al. Near-fatal anaphylaxis to patent blue V. Br J Dermatol 2004;150(5):1037–8.
123. Keller B, Yawalkar N, Pichler C, et al. Hypersensitivity reaction against patent blue during sentinel lymph node removal in three melanoma patients. Am J Surg 2007;193(1):122–4.
124. White PF. Multimodal analgesia: its role in preventing postoperative pain. Curr Opin Investig Drugs 2008;9(1):76–82.
125. Palikhe NS, Kim SH, Park HS. What do we know about the genetics of aspirin intolerance? J Clin Pharm Ther 2008;33(5):465–72.
126. Kim SH, Hur GY, Choi JH, et al. Pharmacogenetics of aspirin-intolerant asthma. Pharmacogenomics 2008;9(1):85–91.
127. Jenneck C, Juergens U, Buecheler M, et al. Pathogenesis, diagnosis, and treatment of aspirin intolerance. Ann Allergy Asthma Immunol 2007;99(1):13–21.
128. Leimgruber A. Allergische Reaktionen auf anti-inflammatorische medikamente [Allergic reactions to nonsteroidal anti-inflammatory drugs]. Rev Med Suisse 2008;4(140):100–3 [in German].
129. Knowles SR, Drucker AM, Weber EA, et al. Management options for patients with aspirin and nonsteroidal antiinflammatory drug sensitivity. Ann Pharmacother 2007;41(7):1191–200.

130. Kong JS, Teuber SS, Gershwin ME. Aspirin and nonsteroidal anti-inflammatory drug hypersensitivity. Clin Rev Allergy Immunol 2007;32(1):97–110.
131. de Weck AL, Gamboa PM, Esparza R, et al. Hypersensitivity to aspirin and other nonsteroidal anti-inflammatory drugs (NSAIDs). Curr Pharm Des 2006;12(26): 3347–58.
132. Sanz ML, Gamboa PM, Mayorga C. Basophil activation tests in the evaluation of immediate drug hypersensitivity. Curr Opin Allergy Clin Immunol 2009;9(4): 298–304.
133. Bousquet PJ, Gaeta F, Bousquet-Rouanet L, et al. Provocation tests in diagnosing drug hypersensitivity. Curr Pharm Des 2008;14(27):2792–802.
134. Viola M, Quaratino D, Gaeta F, et al. Cross-reactive reactions to nonsteroidal anti-inflammatory drugs. Curr Pharm Des 2008;14(27):2826–32.
135. Kober BJ, Scheule AM, Voth V, et al. Anaphylactic reaction after systemic application of aprotinin triggered by aprotinin-containing fibrin sealant. Anesth Analg 2008;107(2):406–9.
136. Levy JH, Adkinson NF Jr. Anaphylaxis during cardiac surgery: implications for clinicians. Anesth Analg 2008;106(2):392–403.
137. Dietrich W, Ebell A, Busley R, et al. Aprotinin and anaphylaxis: analysis of 12,403 exposures to aprotinin in cardiac surgery. Ann Thorac Surg 2007;84(4):1144–50.
138. Garvey LH, Kroigaard M, Poulsen LK, et al. IgE-mediated allergy to chlorhexidine. J Allergy Clin Immunol 2007;120(2):409–15.
139. Nybo M, Madsen JS. Serious anaphylactic reactions due to protamine sulfate: a systematic literature review. Basic Clin Pharmacol Toxicol 2008;103(2):192–6.
140. Dunser MW, Torgersen C, Wenzel V. Treatment of anaphylactic shock: where is the evidence? Anesth Analg 2008;107(2):359–61.
141. The diagnosis and management of anaphylaxis: an updated practice parameter. J Allergy Clin Immunol 2005;115(3 Suppl 2):S483–523.
142. Muraro A, Roberts G, Clark A, et al. The management of anaphylaxis in childhood: position paper of the European academy of allergology and clinical immunology. Allergy 2007;62(8):857–71.
143. Soar J, Pumphrey R, Cant A, et al. Emergency treatment of anaphylactic reactions–guidelines for healthcare providers. Resuscitation 2008;77(2):157–69.
144. Soar J, Deakin CD, Nolan JP, et al. European Resuscitation Council guidelines for resuscitation 2005. Section 7. Cardiac arrest in special circumstances. Resuscitation 2005;67(Suppl 1):S135–70.
145. Pumphrey RS. Lessons for management of anaphylaxis from a study of fatal reactions. Clin Exp Allergy 2000;30(8):1144–50.
146. Hussain AM, Yousuf B, Khan MA, et al. Vasopressin for the management of catecholamine-resistant anaphylactic shock. Singapore Med J 2008;49(9):e225–8.
147. Kill C, Wranze E, Wulf H. Successful treatment of severe anaphylactic shock with vasopressin. Two case reports. Int Arch Allergy Immunol 2004;134(3):260–1.
148. Meng L, Williams EL. Case report: treatment of rocuronium-induced anaphylactic shock with vasopressin. Can J Anaesth 2008;55(7):437–40.
149. Schummer C, Wirsing M, Schummer W. The pivotal role of vasopressin in refractory anaphylactic shock. Anesth Analg 2008;107(2):620–4.
150. Schummer W, Schummer C. Vasopressin and suspected anaphylactic reactions associated with anaesthesia. Anaesthesia 2009;64(7):783.
151. Schummer W, Schummer C, Wippermann J, et al. Anaphylactic shock: is vasopressin the drug of choice? Anesthesiology 2004;101(4):1025–7.
152. Williams SR, Denault AY, Pellerin M, et al. Vasopressin for treatment of shock following aprotinin administration. Can J Anaesth 2004;51(2):169–72.

153. Dewachter P, Jouan-Hureaux V, Lartaud I, et al. Comparison of arginine vaso-pressin, terlipressin, or epinephrine to correct hypotension in a model of anaphylactic shock in anesthetized brown Norway rats. Anesthesiology 2006; 104(4):734–41.
154. Hiruta A, Mitsuhata H, Hiruta M, et al. Vasopressin may be useful in the treatment of systemic anaphylaxis in rabbits. Shock 2005;24(3):264–9.
155. Del Duca D, Sheth SS, Clarke AE, et al. Use of methylene blue for catechol-amine-refractory vasoplegia from protamine and aprotinin. Ann Thorac Surg 2009;87(2):640–2.

The Complex Clinical Picture of Side Effects to Biologicals

Oliver V. Hausmann, MD[a],*, Michael Seitz, MD[a],
Peter M. Villiger, MD[a], Werner J. Pichler, MD[a,b]

KEYWORDS

- Biological • Monoclonal therapeutic antibodies
- Adverse side effects • Hypersensitivity subclassifications
- Acute infusion reactions • Cytokine dysbalance syndrome

Adverse drug reactions (ADR) are a common phenomenon. For a long time, most drugs were small chemicals called xenobiotics that occasionally caused side effects. These were explained by the pharmacologic action of the drug (type A) or were related to the susceptibility of the individual to the drug (type B, idiosyncratic drug reactions). Most of the type B reactions were immune mediated. In addition, some investigators extended this classification and used type C for (chemical) reactions related to the chemical structure and its metabolism, for example, paracetamol hepatotoxicity; type D, corresponding to delayed reactions that appear after many years of treatment, for example, bladder carcinoma after treatment with cyclophosphamide; and type E (end of treatment) reactions occurring after drug withdrawal, for example, seizures after stopping phenytoin. This subclassification of side effects is focused on small chemical compounds, but is considered less suitable for proteins used as drugs.[1]

Biological response modifiers, commonly abbreviated as "biologicals," represent a new category of drugs designed to be as similar to human proteins as possible.[1] The nomenclature of biologicals seems to be arbitrary at first glance, but it is strictly regulated.[2] Taking infliximab as an example, the first 1 or 2 syllables can be chosen freely; in this case "inf-." The following syllable derives from the target structure or target disease, here "-li-" for immune system. The next syllable denotes the species of origin, "-xi-" for chimeric murine-human origin. The last syllable stands for the therapeutic principle, in this case "-mab" for monoclonal antibody. Alternative final syllables are "-cept" for soluble receptors and "-inib" for receptor antagonists. Biological response modifiers interact specifically with the immune system (**Table 1**) and target distinct cell surface structures, for example, cytokine receptors, tumor-specific

a Department of Rheumatology, Clinical Immunology and Allergology, Inselspital, University of Bern, Bern 3010, Switzerland
b ADR-AC GmbH, Holligenstr. 91, CH-3008 Bern, Switzerland
* Corresponding author.
E-mail address: oliver.hausmann@insel.ch

Med Clin N Am 94 (2010) 791–804
doi:10.1016/j.mcna.2010.03.001
0025-7125/10/$ – see front matter © 2010 Elsevier Inc. All rights reserved.

Table 1
Biologicals grouped according to their therapeutic principle

Biological Group	Examples
Cytokines	INF-α, GM-CSF
Monoclonal antibodies against	
Cytokines	Infliximab (anti–TNF-α)
Cell surface molecules	Rituximab (anti-CD20)
IgE	Omalizumab (anti-IgE)
Tumor antigens	Cetuximab (anti-EGFR)
Fusion proteins	
Soluble cytokine receptors	Etanercept (TNF-α-RII-IgG1)
Soluble cellular ligands	Abatacept (CTLA4-IgG1)

Abbreviations: EGFR, epidermal growth factor; GM-CSF, granulocyte macrophage colony stimulating factor; INF, interferon; TNF, tumor necrosis factor.
Data from Pichler WJ. Adverse side effects to biological agents. Allergy 2006;61(8):912–20.

antigens, or soluble mediators (cytokines, interferons). Biologicals have turned out to be potent and effective therapeutic tools for various inflammatory, autoimmune, and oncologic diseases. Their direct and focused effect renders them superior to classic immunosuppressive or cytotoxic drugs, whose use is often limited by unwanted and frequently severe generalized side effects. In 2006, the molecular targeted therapies in oncology accounted for 44% of the total sales of the top 20 cancer therapy brands, overtaking the cytotoxic therapies for the first time.[3] The side effects seen with classic xenobiotics seem to differ considerably from the ones associated with biologicals concerning their pathogenesis and consequences for future therapy (**Table 2**). It is beyond the scope of this article to cover the adverse side effects of all biologicals in detail. Instead typical clinical manifestations are presented, and general rules for treating these and guiding later allergological workup as well as a possible classification scheme are proposed.

Table 2
Differences between classic xenobiotics and biologicals in view of their ADR

	Xenobiotic	Biological
Structure	Low molecular weight chemical compound	High molecular weight protein
Metabolism	Important (reactive metabolites)	Not metabolized (processing, digestion)
Route of administration	Oral, topical, parenteral	Parenteral
Inherent immunologic activity	No (with exception of immunosuppressive drugs)	Yes
Drug interactions	Common	Rare
Immune response	Mostly cellular (T cells) (pro-) hapten Delayed type reaction	Mostly humoral (antibodies) antigenic itself Immediate type
Examples	Penicillin (amoxicillin)	Monoclonal antibodies (anti-TNF-α) Cytokines (INF-α)

Data from Pichler WJ. Adverse side effects to biological agents. Allergy 2006;61(8):912–20.

ADAPTED CLASSIFICATION FOR ADR TO BIOLOGICALS

With certain modifications but analogous to the aforementioned "type A to E scheme" for xenobiotics, ADR to biologicals can be classified as types α to ε, using the Greek alphabet to distinguish them from xenobiotic-induced side effects (**Fig. 1**). This classification is not based on similarity of clinical symptoms but is an attempt to classify ADR to biologicals according to their pathomechanism. This might help in guiding future therapy concerning reexposure, premedication, and/or switch to an alternative biological.

TYPE α (OVERSTIMULATION)

Most cytokines are produced locally and have a predominant local activity. Thus, for most cytokines, only the local concentration is relatively high.[4,5] If the cytokine is applied therapeutically the situation is reversed: comparatively high systemic concentrations are applied to achieve a sufficiently high concentration locally. Such high systemic concentrations of cytokines can sometimes cause severe side effects limiting their use, for example, flu-like symptoms during interferon (INF)-α therapy. Alternatively, if a monoclonal antibody is directed against a potentially stimulatory receptor like CD3 on T cells (OKT3, muromunab) or CD28 on T cells (TGN1412), a substantial release of different cytokines can occur, which reaches high systemic levels and can cause various occasionally severe symptoms.[6] In the phase 1 clinical trial of TGN1412, the previously mentioned anti-CD28 antibody, this principle led to a near-fatal "cytokine storm" in the first 6 healthy volunteers tested,[7] and the product was withdrawn from further trials.

	Type α Overstimulation	Type β Hypersensitivity / Immunogenicity		Type γ Immunodeviation		Type δ Cross-reactivity	Type ε non-immunologic
mechanism	High cytokine levels (applied, released)	Immediate (IgE, IgG + C')	Delayed (T cells, IgG + C')	Immunodeficiency	immune imbalance	target structure similarity	Additional effects
dose dependent	yes	yes	yes	yes	?	yes	?
related to function	yes	no	no	yes	?	yes	possibly
Clinical picture	acute infusion reactions flu-like symptoms (INFα) multiple organ dysfunction	acute infusion reactions, urticaria anaphylaxis	Loss of effect (IgG) Exanthema (rare)	opportunistic infections	autoimmunity atopic/allergic disorders	depending on target organ	?
Effects on	dependent on cytokine (interferon, interleukin)	mast cells basophils	FcR⁺ cells IgG + complement	granuloma maintenance cell migration	auto Ab (auto-)inflammation	macrophages neutrophils	?
Example	OKT3 ("cytokine release syndrome"), TGN1412 ("cytokine storm"), INFα	cetuximab (CCD-med. anaphylaxis)	infliximab (HACA) Serum sickness	TNFα-Inhibitors (tuberculosis)	atopic eczema, SLE neutrophilic AGEP-like dermatitis	cetuximab (acneiform lesions)	INFα (retinopathy, depression)

Fig. 1. Adapted classification for ADR to biologicals in a simplified illustration, with typical examples of each reaction type (for details see text). AGEP, acute generalized exanthematous pustulosis; HACA, human antichimeric antibodies; INF, interferon; SLE, systemic lupus erythematodes; TNF, tumor necrosis factor. (*Data from* Pichler WJ. Adverse side effects to biological agents. Allergy 2006;61(8):912–20.)

Type α is very similar to the type A side effects of classic xenobiotics, because both are dose dependent, are somehow predictable, and are directly related to the function of the drug.

TYPE β (HYPERSENSITIVITY/IMMUNOGENICITY)

A substantial part of biologicals are monoclonal antibodies (mAbs) produced in cell lines of animal origin, therefore biologicals contain nonhuman parts either in their protein backbone or in their glycosylation pattern (posttranslational protein modification in the Golgi apparatus). Those nonhuman parts are immunogenic by definition, and like all foreign proteins can lead to a predominantly, but not exclusively humoral immune response.[4] The therapeutic application of mAbs of murine origin in human disease was limited by the induction of human antimurine antibodies (HAMA). The generation of chimeric antibodies lessened the murine content to about 25% (Fab antibody portion) with a still considerable rate of human antichimeric antibodies (HACA). Further elimination of rodent sequences enabled the production of humanized mAbs (10% murine), followed by generation of fully human antibodies. Nevertheless, it must be pointed out that even "fully human" mAbs, with a given specificity, possess a unique (foreign) amino acid sequence at their antigen-binding site, which is also called idiotype. Therefore, even fully human mAbs can elicit the production of anti-idiotypic antibodies, also called human-antihuman antibodies (HAHA).

During evolution, antibodies in general developed to enhance the immunogenicity and hence the elimination of foreign proteins by linking them to Fcγ receptors on macrophages and neutrophils as well as through direct activation of the complement cascade, a process called opsonization.[4] Antibody binding to Fcγ receptors and complement activation are mediated by carbohydrate determinants in the Fc region and are most effective in the IgG1 subclass. Hence, the constant region of human IgG1 is preferentially used for mAbs designed for high cytotoxicity, for example, tumor lysis in oncology. For rheumatic diseases, this additional complement activation does not seem to be crucial for the intended effect, but can lead to substantial side effects. In the development of acute infusion reactions, complement activation most probably plays a key role.[8,9] Complement cleavage products such as C3a and C5a are potent mast cell stimulators[4] and can therefore trigger IgE-independent histamine release, which can mimic full-blown allergic shock depending on the number of mast cells involved. On the other hand, serum sickness-like reactions based on complement-binding immune complexes in the course of treatment with various biologicals have been reported.[10–13]

The precise pathogenesis of acute infusion reactions remains unknown, and the term itself is merely descriptive. In principle, an IgE-mediated mechanism is possible, because the relevant Fab portion of mAb contains foreign amino acid sequences and is perfectly bivalent. Those reactions are potentially more dangerous. In most cases, clinical evidence argues against an IgE-mediated mechanism, because many patients can be kept on the same biological therapy with a slower infusion rate and/or premedication with antihistamines and corticosteroids.[14] Only in a few cases have skin tests and/or serologic studies been done, and firm conclusions cannot be drawn from the current data (see section on acute infusion reactions).

In contrast to this, cetuximab (anti-epidermal growth factor receptor (EGFR) in cancer therapy) has been well studied in this regard. Preformed IgE antibodies against an environmental component (galactose-α-1,3-galactose) cross-react with a similar nonhuman part of cetuximab's glycosylation pattern and could be held responsible for the sometimes severe anaphylactic reactions, even when first encountered with cetuximab. Sensitization has probably taken place through cow's milk or meat (skin contact?) and is a phenomenon restricted to certain rural parts of the United States.[15,16]

In certain circumstances, infusion or injection excipients such as carboxymethylcellulose[17,18] or polysorbate 80[17,19–21] could be identified as the culprit elicitors of anaphylactic IgE-mediated or nonimmunologic anaphylactoid reactions; this might be of special importance for the excipient-rich subcutaneous drug formulations. Sensitization may have taken place through the use of the same excipients in various vaccines and cosmetics.

Concerning T-cell–mediated delayed type hypersensitivities, various cutaneous ADR ranging from generalized pruritus without exanthema to single cases of toxic epidermal necrolysis,[22] have been reported. Unfortunately, the underlying pathomechanism has not been studied in detail. In fact, infliximab has even been successfully used in the treatment of toxic epidermal necrolysis.[23] Single case reports, for example, a maculopapular exanthem due to abciximab with a positive intracutaneous test after 48 hours,[24] have been published, which might indicate biological-specific delayed type hypersensitivities (type IV, Coombs and Gell classification). In tumor necrosis factor (TNF)-α blocker treatment, no correlation between the atopic status and the incidence of immediate or delayed type hypersensitivity reactions was found.[25]

TYPE γ (IMMUNODEVIATION)

The immune system has evolved to control infections and to prevent them from becoming harmful for the infected individual. Therefore, it is constantly active without causing clinical symptoms in apparently healthy individuals. The immune system controls invading organisms, for example, intracellular herpes viruses and various intracellular bacteria, and stimulates the innate immunity, especially in border regions such as mucosal surfaces or the skin. Important players in this silent but highly effective control mechanism are cytokines produced predominantly by T cells.

The potent effect of various biologicals in eliminating clinically obvious inflammations in colitis or arthritis also has an effect, beyond any doubt, on this "natural" control mechanism of predominantly intracellular pathogens and border regions. This means that biologicals, which successfully interfere with inflammation, also interfere with the well-balanced control of constantly occurring infections. Consequently, biologicals may cause immune deviations or a cytokine imbalance syndrome, and have an immunosuppressive effect, which may cause an exacerbation of an (opportunistic) infection: a typical example is the exacerbation of tuberculosis due to anti–TNF-α therapy whereby, through diminishing the TNF-α level, not only the intended attenuation of the ongoing colitis or arthritis is achieved but also the crucial TNF-α effect on granuloma maintenance to control this intracellular pathogen is lost, with sometimes fatal consequences.[26]

This immune deviation may not only result in obvious immunodeficiency: cytokines also have a regulatory function, which is also documented for the antagonistic effect of Th2-type cytokines (interleukin [IL]-4, IL-5, IL-10, IL-13) on Th1-immune responses and vice versa.[27] Consequently, a suppression of Th1 responses (TNF-α, INF-γ) may enhance Th2 responses. A patient treated with a biological suppressing the Th1-biased immune response, being the case in most autoimmune diseases, may develop a Th2-related reaction: Months after starting treatment, a hitherto nonallergic patient may develop a new-onset respiratory allergy (house dust mite, pollen).[28] Alternatively, if the shift in cytokine balance resulting from treatment with a given biological possibly results in an inadequate handling of apoptotic cells, the patient may develop autoantibodies to DNA, and rarely even an overt systemic lupus erythematodes.[29–31] The immune deviation or cytokine dysbalance syndrome reflects complex clinical pictures that are far from being understood. The analysis of the effects of a certain biological on the "natural" immunity has rarely been investigated, and the effect on distinct parameters has not yet been analyzed. Moreover, the effect may also be related to the individual predisposition: if a person already has a slightly dysbalanced immune system (without causing symptoms), this person may be more susceptible to a further intervention by a biological, whereas others tolerate the same biological well.

At present, diagnosis of this immune deviation relies on clinical symptoms. Certain laboratory parameters may support the diagnosis of a new autoimmune or allergic disorder. Tests to detect hypersensitivities directed to the biological, such as skin tests with the biological agent itself as well as in vitro detection of antibodies (IgG, IgE) to the biological in question, are negative.

TYPE δ (CROSS-REACTIVITY)

Especially in oncology, the target cell surface structures (over-)expressed on tumor cells are usually to some extent also present on healthy tissues such as skin or intestinal mucosa. Therefore, monoclonal antibodies directed against these shared antigens may lead to considerable "off-target" tissue damage. The well-known phenomenon of acneiform lesions during cetuximab treatment is an illustrative example for this mechanism, because the targeted epidermal growth factor receptor is not only present on carcinoma cells but also plays an important role in epidermal homeostasis.[32]

It cannot be ruled out that some monoclonal antibodies binding to their target structure with high affinity may also bind to others, which are structurally similar but not identical proteins, with lower affinity, thus causing unexpected side effects.

TYPE ε (NONIMMUNOLOGIC SIDE EFFECTS)

Many molecules that are defined as therapeutic target structures on a certain disease background may well be involved in other physiologic functions that are not known until the routine use of a certain biological. Daily clinical practice may actually reveal these to date unknown functions of a targeted molecule. An intense postmarketing surveillance is therefore not only important for patient safety but also for deepening the knowledge of the role of the targeted structure in human physiology.

ADR TO BIOLOGICALS: CLINICAL PICTURE IN DAILY PRACTICE

The presented subclassification of ADR to biologicals may be helpful for physicians using biologicals in their daily clinical practice, especially for allergologists who are trying to clarify the underlying pathomechanism for a firm diagnosis. Depending on the type of reaction, dose adjustments, change of preparation, or stoppage of therapy may be advised based on a balanced evaluation of the pros and cons of the treatment.

The clinician directly involved in the treatment of the affected patient is frequently confronted with acute infusion or injection site reactions and delayed reaction primarily affecting the skin. The clinician has to decide how to treat the acute ADR, primarily irrespective of the often unclear underlying pathomechansim. The clinical presentation and procedures of these acute reactions are dealt with in detail in the next sections.

Acute Infusion Reactions

Case

A 25-year-old woman was treated for her methotrexate-resistant rheumatoid arthritis with infliximab, a TNF-α blocking antibody. During the fifth infusion, she developed a pruritic rash with small isolated urticarial lesions and dyspnea. Infusion was discontinued, and the patient was treated with antihistamines and corticosteroid. After switching to an alternative TNF-α blocker, adalimumab, which was applied every second week subcutaneously, she developed a local urticaria at the injection site after the second application. Immediately after the third exposure, this urticaria spread over the whole body and adalimumab had to be stopped.

Allergological workup revealed intradermal skin test positivity for adalimumab and not for infliximab. Because no serologic test system for IgE to biologicals was available at that time, basophil activation tests were performed, which were negative for infliximab and again positive for adalimumab. Taking into account that the reaction to infliximab occurred only at the highest infusion rate (160 mL/h) and not just after the start of infusion and skin test as well as the basophil activation test (BAT) showed no positivity, the reaction was classified as non-IgE mediated acute infusion reaction (most probably IgG and/or complement mediated). The patient was safely reexposed with a premedication of antihistamines (no corticosteroids) at a maximum infusion rate of 100 mL/h. On the contrary, the reaction to adalimumab was classified as IgE-mediated urticaria specific for adalimumab or its excipients, and a reintroduction was not recommended.

As illustrated by this case, 2 different reaction types within 2 biologicals with the same target (TNF-α inhibitors) can occur in the same patient.

A thorough documentation of the acute reaction type with special attention on a clear-cut differentiation between subjective and objective symptoms is crucial for further workup (**Table 3**). Grading of the reaction severity analogous to hymenoptera venom allergy (I–IV according to Mueller[33]) facilitates the communication with other specialties.

In clinical trials,[34–38] acute infusion reactions were defined as any adverse event occurring during or within 1 to 2 hours after an infusion. This definition comprises everything ranging from a simple headache to dyspnea, cardiovascular symptoms, and loss of consciousness. Hence, there is considerable controversy regarding the optimal emergency treatment of acute infusion reactions. Based on a large clinical experience showing mainly mild reactions, some investigators suggest that stopping the infusion may be sufficient.[39] However, some reactions do not appear clinically harmless: from an allergological and pharmacological point of view as well as in the authors' experience, anaphylactic reactions with rapidly evolving symptoms including

Table 3 Subjective versus objective symptoms in the evaluation of ADR to biologicals		
	Subjective	**Objective**
Skin/Mucosa	Itch	Flush, exanthema, urticaria, angioedema
Eye/Nose	Itch, disturbed vision	Rhinoconjunctivitis
Gastrointestinal Tract	Nausea, crampy pain	Vomiting, diarrhea
Lung	Tightness, dyspnea	Obstruction (peak expiratory flow, lung function)
Heart/Brain	Chest pain, dizziness, vertigo	Hypotension, unconsciousness, incontinence, cardiac arrest

flush and dizziness (vasodilatation) and dyspnea (bronchospasm) should be treated with epinephrine as early as possible (**Fig. 2**).[40] Even if acute reactions to biologicals can occur at any time during the infusion, only the ones starting within the first 10 minutes of infusion are suggestive of an IgE-mediated mechanism. This finding is already well documented in the setting of perioperative anaphylaxis (see the article by Mertes and colleagues elsewhere in this issue for further exploration of this topic), and cannot be avoided with premedication of any kind.[41,42]

The precise role of different premedication schemes (antihistamines + paracetamol ± steroids) is unclear.[43–45] For patient safety and because of the lack of relevant ADR

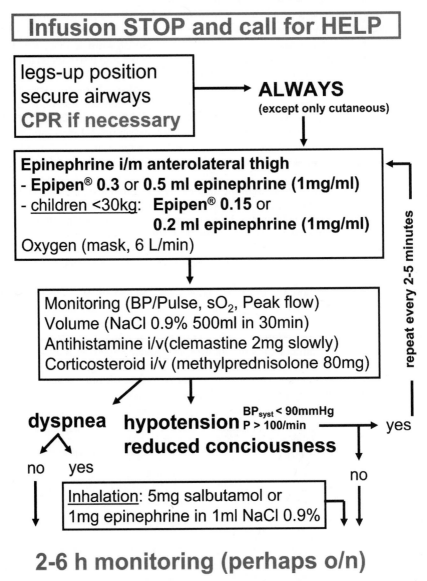

Fig. 2. Proposed algorithm for emergency treatment of acute infusion reactions. BP, blood pressure; CPR, cardiopulmonary resuscitation; i/m, intramuscular; i/v, intravenous; P, pulse.

of this premedication, some clinicians argue for a regular use for all patients regardless of their disease background or comedication. In the setting of autoimmune diseases, most clinicians disapprove a regular premedication because of the resulting difficulties in assigning the therapeutic benefit to the biological or the corticosteroids applied.[39,46] At least 2 open studies on ADR to infliximab suggest that there is no advantage of a routine premedication for patients with no history of a prior infusion reaction,[47] whereas another randomized controlled trial showed a reduction in antibody production against infliximab (HACA) and consecutively also in acute infusion reactions using high-dose intravenous hydrocortisone premedication.[48]

After stabilization of the patient and complete resolution of the symptoms without suspicion of an IgE-mediated mechanism according to symptom severity and timing, a restart of infusion at a slower infusion rate (maximal 60–100 mL/h in the case of infliximab[49]) is usually possible. For further allergological workup, determination of the tryptase level during the acute phase of the reaction (within 90–120 minutes) can help to elucidate the underlying mechanism. This mast cell specific enzyme is released during degranulation and an increase to more than 150% of baseline level, even within normal limits, proves mast cell involvement and is suggestive of an IgE-mediated mechanism.[50] Further investigations (skin test, sIgE, sIgG, BAT), including determination of baseline tryptase levels, should be postponed for 4 to 6 weeks because of the refractory state of unresponsiveness of the effector cells involved (**Fig. 3**). For proven (or highly suggestive) IgE-mediated reactions, several desensitization protocols have been successfully applied.[51–55]

Acute infusion reactions were more common when biological therapy was reinstituted following an extended period without treatment (>16 weeks in the case of infliximab[56,57]). Patients who developed antibodies against infliximab (HACA) had a 2- to 3-fold higher chance of having an acute infusion reaction than patients who did not develop antibodies against infliximab.[58,59] According to recent studies, the use of concomitant immunosuppressive agents such as methotrexate reduced the frequency of antibodies to infliximab and infusion reactions.[59–61]

Injection Site Reactions

Pruritic erythema, swelling, and infiltrated plaques are typical clinical manifestations at the injection site of subcutaneously applied biologicals. These manifestations usually appear within the first 2 days of each treatment cycle, usually within minutes of

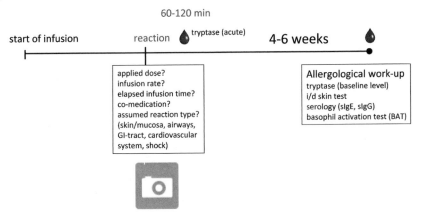

Fig. 3. Schematic course of allergological workup of acute infusion reactions. GI, gastrointestinal.

injection. Most of the time, these are benign and self-limiting on continuation of therapy[62,63]; only in rare cases has an exanthematous dissemination been reported.[64] Studies on injection site reactions are scarce, and case descriptions or small case series dominate the field.[65–67] These studies conclude that further studies with more patients are needed including biopsies of lesions, skin testing and, if available, determination of sIgE and sIgG against the biological in question, to elucidate the precise immune mechanism behind these reactions.

Of note, similar large local reactions following hymenoptera stings are frequently observed in patients with sIgE and sIgG against the respective venoms.[68]

SUMMARY

The clinical picture of ADR to biologicals can be misleading with regard to pathogenesis of the reaction, because different pathomechanisms may lead to similar symptoms. This is especially important for acute infusion reactions, whereby no clear clinical distinction between allergic, IgE-mediated, and the more frequent nonallergic, most probably complement-mediated reactions is possible. Emergency treatment of those reactions is identical, but they differ substantially according to their further management, because only an IgE-mediated mechanism necessitates a strict avoidance or a repetitive desensitization procedure. The authors have therefore proposed a classification of the ADR to biologicals based on their pathomechanism, and suggest a strong effort for classifying preferably every ADR encountered in collaboration with the local allergologists, if necessary and possible. For the patients, the advantage is a precise advice for safe future application concerning threshold infusion rates (eg, 60–100 mL/h for infliximab), a meaningful premedication (antihistamines without repetitive corticosteroids), a possible desensitization procedure, or a switch to an alternative biological. For the scientific community, the understanding of these complex phenomena would grow, and allow for safe future treatments and drug development.

KEY MESSAGES

- Biologicals differ from classic drugs in their mode of action and ADR
- ADR to biologicals are a common phenomenon but not well understood
- Acute infusion reactions and injection site reactions are the most common clinical presentation
- Not all acute infusion reactions are allergic (on the contrary, it seems to be the exception rather than the rule)
- Most acute infusion reactions are mild, and the culprit biological can be restarted at a slower infusion rate
- For proven or highly suggestive IgE-mediated allergic reactions, desensitization protocols allow for a safe reexposure with the culprit biological
- The role of a premedication with corticosteroids or antihistamines is still a matter of debate.

REFERENCES

1. Pichler WJ. Adverse side effects to biological agents. Allergy 2006;61(8):912–20.
2. Saxon A. Who-mab's on first and what-cept's on second. I don't know—third base. Clin Immunol 2008;127(3):267.

3. Friedmann B. Commercial insight: top 20 cancer therapy brands—sales of targeted therapies overtake cytotoxics in 2006. A Datamonitor 2007. Product Code DMHC2299. 2007. Available at: http://www.datamonitor.com. Accessed March 9, 2010.

4. Abbas AK, Lichtman AH. Cellular and molecular immunology. 6th edition. Philadelphia: Saunders; 2009. Accessed March 9, 2010.

5. Desgeorges A, Gabay C, Silacci P, et al. Concentrations and origins of soluble interleukin 6 receptor-alpha in serum and synovial fluid. J Rheumatol 1997; 24(8):1510–6.

6. Vasquez EM, Fabrega AJ, Pollak R. OKT3-induced cytokine-release syndrome: occurrence beyond the second dose and association with rejection severity. Transplant Proc 1995;27(1):873–4.

7. Suntharalingam G, Perry MR, Ward S, et al. Cytokine storm in a phase 1 trial of the anti-CD28 monoclonal antibody TGN1412. N Engl J Med 2006;355(10):1018–28.

8. van der Kolk LE, Grillo-Lopez AJ, Baars JW, et al. Complement activation plays a key role in the side effects of rituximab treatment. Br J Haematol 2001; 115(4):807–11.

9. Raasveld MH, Bemelman FJ, Schellekens PT, et al. Complement activation during OKT3 treatment: a possible explanation for respiratory side effects. Kidney Int 1993;43(5):1140–9.

10. Lees CW, Ali AI, Thompson AI, et al. The safety profile of anti-tumour necrosis factor therapy in inflammatory bowel disease in clinical practice: analysis of 620 patient-years follow-up. Aliment Pharmacol Ther 2009;29(3):286–97.

11. Medeot M, Zaja F, Vianelli N, et al. Rituximab therapy in adult patients with relapsed or refractory immune thrombocytopenic purpura: long-term follow-up results. Eur J Haematol 2008;81(3):165–9.

12. Pilette C, Coppens N, Houssiau FA, et al. Severe serum sickness-like syndrome after omalizumab therapy for asthma. J Allergy Clin Immunol 2007;120(4):972–3.

13. Gamarra RM, McGraw SD, Drelichman VS, et al. Serum sickness-like reactions in patients receiving intravenous infliximab. J Emerg Med 2006;30(1):41–4.

14. Cheifetz A, Smedley M, Martin S, et al. The incidence and management of infusion reactions to infliximab: a large center experience. Am J Gastroenterol 2003;98(6):1315–24.

15. Arnold DF, Misbah SA. Cetuximab-induced anaphylaxis and IgE specific for galactose-alpha-1,3-galactose. N Engl J Med 2008;358(25):2735 [author reply: 2735–6].

16. Chung CH, Mirakhur B, Chan E, et al. Cetuximab-induced anaphylaxis and IgE specific for galactose-alpha-1,3-galactose. N Engl J Med 2008;358(11):1109–17.

17. Grims RH, Kranke B, Aberer W. Pitfalls in drug allergy skin testing: false-positive reactions due to (hidden) additives. Contact Dermatitis 2006;54(5):290–4.

18. Steiner UC, Gentinetta T, Hausmann O, et al. IgE-mediated anaphylaxis to intra-articular glucocorticoid preparations. AJR Am J Roentgenol 2009;193(2): W156–157.

19. Coors EA, Seybold H, Merk HF, et al. Polysorbate 80 in medical products and nonimmunologic anaphylactoid reactions. Ann Allergy Asthma Immunol 2005; 95(6):593–9.

20. Price KS, Hamilton RG. Anaphylactoid reactions in two patients after omalizumab administration after successful long-term therapy. Allergy Asthma Proc 2007; 28(3):313–9.

21. Steele RH, Limaye S, Cleland B, et al. Hypersensitivity reactions to the polysorbate contained in recombinant erythropoietin and darbepoietin. Nephrology (Carlton) 2005;10(3):317–20.

22. Lin WL, Lin WC, Yang JY, et al. Fatal toxic epidermal necrolysis associated with cetuximab in a patient with colon cancer. J Clin Oncol 2008;26(16): 2779–80.

23. Fischer M, Fiedler E, Marsch WC, et al. Antitumour necrosis factor-alpha antibodies (infliximab) in the treatment of a patient with toxic epidermal necrolysis. Br J Dermatol 2002;146(4):707–9.

24. Moneret-Vautrin DA, Morisset M, Vignaud JM, et al. T cell mediated allergy to abciximab. Allergy 2002;57(3):269–70.

25. Benucci M, Manfredi M, Saviola G, et al. Correlation between atopy and hypersensitivity reactions during therapy with three different TNF-alpha blocking agents in rheumatoid arthritis. Clin Exp Rheumatol 2009;27(2):333–6.

26. Clay H, Volkman HE, Ramakrishnan L. Tumor necrosis factor signaling mediates resistance to mycobacteria by inhibiting bacterial growth and macrophage death. Immunity 2008;29(2):283–94.

27. Abbas AK, Murphy KM, Sher A. Functional diversity of helper T lymphocytes. Nature 1996;383(6603):787–93.

28. Bennett AN, Wong M, Zain A, et al. Adalimumab-induced asthma. Rheumatology (Oxford) 2005;44(9):1199–200.

29. Gonnet-Gracia C, Barnetche T, Richez C, et al. Anti-nuclear antibodies, anti-DNA and C4 complement evolution in rheumatoid arthritis and ankylosing spondylitis treated with TNF-alpha blockers. Clin Exp Rheumatol 2008;26(3):401–7.

30. Krause I, Valesini G, Scrivo R, et al. Autoimmune aspects of cytokine and anticytokine therapies. Am J Med 2003;115(5):390–7.

31. Costa MF, Said NR, Zimmermann B. Drug-induced lupus due to anti-tumor necrosis factor alpha agents. Semin Arthritis Rheum 2008;37(6):381–7.

32. Perez-Soler R, Saltz L. Cutaneous adverse effects with HER1/EGFR-targeted agents: is there a silver lining? J Clin Oncol 2005;23(22):5235–46.

33. Mueller HL. Diagnosis and treatment of insect sensitivity. J Asthma Res 1966;3(4): 331–3.

34. Sands BE, Anderson FH, Bernstein CN, et al. Infliximab maintenance therapy for fistulizing Crohn's disease. N Engl J Med 2004;350(9):876–85.

35. Fidder H, Schnitzler F, Ferrante M, et al. Long-term safety of infliximab for the treatment of inflammatory bowel disease: a single-centre cohort study. Gut 2009;58(4):501–8.

36. Schnitzler F, Fidder H, Ferrante M, et al. Long-term outcome of treatment with infliximab in 614 patients with Crohn's disease: results from a single-centre cohort. Gut 2009;58(4):492–500.

37. Rutgeerts P, Sandborn WJ, Feagan BG, et al. Infliximab for induction and maintenance therapy for ulcerative colitis. N Engl J Med 2005;353(23):2462–76.

38. Maini R, St Clair EW, Breedveld F, et al. Infliximab (chimeric anti-tumour necrosis factor alpha monoclonal antibody) versus placebo in rheumatoid arthritis patients receiving concomitant methotrexate: a randomised phase III trial. ATTRACT study group. Lancet 1999;354(9194):1932–9.

39. Prupas M. Reactions to infliximab in patients with rheumatoid arthritis. J Rheumatol 2005;32(7):1411 [author reply: 1411].

40. Kemp SF, Lockey RF, Simons FE. Epinephrine: the drug of choice for anaphylaxis. A statement of the World Allergy Organization. Allergy 2008;63(8): 1061–70.

41. Sany J, Kaiser MJ, Jorgensen C, et al. Study of the tolerance of infliximab infusions with or without betamethasone premedication in patients with active rheumatoid arthritis. Ann Rheum Dis 2005;64(11):1647–9.

42. Tramer MR, von Elm E, Loubeyre P, et al. Pharmacological prevention of serious anaphylactic reactions due to iodinated contrast media: systematic review. BMJ 2006;333(7570):675.

43. Lenz HJ. Management and preparedness for infusion and hypersensitivity reactions. Oncologist 2007;12(5):601–9.

44. Chung CH. Managing premedications and the risk for reactions to infusional monoclonal antibody therapy. Oncologist 2008;13(6):725–32.

45. Augustsson J, Eksborg S, Ernestam S, et al. Low-dose glucocorticoid therapy decreases risk for treatment-limiting infusion reaction to infliximab in patients with rheumatoid arthritis. Ann Rheum Dis 2007;66(11):1462–6.

46. Wasserman MJ, Weber DA, Guthrie JA, et al. Infusion-related reactions to infliximab in patients with rheumatoid arthritis in a clinical practice setting: relationship to dose, antihistamine pretreatment, and infusion number. J Rheumatol 2004; 31(10):1912–7.

47. Ricart E, Panaccione R, Loftus EV, et al. Infliximab for Crohn's disease in clinical practice at the Mayo Clinic: the first 100 patients. Am J Gastroenterol 2001;96(3): 722–9.

48. Farrell RJ, Alsahli M, Jeen YT, et al. Intravenous hydrocortisone premedication reduces antibodies to infliximab in Crohn's disease: a randomized controlled trial. Gastroenterology 2003;124(4):917–24.

49. Lequerre T, Vittecoq O, Klemmer N, et al. Management of infusion reactions to infliximab in patients with rheumatoid arthritis or spondyloarthritis: experience from an immunotherapy unit of rheumatology. J Rheumatol 2006;33(7): 1307–14.

50. Borer-Reinhold M, Haeberli G, Bitzenhofer M, et al. A definite increase of serum tryptase within normal limits indicates a systemic allergic reaction [abstract 14]. Abstracts of the XXVIII EAACI Congress of the European Academy of Allergy and Clinical Immunology, Warszawa, Poland, 6–10 June 2009. Allergy 2009; 64(Suppl 90):7.

51. Puchner TC, Kugathasan S, Kelly KJ, et al. Successful desensitization and therapeutic use of infliximab in adult and pediatric Crohn's disease patients with prior anaphylactic reaction. Inflamm Bowel Dis 2001;7(1):34–7.

52. Lelong J, Duburque C, Fournier C, et al. [Desensitisation to infliximab in patients with Crohn's disease]. Rev Mal Respir 2005;22(2 Pt 1):239–46 [in French].

53. Duburque C, Lelong J, Iacob R, et al. Successful induction of tolerance to infliximab in patients with Crohn's disease and prior severe infusion reactions. Aliment Pharmacol Ther 2006;24(5):851–8.

54. Jerath MR, Kwan M, Kannarkat M, et al. A desensitization protocol for the mAb cetuximab. J Allergy Clin Immunol 2009;123(1):260–2.

55. Brennan PJ, Rodriguez Bouza T, Hsu FI, et al. Hypersensitivity reactions to mAbs: 105 desensitizations in 23 patients, from evaluation to treatment. J Allergy Clin Immunol 2009;124(6):1259–66.

56. Hanauer SB, Wagner CL, Bala M, et al. Incidence and importance of antibody responses to infliximab after maintenance or episodic treatment in Crohn's disease. Clin Gastroenterol Hepatol 2004;2(7):542–53.

57. Kavanaugh A, Cush J, Clair ES. Anti-TNF-alpha monoclonal antibody (mAb) treatment of rheumatoid arthritis (RA) patients with active disease on methotrexate (MTX): results of open label, repeated dose administration following a single dose double-blind, placebo controlled trial [abstract]. Arthritis Rheum 1996; 39(Suppl 9):1296.

58. Hanauer SB, Feagan BG, Lichtenstein GR, et al. Maintenance infliximab for Crohn's disease: the ACCENT I randomised trial. Lancet 2002;359(9317):1541–9.

59. Baert F, Noman M, Vermeire S, et al. Influence of immunogenicity on the long-term efficacy of infliximab in Crohn's disease. N Engl J Med 2003;348(7):601–8.

60. Sandborn WJ. Preventing antibodies to infliximab in patients with Crohn's disease: optimize not immunize. Gastroenterology 2003;124(4):1140–5.

61. Vermeire S, Noman M, Van Assche G, et al. Effectiveness of concomitant immunosuppressive therapy in suppressing the formation of antibodies to infliximab in Crohn's disease. Gut 2007;56(9):1226–31.

62. Dore RK, Mathews S, Schechtman J, et al. The immunogenicity, safety, and efficacy of etanercept liquid administered once weekly in patients with rheumatoid arthritis. Clin Exp Rheumatol 2007;25(1):40–6.

63. Weinblatt ME, Keystone EC, Furst DE, et al. Adalimumab, a fully human anti-tumor necrosis factor alpha monoclonal antibody, for the treatment of rheumatoid arthritis in patients taking concomitant methotrexate: the ARMADA trial. Arthritis Rheum 2003;48(1):35–45.

64. Vila AT, Puig L, Fernandez-Figueras MT, et al. Adverse cutaneous reactions to anakinra in patients with rheumatoid arthritis: clinicopathological study of five patients. Br J Dermatol 2005;153(2):417–23.

65. Zeltser R, Valle L, Tanck C, et al. Clinical, histological, and immunophenotypic characteristics of injection site reactions associated with etanercept: a recombinant tumor necrosis factor alpha receptor: Fc fusion protein. Arch Dermatol 2001; 137(7):893–9.

66. Winfield H, Lain E, Horn T, et al. Eosinophilic cellulitis-like reaction to subcutaneous etanercept injection. Arch Dermatol 2006;142(2):218–20.

67. Benucci M, Manfredi M, Demoly P, et al. Injection site reactions to TNF-alpha blocking agents with positive skin tests. Allergy 2008;63(1):138–9.

68. Severino M, Bonadonna P, Passalacqua G. Large local reactions from stinging insects: from epidemiology to management. Curr Opin Allergy Clin Immunol 2009;9(4):334–7.

The Complex Clinical Picture of β-Lactam Hypersensitivity: Penicillins, Cephalosporins, Monobactams, Carbapenems, and Clavams

Maria J. Torres, MD, PhD*, Miguel Blanca, MD, PhD

KEYWORDS

- β-Lactam • Skin test • Drug provocation test • Management

β-Lactam (BL) antibiotics are the most frequent elicitors of drug hypersensitivity reactions. Benzylpenicillin (BP) was the first reported BL involved, followed over the years by different penicillins and cephalosporins, with amoxicillin (AX) now being the drug most frequently inducing reactions.[1] The BLs involved in hypersensitivity will increase over the years as new compounds of this family become available. Hypersensitivity has already occurred with the new cephalosporins and also recently with clavulanic acid.[1,2]

Hypersensitivity reactions can lead to any of the 4 immunologic effector mechanisms described by Coombs and Gell (**Table 1**).[3] Type I (immediate) reactions occur less than 1 hour after drug administration and are mediated by drug-specific IgE antibodies, with the typical clinical manifestations being urticaria and anaphylaxis. Type II (cytotoxic) and type III (immunocomplex) reactions are mediated by drug-specific, complement-fixing IgG or IgM antibodies, with typical symptoms being hemolytic

This work was supported by Fondo de Invetigaciones Sanitarias (FIS)-Thematic Networks and Co-operative Research Centres: Red de Investigación de Reacciones Adversas a Alergenos y Fármacos (RD07/0064), FIS (PS09/01768) and Junta de Andalucia (PI-0243/2007).

The authors have nothing to disclose.

Allergy Service, Plaza del Hospital Civil s/n, Pabellón 5 Sótano, Carlos Haya Hospital (Pabellon C), Málaga 29009, Spain

* Corresponding author.

E-mail address: mjtorresj@gmail.com

Med Clin N Am 94 (2010) 805–820

doi:10.1016/j.mcna.2010.04.006

Immediate Reactions

Skin testing

The recommended procedure is skin testing with penicilloyl polylysine (PPL) (PRE-PEN) and with MDM consisting of BP and benzylpenilloic acid.[5] However, in countries where AX is the most important drug involved in sensitization, this determinant is also required for diagnosis.[61,62] Furthermore, when any other BL is involved in the reaction and the results of skin tests for PPL, MDM, and AX are negative, skin testing with the culprit BL, such as cephalosporin or clavulanic acid, can be done if it is available.[2,61,62]

For the procedure, it is recommended to do prick testing first, and if results are negative, the intradermal test can be performed. General procedures have been described by the European Academy of Allergy and Clinical Immunology.[61–63] Positive prick and intradermal test results are shown in **Fig. 2**, and the doses recommended for skin testing are shown in **Table 3**.

Rates of 1.3% of systemic symptoms in all tested patients and 8.8% in those with a positive skin test result and a history of anaphylaxis have been reported.[52] Consequently, precautions must be taken, particularly in severe cases, reducing the hapten concentration by as much as 1000-fold dilution, using each determinant separately in time, or even considering performing an in vitro test first.

In vitro testing

For immediate reactions, methods widely used for detecting BL-specific IgE are antibody-based immunoassays that use solid phases (agarose [Sepharose], cellulose discs), carrier molecules (human serum albumin, aliphatic spacers, or PLL), and different determinants such as BP, AX, and cephalosporins.[64,65] A commercial platform for routine analysis is the CAP System FEIA (fluorescense immunoassay) method (Phadia AB, Uppsala, Sweden), which works by a high surface-capacity solid-phase assay using a secondary fluorolabeled antibody. The specificity of this method ranges from 83.3% to 100% and the sensitivity from 12.5% to 45%, depending on the clinical manifestations.[66–68]

Another procedure being progressively used is the basophil activation test, which is based on the capacity of basophils to release histamine or to upregulate activation markers such as CD63 or CD203c after activation. How surface-bound drug-specific IgE is cross-linked if a free drug is added is not yet clear. The method has a sensitivity

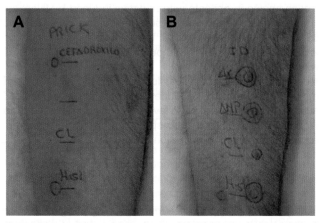

Fig. 2. Immediate skin test results positive for BL. (*A*) Prick test results positive for cefadroxil. (*B*) Intradermal test results positive for AX and AM.

Table 3
Reagents and concentrations recommended for prick and intradermal skin testing and DPT

Reagent	Skin Testing	DPT
PPL	5×10^{-5} mmol/L	Not done
MDM	2×10^{-2} mmol/L	Not done
BP	10,000 IU/mL	10^3, 10^4, 10^5, 5×10^5 IU/mL Cumulative dose (6×10^5 IU/mL)
AX	20 mg/mL	5, 50, 100, 150, 200 mg Cumulative dose (500 mg)
Ampicillin	20 mg/mL	5, 50, 100, 150, 200 mg Cumulative dose (500 mg)
Cephalosporins	2 mg/mL	5, 50, 100, 150, 200 mg Cumulative dose (500 mg)

Abbreviation: DPT, drug provocation testing.

of 48.6% and a specificity of 93%.[67,68] Both in vitro tests, although less sensitive than skin testing, have proved to be complementary, and some cases have tested negative for the skin test and positive for the in vitro test.[69]

Drug provocation testing

Drug provocation testing (DPT) can be considered for those patients who have tested negative for the skin test and in vitro test, who have no risk factors, and for whom diagnosis is mandatory.[70] In contrast to earlier investigations, where a sensitivity of 95% was found, recent research suggests the sensitivity of penicillin tests to be substantially lower, and European researchers have estimated that up to 30% of patients with immediate allergic reactions to BL will fail to be diagnosed if DPT is not done.[70,71]

The general guidelines for performing a DPT are a single-blind placebo-controlled test under strict hospital surveillance with emergency room facilities.[61,62] The drug is administered at increasing doses, with a minimum interval of 30 to 60 minutes between each administration if good tolerance is established at the previous dose, until the full therapeutic dose is reached. In patients with a history of severe reactions, this dose can be as low as 0.1 to 5 mg. The doses recommended for DPT is shown in **Table 3**.

Nonimmediate Reactions

Skin testing

Results of skin testing with immediate readings are often negative in nonimmediate reactions like many forms of exanthemas. However, this does not rule out a delayed, mainly T-cell–based reaction. Intradermal and/or patch tests with a late reading at 24 to 48 hours have usually been recommended for the diagnosis of nonimmediate reactions to BL, such as nonimmediate exanthematic reactions or delayed-appearing urticarial reactions. Some evidence indicates that the former test has a higher sensitivity, and patch testing is recommended for BLs where no preparation for parenteral use is available.[70]

Intradermal testing is done in the same way as for immediate reactions. Readings are taken at 48 and 72 hours, and any infiltrated erythema with a diameter greater than 5 mm is considered as a positive result (**Fig. 3**).[72] These reactions should be documented by the diameter of the erythema and the papulation or infiltrate, as well

In the case of nonimmediate reactions to BLs, sensitivity seems to be maintained over time, although the possibility of a decrease in the response also exists.[12,13,16,17]

DESENSITIZATION

Desensitization has been shown to be useful in BL hypersensitivity, especially in immediate reactions. Oral and parenteral protocols have been published.[79] Desensitization is indicated when a BL cannot be replaced or when a particular BL is more effective or has fewer side effects than other alternatives. Before desensitization, an accurate diagnosis needs to be done, and the benefits must outweigh the risks.

SUMMARY

The world of BLs has changed over the years, with more BLs becoming involved, although penicillin, the initial sensitizing agent, is now less involved. Other BLs are taking on a relevant role, and AX is the drug most frequently involved. Sensitization is related with patterns of consumption. The latest widely used BL reported to produce allergic reactions is clavulanic acid. Any BL can induce a hypersensitivity response. Diagnosis in immediate reactions is less sensitive than earlier because the BP molecule is not responsible for the allergic reaction and the BPO group is therefore less relevant. In addition to IgE responses such as anaphylaxis and urticaria, nonimmediate reactions occur, of which the most common are exanthematic or nonimmediate urticaria.

Improvement of diagnostic tests is based on the use of the relevant BL that induces sensitization and on the progress of research to identify the relevant proteins to which BLs are bound in the body. Allergy to these antibiotics will always exist, and as new molecules are introduced, they can be considered as putative causes of drug hypersensitivity. This assumption is related with consumption and other currently unknown genetic factors.

REFERENCES

1. Blanca M. Allergic reactions to penicillins. A changing world? Allergy 1995;50: 777–82.
2. Torres MJ, Ariza A, Mayorga C, et al. Clavulanic acid can be the component in amoxicillin-clavulanic acid responsible for immediate hypersensitivity reactions. J Allergy Clin Immunol 2010;125:502–5.
3. Coombs PR, Gell PG. Classification of allergic reactions responsible for clinical hypersensitivity and disease. In: Gell RR, editor. Clinical aspects of immunology. Oxford (UK): Oxford University Pess; 1968. p. 575–96.
4. Levine B. Immunological mechanisms of penicillin allergy. A haptenic model system for the study of allergic diseases in man. N Engl J Med 1966;275: 1115–25.
5. Weiss ME, Adkinson NF. Immediate hypersensitivity reactions to penicillin and related antibotics. Clin Allergy 1988;18:515–40.
6. Ahlstedt S. Penicillin allergy. Can the incidence be reduced? Allergy 1984;39: 151–64.
7. Rebelo-Gomes E, Demoly P. Epidemiology of hypersensitivity drug reactions. Curr Opin Allergy Clin Immunol 2005;5:309–16.
8. Idsoe O, Guthe T, Wilcox RR, et al. Nature and extent of penicillin side reactions, with particular reference to fatalities from anaphylactic shock. Bull World Health Organ 1968;38:159–88.

9. Gadde J, Spence M, Wheeler B, et al. Clinical experience with penicillin skin testing in a large inner-city STD clinic. JAMA 1993;27:2456–63.

10. Blanca M, Vega JM, García J, et al. New aspects of allergic reactions to betalactams. Cross-reactions and unique specificities. Clin Exp Allergy 1994;24:407–15.

11. Torres MJ, Mayorga C, Pamies R, et al. Immunologic response to different determinants of benzylpenicillin, amoxicillin, and ampicillin. Comparison between urticaria and anaphylactic shock. Allergy 1999;54:936–43.

12. Padial A, Antunez C, Blanca-Lopez N, et al. Non-immediate reactions to beta-lactams: diagnostic value of skin testing and drug provocation test. Clin Exp Allergy 2008;38:822–8.

13. Blanca-Lopez N, Zapatero L, Alonso E, et al. Skin testing and drug provocation tests in the diagnosis of non immediate reactions to aminopenicillins in children. Allergy 2009;64:229–33.

14. Warrington RJ, Silviu-Dan F, Magro C. Accelerated cell-mediated immune reactions in penicillin allergy. J Allergy Clin Immunol 1993;92:626–8.

15. Mayorga C, Torres MJ, Fernandez J, et al. Cutaneous symptoms in drug allergy: what have we learnt? Curr Opin Allergy Clin Immunol 2009;9:431–6.

16. Romano A, Di Fonso M, Papa G, et al. Evaluation of adverse cutaneous reactions to aminopenicillins with emphasis on those manifested by maculopapular rashes. Allergy 1995;50:113–8.

17. Terrados S, Blanca M, Garcia J, et al. Non-immediate reactions to betalactams: prevalence and role of the different penicillins. Allergy 1995;50:563–7.

18. Doña I, Chaves P, Gómez E, et al. Drug rash with eosinophilia and systemic symptoms after penicillin V administration in a patient with acquired C1 inhibitor acquired deficiency. J Investig Allergol Clin Immunol 2009;19:325–7.

19. Liberopoulos EN, Liamis GL, Elisaf MS. Possible cefotaxime-induced Stevens-Johnson syndrome. Ann Pharmacother 2003;37:812–4.

20. Saenz de San Pedro Morera B, Enriquez JQ, López JF. Fixed drug eruptions due to betalactams and other chemically unrelated antibiotics. Contact Dermatitis 1999;40:220–1.

21. Clark BM, Kotti GH, Shah AD, et al. Severe serum sickness reaction to oral and intramuscular penicillin. Pharmacotherapy 2006;26:705–8.

22. Arndt PA. Practical aspects of investigating drug-induced immune haemolytic anemia due to cefotetan or ceftriaxone-a case study approach. Immunohematology 2002;18:27–32.

23. Leger RM, Arndt PA, Garratty G. Serological studies of piperacillin antibodies. Transfusion 2008;48:2429–34.

24. Arndt PA, Garratty G. The changing spectrum of drug-induced immune hemolytic anemia. Semin Hematol 2005;42:137–44.

25. Olaison L, Belin L, Hogevik H, et al. Incidence of beta-lactam-induced delayed hypersensitivity and neutropenia during treatment of infective endocarditis. Arch Intern Med 1999;159:607–15.

26. Gielen K, Goosens A. Occupational allergic contact dermatitis from drug healthy healthcare workers. Contact Dermatitis 2001;45:273–9.

27. Stricker BH, Van den Broek JW, Keuning J, et al. Cholestatic hepatitis due to antibacterial combination of amoxicillin and clavulanic acid (augmentin). Dig Dis Sci 1989;34:1576–80.

28. Andrews E, Daly AK. Flucloxacillin-induced liver injury. Toxicology 2008;254:158–63.

29. Castell JV, Castell M. Allergic hepatitis induced by drugs. Curr Opin Allergy Clin Immunol 2006;6:258–65.

30. Gresser U. Amoxicillin-clavulanic acid therapy may be associated with severe side effects—review of the literature. Eur J Med Res 2001;6:139–49.
31. Daly AK, Donaldson PT, Bhatnagar P, et al. HLA-B*5701 genotype is a major determinant of drug-induced liver injury due to flucloxacillin. Nat Genet 2009; 41:816–9.
32. Spanou Z, Keller M, Britschgi M, et al. Involvement of drug-specific T cells in acute drug-induced interstitial nephritis. J Am Soc Nephrol 2006;17:2919–27.
33. Sammett D, Greben C, Sayeed-Shah U. Acute pancreatitis caused by penicillin. Dig Dis Sci 1998;43:1778–83.
34. Yonemaru M, Mizuguchi Y, Kasuga I, et al. Hilar and mediastinal lymphadenopathy with hypersensitivity pneumonitis induced by penicillin. Chest 1992;102: 1907–9.
35. Burke AP, Saenger J, Mullick F, et al. Hypersensitivity myocarditis. Arch Pathol Lab Med 1991;115:764–9.
36. Levine BB, Ovary Z. Studies of the mechanism of the formation of the penicillin antigen. III. The N-(D-alpha-benzylpenicilloyl) group as an antigenic determinant responsible for hypersensitivity to penicillin G. J Exp Med 1961;114:875–904.
37. Dewdney JM. Immunology of the antibiotics. In: Sela M, editor, The antigens, vol. 4. New York: Academic Press; 1977. p. 114–22.
38. Warbrick EV, Thomas AL, Stejkal V, et al. An analysis of betalactam derived antigens on spleen cells and serum proteins by ELISA and Western blotting. Allergy 1995;50:910–7.
39. Adkinson NF Jr, Thompson WL, Maddrey WC, et al. Routine use of penicillin skin testing on an inpatient service. N Engl J Med 1971;285:22–4.
40. Parker CW, de Weck AL, Shapiro J, et al. The preparation and some properties of penicillenic acid derivatives relevant to penicillin hypersensitivity. J Exp Med 1962;115:803–19.
41. Levine BB, Redmond AP. Minor haptenic determinant specific reagins of penicillin hypersensitivity in man. Int Arch Allergy Appl Immunol 1969;35:445–55.
42. Perez-Inestrosa E, Suau R, Montañez MI, et al. Cephalosporin chemical reactivity and its immunological implications. Curr Opin Allergy Clin Immunol 2005;5:323–30.
43. Romano A, Mayorga C, Torres MJ, et al. Immediate allergic reactions to cephalosporins: cross-reactivity and selective responses. J Allergy Clin Immunol 2000;106:1177–83.
44. Antúnez C, Blanca-López N, Torres MJ, et al. Immediate allergic reactions to cephalosporins: evaluation of cross-reactivity with a panel of penicillins and cephalosporins. J Allergy Clin Immunol 2006;117:404–10.
45. De Haan P, Jonge AJ, Verbrugge E, et al. Three epitope-specific monoclonal antibodies against the hapten penicillin. Int Arch Allergy Appl Immunol 1985;76: 42–6.
46. Mayorga C, Obispo T, Jimeno L, et al. Epitope mapping of betalactam antibiotics with the use of monoclonal antibodies. Toxicology 1995;97:225–34.
47. Nagakura N, Souma S, Shimizu T, et al. Antiampicillin monoclonal antibodies and their cross-reactivities to various ß-lactams. J Antimicrob Chemother 1991;28: 357–68.
48. Nagakura N, Shimizu T, Masuzawa T, et al. Anti-cephalexin monoclonal antibodies and their cross-reactivities to cephems and penams. Int Arch Allergy Appl Immunol 1990;93:126–32.
49. Shimizu T, Souma S, Nagakura N, et al. Epitope analysis of aztreonam by antiaztreonam monoclonal antibodies and possible consequences in beta-lactams hypersensitivity. Int Arch Allergy Immunol 1992;98:392–7.

50. Moreno F, Blanca M, Mayorga C, et al. Studies of the specificities of IgE anti-bodies found in sera from subjects with allergic reactions to penicillins. Int Arch Allergy Appl Immunol 1995;108:74–81.
51. Blanca M, Garcia J, Vega JM, et al. Anaphylaxis to penicillins after non-thera-peutic exposure: an immunological investigation. Clin Exp Allergy 1996;26: 335–40.
52. Co Minh HB, Bousquet PJ, Fontaine C, et al. Systemic reactions during skin tests with betalactams: a risk factor analysis. J Allergy Clin Immunol 2006; 117:466–8.
53. Antúnez C, Fernández T, Blanca-Lopez N, et al. IgE antibodies to betalactams: relationship between the triggering hapten and the specificity of the immune response. Allergy 2006;61:940–6.
54. Blanca M, Torres MJ, García JJ, et al. Natural evolution of skin test sensitivity in patients allergic to beta-lactam antibiotics. J Allergy Clin Immunol 1999;103: 918–24.
55. Fernández TD, Torres MJ, Blanca-López N, et al. Negativization rates of IgE radioimmunoassay and basophil activation test in immediate reactions to penicil-lins. Allergy 2009;64:242–8.
56. Pichler WJ, Schnyder B, Zanni M, et al. Role of T cells in drug allergies. Allergy 1998;53:225–32.
57. Pichler WJ. Delayed drug hypersensitivity reactions. Ann Intern Med 2003;39: 683–93.
58. Rozieres A, Vocanson M, Saïd BB, et al. Role of T cells in nonimmediate allergic drug reactions. Curr Opin Allergy Clin Immunol 2009;9:305–10.
59. Torres MJ, Sanchez-Sabate E, Alvarez J, et al. Skin test evaluation in non-imme-diate allergic reactions to penicillins. Allergy 2004;59:219–24.
60. Carey MA, van Pelt FN. Immunochemical detection of flucloxacillin adducts formation in livers of treated rats. Toxicology 2005;216:41–8.
61. Blanca M, Romano A, Torres MJ, et al. Update on the evaluation of hypersensi-tivity reactions to betalactams. Allergy 2009;64:183–93.
62. Torres MJ, Blanca M, de Weck A, et al. Diagnosis of immediate allergic reactions to betalactam antibiotics. Allergy 2003;58:854–63.
63. Brockow K, Romano A, Blanca M, et al. General considerations for skin test procedures in the diagnosis of drug hypersensitivity. Allergy 2002;57:45–51.
64. Blanca M, Mayorga C, Perez E, et al. Determination of IgE antibodies to the ben-zylpenicilloyl determinant. A comparison between poly-L-lysine and human serum albumin as carriers. J Immunol Methods 1992;153:99–105.
65. Garcia JJ, Blanca M, Moreno F, et al. Determination of IgE antibodies to the ben-zylpenicilloyl determinant: a comparison of the sensitivity and specificity of three radio allergo sorbent test methods. J Clin Lab Anal 1997;11:251–7.
66. Blanca M, Mayorga C, Torres MJ, et al. Clinical evaluation of Pharmacia CAP System RAST FEIA amoxicilloyl and benzylpenicilloyl in patients with penicillin allergy. Allergy 2001;56:862–70.
67. Torres MJ, Padial A, Mayorga C, et al. The diagnostic interpretation of basophil activation test in immediate allergic reactions to betalactams. Clin Exp Allergy 2004;34:1768–75.
68. Sanz ML, Gamboa PM, Antepara I, et al. Flow cytometric basophil activation test by detection of CD63 expression in patients with immediate-type reactions to be-talactam antibiotics. Clin Exp Allergy 2002;32:277–86.
69. Torres MJ, Mayorga C, Cornejo-García JA, et al. IgE antibodies to penicillin in skin test negative patients. Allergy 2002;57:965.

70. Bousquet PJ, Pipet A, Bousquet-Rouanet L, et al. Oral challenges are needed in the diagnosis of beta-lactam hypersensitivity. Clin Exp Allergy 2008;38:185–90.
71. Torres MJ, Romano A, Mayorga C, et al. Diagnostic evaluation of a large group of patients with immediate allergy to penicillins: the role of skin testing. Allergy 2001; 56:850–6.
72. Romano A, Blanca M, Torres MJ, et al. Diagnosis of nonimmediate reactions to beta-lactam antibiotics. Allergy 2004;59:1153–60.
73. Nyfeler B, Pichler WJ. The lymphocyte transformation test for the diagnosis of drug allergy: sensitivity and specificity. Clin Exp Allergy 1997;27:175–81.
74. Luque I, Leyva L, Torres MJ, et al. In vitro T lymphocyte responses to betalactam drugs in immediate and nonimmediate allergic reactions. Allergy 2001;56:611–8.
75. Romano A, Gueant-Rodriguez RM, Viola M, et al. Cross-reactivity and tolerability of cephalosporins in patients with immediate hypersensitivity to penicillins. Ann Intern Med 2004;141:16–22.
76. Miranda A, Blanca M, Vega JM, et al. Cross-reactivity between a penicillin and a cephalosporin with the same side chain. J Allergy Clin Immunol 1996;98:671–7.
77. Romano A, Viola M, Gueant-Rodriguez RM, et al. Imipenem in patients with immediate hypersensitivity to penicillins. N Engl J Med 2006;354:2835–7.
78. Vega JM, Blanca M, García JJ, et al. Tolerance to aztreonam in patients allergic to beta-lactam antibiotics. Allergy 1991;46:196–202.
79. Castells M. Rapid desensitization for hypersensitivity reactions to medications. Immunol Allergy Clin North Am 2009;29:585–606.

The Complex Clinical Picture of Side Effects to Anticoagulation

Axel Trautmann, MD[a],*, Cornelia S. Seitz, MD[b]

KEYWORDS

- Adverse drug reaction • Coumarin • Heparin
- Hypersensitivity • Skin necrosis • Thrombocytopenia

Antithrombotics are used to prevent intravasal thrombus formation or dissolve blood clots by influencing the coagulation cascade, thrombolysis, or thrombocyte function. Accordingly, 3 main groups of substances are differentiated: anticoagulants (inhibiting fibrin formation), thrombolytic drugs (dissolving fibrin), and thrombocyte aggregation inhibitors.

Anticoagulants are used for prophylaxis and therapy for thromboembolic complications. According to the mechanism of action, direct anticoagulants interacting directly with coagulation factors such as heparins, heparinoids, hirudins, and thrombin inhibitors are distinguished from indirect anticoagulants, which interfere with the synthesis of clotting factors (vitamin K antagonists). Side effects of anticoagulants may be caused by predictable pharmacologic effects (type A reactions, a = augmented) or be caused by unpredictable events such as immune reactions and individual disposition (type B reactions, b = bizarre) (**Fig. 1**). Heparin is still the most commonly used anticoagulant for hospitalized patients but its usage has also increased in outpatient settings.[1] Cost pressure on hospitals has led to earlier discharge of patients or ambulatory surgeries so that side effects of heparin treatment are nowadays increasingly observed in outpatients.

Following a summary of the coagulation physiology and common anticoagulant drugs, the focus of this review is on the clinical appearance, diagnostics, and therapy for anticoagulant-induced type B reactions.

PHARMACOLOGY OF COAGULATION

According to current knowledge, blood coagulation does not simply consist of 2 converging cascades (intrinsic and extrinsic pathways) as previously believed but

There are no conflicts of interest and no funding.
[a] Allergy Unit, Department of Dermatology, Venereology, and Allergology, University of Würzburg, Josef Schneider Strasse 2, 97080 Würzburg, Germany
[b] Department of Dermatology, Venereology, and Allergology, University of Göttingen, Von Siebold Strasse 3, 37075 Göttingen, Germany
* Corresponding author.
E-mail address: trautmann_a@klinik.uni-wuerzburg.de

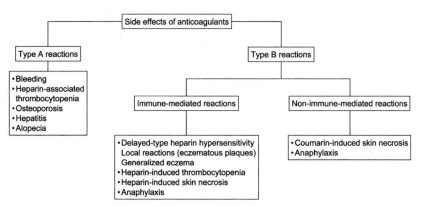

Fig. 1. Type A and type B reactions to anticoagulants.

rather is a chronology of 3 coagulation phases.[2] (1) In the initiation phase, injury of the endothelium leads to interaction of circulating active factor VII (FVIIa) with an endothelial cell-bound transmembrane glycoprotein (tissue factor [TF]) with formation of a catalytic complex (FVIIa/TF). This FVIIa/TF complex activates FX to FXa resulting in the production of small amounts of thrombin (FIIa). (2) In the amplification phase, thrombin itself promotes molecular and cellular changes for generation of greater thrombin amounts. (3) In the following propagation phase, thrombin efficiently binds to the surface of activated thrombocytes, which is followed by fibrin polymerization and development of stable fibrin clots.

Pharmacologic interference of coagulation principally aims to inhibit thrombin (FIIa), which is the key molecule of homeostasis. This aim may be achieved by interference with all coagulation phases or by inhibition of single clotting factors.[3]

Heparin

Heparins are naturally occurring polysaccharides that contain multiple carboxyl and sulfate groups. Their anticoagulation capacity depends on the anionic charge of these carboxyl and sulfate groups. High molecular weight and negative charge prevent resorption after oral administration and therefore parenteral application of heparins is mandatory. The crucial mechanism of action is the activation of antithrombin by binding to a specific pentasaccharide sequence of the heparin polymer.[4] For thrombin inhibition it is essential that the heparin polymer consists of at least 18 monomers allowing formation of a complex of heparin, antithrombin, and thrombin. For inhibition of FXa only the pentasaccharide sequence is necessary. Therefore, unfractionated heparin (UFH) inhibits thrombin and FXa, whereas low-molecular-weight heparin (LMWH) exerts its anticoagulation effect mainly by blockade of FXa.

UFH

Pharmaceutical heparin preparations are extracted from porcine intestinal mucosa. During processing they are partially fractionated and depolymerized.[5] Therefore, UFH preparations are not pure substances but a composite of heterogeneous molecules varying in size and chemical structure. For this reason, the dose of UFH is not recorded in milligrams but in international units (IU). The average molecular weight of UFH is 15 kDa corresponding to 40 to 50 monomers. Generally, long-chain heparins are eliminated faster than short-chain heparins. In addition, only 30% to 40% of UFH contain the specific pentasaccharide sequence that is responsible for the anticoagulant effect, which makes it is difficult to exactly predict the influence on coagulation and makes monitoring mandatory. Like other anionic polysaccharides, UFH unspecifically binds to plasma and tissue macromolecules resulting in bioavailability of 15% to 30% after subcutaneous application.

LMWH

Controlled extensive fractionation of native heparin leads to LMWH with an average molecular weight of 4 to 6 kDa corresponding to 13 to 22 monomers.[6,7] Available LMWH such as enoxaparin (4.2 kDa), reviparin (3.9 kDa), dalteparin (6.1 kDa), nadroparin (5.5 kDa), tinzaparin (4.5 kDa), and certoparin (6 kDa) have a significantly decreased unspecific binding capacity resulting in almost 100% bioavailability after subcutaneous application. The relative fraction of the relevant pentasaccharide sequence is higher compared with UFH, the anticoagulant effect is therefore better predictable, and monitoring is only indicated in patients with renal insufficiency.

Fondaparinux

Fondaparinux (1.7 kDa) is a chemically synthesized sulfated pentasaccharide specifically inhibiting FXa.[8] In contrast to heparins and heparinoids, fondaparinux is a chemically defined molecule without unspecific binding characteristics and with fast and complete resorption after subcutaneous injection (100% bioavailability).

Heparinoids

Heparinoids are sulfated polysaccharides with antithrombotic effects similar to heparins. Danaparoid (average molecular weight 6 kDa) is a mixture of heparan sulfate (84%), dermatan sulfate (12%), and chondroitin sulfate (4%). Pentosan polysulfate (average molecular weight 6 kDa) is a semi-synthetically produced polysaccharide, derived from pentosan extracted from the bark of the beech tree. Although pentosan polysulfate is approved for thrombosis prophylaxis, it is not mentioned in international treatment guidelines.[7]

Hirudins

Hirudins are polypeptides originally extracted from the leech *Hirudo medicinalis* and function as direct thrombin inhibitors without affecting antithrombin.[9] There are multiple hirudin variants (average molecule weight 7 kDa). Recently, recombinant hirudins and hirudin variants such as lepirudin, desirudin, and bivalirudin were approved as antithrombotic substances. Lepirudin is indicated for the treatment of thromboembolic complications and heparin-induced thrombocytopenia (HIT).[10] In Germany, desirudin and bivalirudin are only approved for limited indications: desirudin is approved for prophylaxis of deep vein thrombosis after hip and knee replacement surgeries, and bivalirudin is indicated as an anticoagulant in patients undergoing percutaneous coronary intervention.

Synthetic Direct Thrombin Inhibitors

Argatroban is a direct thrombin inhibitor, approved for parenteral anticoagulation of adults with HIT. Dabigatran and rivaroxaban are orally active thrombin inhibitors approved for prophylaxis of deep vein thrombosis after total hip and total knee arthroplasty.[11] The main reason for these application limits is the relatively narrow therapeutic index of these drugs.

Vitamin K Antagonists

Vitamin K antagonists (phenprocoumon, warfarin, and acenocoumarol) are widely used for long-term primary and secondary prevention of thromboembolic disorders.

These highly effective anticoagulants lead to inhibition of vitamin K-dependent coagulation factors (ie, FII, FVII, FIX, FX).[12] They are administered orally, metabolized by hepatic cytochrome enzymes (mainly isoform CYP2C9) and excreted as inactive metabolites into the bile. Disadvantages of vitamin K antagonists include delayed onset of action, narrow therapeutic index (bleeding complications) as well as numerous interactions with drugs and foods.

In summary, despite some progress, the therapeutic options for anticoagulation remain unsatisfactory. Compared with UFH, LMWH have several advantages but are chemically not clearly defined, act antithrombin-dependently, and have to be applied parenterally. Because of lack of antidotes for neutralization, application of direct thrombin inhibitors is always associated with increased risk of bleeding complications. Therefore, despite the development and approval of these new anticoagulants (direct thrombin inhibitors, FXa inhibitors), heparin remains the medication of first choice especially for intravenous anticoagulation.[13] Current development of new anticoagulants is based on the improved understanding of coagulation physiology and is dominated by the search for orally active direct anticoagulants.[3,14]

DELAYED-TYPE HEPARIN HYPERSENSITIVITY

In case of DTH to subcutaneously injected heparins, itchy erythematous or eczematous plaques develop around injection sites (**Fig. 2**A).[15–20] The usual latency for development of characteristic lesions during ongoing therapy is 7 to 10 days; in cases of previous sensitization and re-exposure, skin lesions appear within 1 to 3 days. The spectrum of skin lesions ranges from mild erythema with little infiltration to typical eczematous plaques with papulovesicles located on an infiltrated erythematous

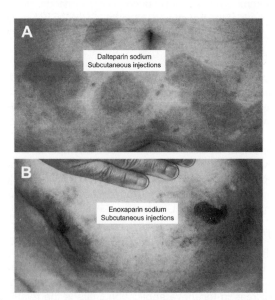

Fig. 2. DTH to subcutaneously applied heparins and heparin-induced skin necrosis. (*A*) Itchy erythematous and eczematous plaques 12 days after initiation of subcutaneously applied dalteparin. (*B*) Painful heparin-induced skin necrosis at injection sites 10 days after initiation of subcutaneous enoxaparin injections. (*Reproduced from* Gaigl Z, Klein CE, Großmann R et al. [Managing allergy to heparins]. Dtsch Arztebl 2006;103:2878 [in German]; with permission.)

ground. Less frequently, in cases with continuation of subcutaneous injections despite local reactions, a generalized eczema or exanthema with accentuation around injection sites may be observed.[21–25] In early erythematous lesions, histopathologic examination reveals a dense mononuclear infiltrate of predominantly $CD4^+$ lymphocytes with scattered eosinophils. Eczematous lesions additionally show epidermal spongiosis.[15,18,22,26] These findings are consistent with an immunologically mediated DTH reaction of the skin. However, potential antigenic determinants of the heparin molecule have not yet been determined. DTH reactions to subcutaneously injected heparin are mostly described in obese women.[27,28] Therefore, gender and obesity seem to be risk factors for the development of DTH to heparin. It is tempting to speculate that hormonal and metabolic influences may play a role in the pathogenesis.[29]

The differential diagnosis of erythematous and eczematous plaques after subcutaneous heparin administration includes hematomas, local infections, and eczema caused by skin disinfectants.[30] However, the most important differential diagnosis is heparin-induced skin necrosis (**Table 1**).[30,31] In most cases the allergologist does not see the lesions and the presumptive diagnosis relies on the description by referring physicians or patients. Moreover, nondermatologists and/or nonallergologists may confuse the clinically distinct signs of skin necrosis, that is, redness of the skin is assumed to be the same as eczema or dermatitis.

Allergologic Testing

Patients with suspected DTH to heparins should be subjected to an allergologic workup including skin tests and subcutaneous challenge tests. In cases in whom DTH to heparins is verified, intravenous challenge tests should be done (**Fig. 3**). The

Table 1
Comparison of heparin-induced DTH and HIT-associated skin necrosis

	DTH	HIT
Incidence	1%–5%	UFH: up to 3% LMWH: <0.1%
Latency	7–10 days (sensitization) 1–3 days (re-exposure)	5–14 d (sensitization) 3–5 d (re-exposure within 100 d)
Symptoms	Itching	Pain
Gross appearance	Erythema, plaque, eczema (dermatitis)	Necrosis, hemorrhagic rim
Histology	Dermal mononuclear infiltrate of lymphocytes, spongiosis	Thrombosis of skin vessels without signs of vasculitis
Associated features	None	Thromboembolic complications (white-clot syndrome)
Prognosis	Good	Poor, if thromboembolism occurs
Pathogenesis	T cell–mediated allergic hypersensitivity	Immune complexes composed of heparin, platelet factor 4, and specific IgG antibodies activating thrombocytes
Allergologic testing	Skin test, s.c. provocation, i.v. provocation	Contraindicated
Recommendations	Fondaparinux s.c. Heparin i.v. Topical steroids	Danaparoid, hirudins Re-exposure to heparins has to be avoided

Abbreviations: i.v., intravenous; s.c., subcutaneous.

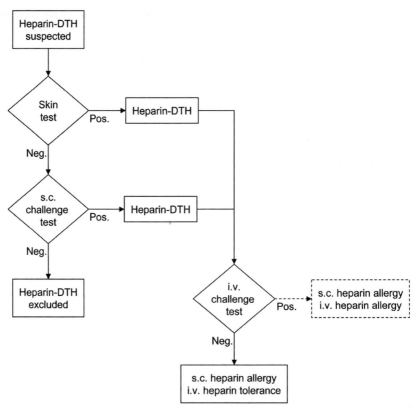

Fig. 3. Recommended steps of the allergologic workup in patients with a history of DTH to subcutaneously injected heparins. Diagnosis in case of a positive intravenous challenge test is depicted in dotted lines because this has not occurred in our studies where all patients tolerated intravenous challenge tests. i.v., intravenous; s.c., subcutaneous. (*Reproduced from* Trautmann A, Seitz CS. Heparin allergy: delayed-type non-IgE-mediated allergic hypersensitivity to subcutaneous heparin injection. Immunol Allergy Clin N Am 2009;29:473; with permission.)

authors perform intradermal tests on the volar forearm and patch tests on the upper back with a panel of heparin and heparinoid preparations, including an UFH, as well as LMWHs (nadroparin, dalteparin, and enoxaparin), heparinoids (danaparoid and pentosan polysulfate), and fondaparinux. Allergologic testing of patients with a panel of different heparin preparations reveals cross-reactivity among heparins and excludes a causal role of the preservatives sometimes added to heparin multidose products, such as sodium metabisulfite, benzyl alcohol, or chlorocresol. However, most single-dose heparin products contain salts, acids, or bases for pH adjustment, but no preservatives. As a rule, multiple positive reactions throughout the test panel of UFHs and LMWHs do reflect extensive cross-reactivity. Single negative skin test reactions are usually false-negative and subsequent subcutaneous challenge proves cross-reactivity.

Immediate-type reactions may be observed in approximately 10% of intradermal tests despite the 1:10 dilution of heparin solutions. These immediate wheal-and-flare responses are mainly caused by histamine liberation and contamination of the heparin preparation and should therefore not be interpreted naively as proof of an IgE-mediated allergy. These unspecific histamine-mediated reactions may be discriminated from extremely rare allergic reactions by negative intradermal tests with further dilutions (1:100, 1:1000), whereas true allergic reactions still produce positive skin test results with these lower concentrations. Anaphylaxis symptoms and/or immediate-type skin test reactions may also be caused by accidental or deliberate contaminants (eg, oversulfated chondroitin sulfate [OSCS]) during the processing of heparins.[32–34]

Subcutaneous Allergy and Intravenous Tolerance

In cases of DTH to subcutaneously injected heparin, intravenous application of this drug theoretically implies the risk of a generalized eczematous reaction. However, evidence that intravenous administration of heparin is tolerated despite DTH was previously observed in single patients.[35–38] In 2 prospective studies, the authors showed that intravenous administration of heparin was well tolerated without side effects in 64 patients who developed eczema-like infiltrated plaques after subcutaneous injection of heparin.[28,39] Therefore, intravenous application of heparin is a safe alternative for anticoagulation in these patients. Furthermore, in cases of therapeutic necessity, the shift from subcutaneous to intravenous heparin administration without previous tests may be justified even in cases with generalized eczema.[22]

Currently it is unknown why some patients develop an immune reaction after subcutaneous application of UFH and LMWH, but still tolerate intravenous administration of UFH. Eczematous plaques after subcutaneously injected heparins are likely real DTH, caused by heparin-specific T lymphocytes. Subtle differences in the absorption of heparin from the skin and differential processing/presentation of antigens depending on the route of application may be responsible factors.

Cross-reactivity and Alternative Anticoagulation

Typical for DTH against subcutaneously administered heparins is the extensive cross-reactivity among all UFH and LMWH. Potential alternative antithrombotic compounds are the heparinoids, danaparoid and pentosan polysulfate.[40] Heparinoids were initially developed as alternatives in case of antibody-mediated HIT. Although danaparoid shows a low cross-reactivity with heparin in terms of heparin-induced antibody binding, it often cross reacts with heparin in case of DTH. Tolerance of a single subcutaneous challenge test should not be over interpreted. Several of our patients developed eczematous plaques around injection sites despite an initial negative subcutaneous challenge test to heparinoids after a longer anticoagulation period and increasing number of heparinoid injections. As already suggested by the chemical structure, cross-reactivity between heparinoids and heparins is common.[26]

Fondaparinux has been considered as a potential alternative anticoagulant compound.[41,42] However, in 1 of our studies we observed positive skin tests with fondaparinux in 6 out of 16 patients with DTH to subcutaneously applied heparins. Meanwhile several studies confirmed that only up to 50% of patients with DTH to subcutaneous heparins tolerate fondaparinux.[43–46] This is not surprising because fondaparinux is an anionic polysaccharide like heparin and therefore cross-reactivity may develop after continued anticoagulation for a longer period of time despite initial tolerance of the compound in skin and subcutaneous challenge tests.

HIT

Nonimmune-mediated thrombocytopenia is a common side effect of heparin treatment, occurring in up to 25% of patients. It is clinically characterized by a minor decrease of thrombocytes (<30%) within the first 2 days of treatment.[47] In cases of nonimmune-mediated heparin-associated thrombocytopenia, the highly negatively charged polysaccharide heparin binds unspecifically to positively charged proteins on thrombocytes leading to a moderate decrease of thrombocytes.[48] With continued heparin application, the thrombocyte count spontaneously normalizes in these patients. In contrast, immune-mediated HIT is caused by heparin-induced antibodies that activate thrombocytes leading to a prothrombotic condition. This results in thrombocytopenia and increased thrombin generation with risk for venous and arterial thromboembolism.

HIT is the most common serious immune-mediated side effect of heparin treatment.[49] Clinical symptoms and laboratory data are crucial for diagnosis. The usual latency for development of characteristic symptoms during ongoing therapy is 5 to 14 days; in cases of prior sensitization (exposure to heparins within the past 100 days) and re-exposure, symptoms appear within 3 to 5 days. Functional assays (serotonin-release test, platelet activation test) and antigen assays (ELISA) may confirm the clinical diagnosis of HIT.[50]

Patients undergoing hip arthroplasty and thoracic or coronary artery bypass surgery have a risk of 2.5% to 3% for developing HIT. UFH have a 10-fold risk of HIT compared with LMWH.[51] Immune complexes composed of heparin, platelet factor 4, and specific antibodies activate thrombocytes and induce the characteristic decline of thrombocytes of more than 50% or a decrease to less than 100,000/μL. In case of HIT, thromboembolic complications occur despite thrombocytopenia as deep vein thrombosis and pulmonary embolism or arterial thrombosis leading to ischemia of extremities, cerebrovascular insult, or myocardial infarction (thrombi consist mostly of platelets and fibrin, the so-called white-clot syndrome). Arterial embolisms are often the result of the false diagnosis of thrombosis despite anticoagulation with subsequent increase of heparin dosage.

Heparin-induced skin necrosis is the cutaneous manifestation of HIT.[52–55] Typically a painful, mildly infiltrated erythema is followed by a central bullous and necrotic area surrounded by a hemorrhagic rim (see **Fig. 2**B). Skin necrosis developing only at the sites of subcutaneous injection is interpreted as a local manifestation of HIT. However, skin necrosis is not restricted to heparin application sites but may also occur at distant sites with a predilection for locations with increased subcutaneous fat tissue such as mammae, abdomen, buttock, and thighs.[56] Skin biopsies of lesions show thrombosis of skin vessels without signs of vasculitis. In cases of suspected HIT, immediate discontinuation of heparin treatment is required and alternative compounds such as danaparoid or hirudins are indicated for treatment of thromboembolic complications.[57,58] Re-exposure to heparins has to be strictly avoided in the future.

Only patients who have received heparin within the past 100 days are at risk of a rapid onset of HIT (<5 days). In life-threatening situations, for example, open heart surgery requiring cardiopulmonary bypass, patients with a history of HIT longer than 100 days may be exposed to heparin during surgery provided that no circulating HIT antibodies are detectable and pre- and postoperative heparin application is strictly avoided.[59,60] With this approach, bleeding complications from alternative anticoagulants (hirudins, danaparoid) without known antidotes during surgery requiring cardiopulmonary bypass may be avoided.[61,62]

ANAPHYLAXIS

Anaphylaxis, a severe, generalized, or systemic hypersensitivity reaction is subclassified as allergic anaphylaxis when the reaction is mediated by an immunologic mechanism, or nonallergic anaphylaxis of whatever nonimmunologic cause (formerly anaphylactoid reaction). Evidence for IgE- or IgG-mediated allergic anaphylaxis to anticoagulants such as heparin and lepirudin is rarely reported in the literature. One case report suggests IgE-mediated allergy to subcutaneously administered dalte-parin.[63] Such reactions to heparin preparations were also attributed to preservatives and protein contaminants of animal origin during the production process.[64] Minutes after initiation of intravenous lepirudin application, anaphylactic reactions with erythema, urticaria, angioedema, bronchospasm, laryngeal edema, hypotension, shock, and cardiorespiratory arrest were described. In 2 patients with anaphylaxis symptoms, lepirudin-specific IgG antibodies could be detected.[65–67]

On the other hand, symptoms of nonallergic anaphylaxis may be caused by direct histamine release from mast cells and basophils by nonspecific binding of contaminants on membrane receptors or indirectly by complement/kinin activation. At the beginning of 2008 the Centers for Disease Control and Prevention registered a cluster of heparin-associated anaphylaxis reactions. Among patients receiving UFH during hemodialysis, reactions included dyspnoea, facial edema, urticaria, nausea or vomiting, tachycardia and hypotension, and life-threatening shock. In test samples of 1 heparin manufacturer, spectroscopy identified OSCS as well as dermatan sulfate, a known contaminant of heparin.[32] Although chondroitin sulfate is a natural substance derived from animal cartilage, its oversulfated form (OSCS) does not occur naturally. OSCS exerts its effects by activation of the kinin-kallikrein system leading to generation of bradykinin, and activation of C3a and C5a, which are potent anaphylatoxins.[34,68] The contaminated heparin could be traced back to China, where heparins are regularly processed by small, often unregistered plants. However, until now, it was not clear where the contamination occurred.

COUMARIN-INDUCED SKIN NECROSIS

Coumarin-induced skin necrosis is a rare (0.01%–0.1% of treated patients) complication of anticoagulant therapy with coumarin and its derivatives (phenprocoumon, warfarin/coumadin, and acenocoumarol) associated with significant morbidity and even mortality.[69–71] Predilection sites of coumarin necrosis are areas of increased subcutaneous fat tissue such as breasts, abdomen, thighs, and buttocks.[72] Typically, coumarin-induced skin necrosis develops in middle-aged women symmetrically within the first week of coumarin therapy (range 1–10 days); severe lesions appear between the third and sixth day. The first symptoms of coumarin-induced skin necrosis are paresthesia and circumscribed, livedo-like livid maculae coalescing into large hemorrhagic lesions with secondary blister formation. Within days these skin lesions become necrotic and deep painful ulcerations develop.

Coumarin-induced skin necrosis may occur because of a hereditary defect or in patients with acquired and transient protein C and/or S deficiency.[73,74] Chronic liver disease, chronic renal failure and dialysis, acute leukemia, autoimmune diseases (lupus, antiphospholipid syndrome), infections (Epstein-Barr virus), acute respiratory distress syndrome, and plasmapheresis are all conditions with acquired protein C deficiency. Coumarin not only inhibits the synthesis and functional activity of the vitamin K-dependent clotting factors FII, FVII, FIX and FX but it also inhibits the anti-coagulant proteins C and S. Protein C is an endogenous vitamin K-dependent anticoagulant, which decreases at the initiation of coumarin therapy faster (6–8 hours) than other coagulation factors (2–5 days). Especially in patients with protein C deficiency or initial high doses of coumarins, this disequilibrium results in temporary hypercoagulability leading to thrombotic occlusions of the microvasculature with consecutive skin necrosis. Coumarin necrosis is a severe but self-limiting local complication that slowly

Table 2
Comparison of heparin- and coumarin-induced skin necrosis

	Heparin-induced Skin Necrosis	Coumarin-induced Skin Necrosis
Latency	5–14 d (sensitization) 3–5 d (re-exposure within 100 d)	1–10 d
Gross appearance	Indistinguishable	
Histology	Indistinguishable	
Associated features	Thrombocytopenia Arterial and venous thromboembolic complications	None
Effect of continuing drug	Fatal thromboembolic complications New skin necrosis, extension of current skin necrosis	Lesions do not progress
Need to stop anticoagulant	Yes	No

Data from Yates P, Jones S. Heparin skin necrosis – an important indicator of potentially fatal heparin hypersensitivity. Clin Exp Dermatol 1993;18:140.

resolves within several weeks but sometimes requires surgical debridement. Replacement therapy with recombinant protein C concentrate seems to block progression of the lesions and enhances healing.[69] After prompt withdrawal of coumarin it is recommended to start heparin treatment immediately. Reintroduction of coumarin should only be performed with caution starting with low doses and only gradually increasing the dose.[75] Heparin may be discontinued 3 days after reaching the therapeutic level of coumarin.

Differential diagnoses of coumarin-induced skin necrosis including calciphylaxis, microembolization (septic emboli, cholesterol emboli), heparin-induced skin necrosis, disseminated intravascular coagulation, necrotizing fasciitis and cryoglobulinemia, were recently reviewed in detail.[71] The gross appearance of the lesions and the histology of coumarin-induced and heparin-induced skin necrosis are identical. However, there are some differences between the 2 conditions that are summarized in **Table 2**. In coumarin-induced skin necrosis, therapy can be continued or restarted at a lower dose, but heparin-induced skin necrosis should lead to the immediate cessation of the drug.

REFERENCES

1. Hirsh J, Raschke R. Heparin and low-molecular-weight heparin: the seventh ACCP conference on antithrombotic and thrombolytic therapy. Chest 2004;126: 188–203.
2. Monroe DM, Hoffman M, Roberts HR. Platelets and thrombin generation. Arterioscler Thromb Vasc Biol 2002;22:1381–9.
3. Bauer KA. New anticoagulants. Curr Opin Hematol 2008;15:509–15.
4. Al Dieri R, Wagenvoord R, van Dedem GW, et al. The inhibition of blood coagulation by heparins of different molecular weight is caused by a common functional motif–the C-domain. J Thromb Haemost 2003;1:907–14.

5. Hirsh J, Warkentin TE, Shaughnessy SG, et al. Heparin and low-molecular-weight heparin: mechanisms of action, pharmacokinetics, dosing, monitoring, efficacy, and safety. Chest 2001;119:64–94.

6. Blann AD, Landray MJ, Lip GY. ABC of antithrombotic therapy: an overview of antithrombotic therapy. BMJ 2002;325:762–5.

7. Geerts WH, Bergqvist D, Pineo GF, et al. Prevention of venous thromboembolism: American College of Chest Physicians evidence-based clinical practice guidelines (8th edition). Chest 2008;133:381–453.

8. Keam SJ, Goa KL. Fondaparinux sodium. Drugs 2002;62:1673–85.

9. Weitz JI, Crowther M. Direct thrombin inhibitors. Thromb Res 2002;106:275–84.

10. Kam PC, Kaur N, Thong CL. Direct thrombin inhibitors: pharmacology and clinical relevance. Anaesthesia 2005;60:565–74.

11. Gerotziafas GT, Samama MM. Heterogeneity of synthetic factor Xa inhibitors. Curr Pharm Des 2005;11:3855–76.

12. Ansell J, Hirsh J, Poller L, et al. The pharmacology and management of the vitamin K antagonists: the seventh ACCP conference on antithrombotic and thrombolytic therapy. Chest 2004;126:204–33.

13. Hyers TM. Management of venous thromboembolism: past, present, and future. Arch Intern Med 2003;163:759–68.

14. Lassen MR, Laux V. Emergence of new oral antithrombotics: a critical appraisal of their clinical potential. Vasc Health Risk Manag 2008;4:1373–86.

15. Klein GF, Kofler H, Wolf H, et al. Eczema-like, erythematous, infiltrated plaques: a common side effect of subcutaneous heparin therapy. J Am Acad Dermatol 1989;21:703–7.

16. Trautmann A, Seitz CS. Heparin allergy: delayed-type non-IgE-mediated allergic hypersensitivity to subcutaneous heparin injection. Immunol Allergy Clin North Am 2009;29:469–80.

17. Trautmann A, Hamm K, Bröcker EB, et al. [Delayed hypersensitivity to heparins. Clinical signs, diagnosis, therapeutic alternatives]. Z Hautkr 1997;72:447–50 [in German].

18. Bircher AJ, Flückiger R, Buchner SA. Eczematous infiltrated plaques to subcutaneous heparin: a type IV allergic reaction. Br J Dermatol 1990;123:507–14.

19. Guillet G, Delaire P, Plantin P, et al. Eczema as a complication of heparin therapy. J Am Acad Dermatol 1989;20:1130–2.

20. Korstanje MJ, Bessems PJ, Hardy E, et al. Delayed-type hypersensitivity reaction to heparin. Contact Dermatitis 1989;20:383–4.

21. Kim KH, Lynfield Y. Enoxaparin-induced generalized exanthema. Cutis 2003;72: 57–60.

22. Seitz CS, Bröcker EB, Trautmann A. Management of allergy to heparins in postoperative care: subcutaneous allergy and intravenous tolerance. Dermatol Online J 2008;14:4.

23. Patrizi A, DiLernia V, Patrone P. Generalized reaction to subcutaneous heparin. Contact Dermatitis 1989;20:309–10.

24. Greiner D, Schöfer H. [Allergic drug exanthema to heparin. Cutaneous reactions to high molecular and fractionated heparin]. Hautarzt 1994;45:569–72 [in German].

25. Estrada Rodriguez JL, Gozalo RF, Ortiz U, et al. Generalized eczema induced by nadroparin. J Investig Allergol Clin Immunol 2003;13:69–70.

26. Grassegger A, Fritsch P, Reider N. Delayed-type hypersensitivity and cross-reactivity to heparins and danaparoid: a prospective study. Dermatol Surg 2001;27: 47–52.

27. Mendez J, Sanchis ME, de la Fuente R, et al. Delayed-type hypersensitivity to subcutaneous enoxaparin. Allergy 1998;53:999–1003.

28. Gaigl Z, Pfeuffer P, Raith P, et al. Tolerance to intravenous heparin in patients with delayed-type hypersensitivity to heparins: a prospective study. Br J Haematol 2005;128:389–92.

29. Kroon C, de Boer A, Kroon JM, et al. Influence of skinfold thickness on heparin absorption. Lancet 1991;337:945–6.

30. Bircher AJ, Harr T, Hohenstein L, et al. Hypersensitivity reactions to anticoagulant drugs: diagnosis and management options. Allergy 2006;61:1432–40.

31. Jappe U. Allergy to heparins and anticoagulants with a similar pharmacological profile: an update. Blood Coagul Fibrinolysis 2006;17:605–13.

32. Guerrini M, Beccati D, Shriver Z, et al. Oversulfated chondroitin sulfate is a contaminant in heparin associated with adverse clinical events. Nat Biotechnol 2008;26:669–75.

33. Hermann K, Frank G, Ring J. Contamination of heparin by histamine: measurement and characterization by high-performance liquid chromatography and radioimmunoassay. Allergy 1994;49:569–72.

34. Kishimoto TK, Viswanathan K, Ganguly T, et al. Contaminated heparin associated with adverse clinical events and activation of the contact system. N Engl J Med 2008;358:2457–67.

35. Liew G, Campbell C, Thursby P. Delayed-type hypersensitivity to subcutaneous heparin with tolerance of i.v. administration. ANZ J Surg 2004;74:1020–1.

36. Boehncke WH, Weber L, Gall H. Tolerance to intravenous administration of heparin and heparinoid in a patient with delayed-type hypersensitivity to heparins and heparinoids. Contact Dermatitis 1996;35:73–5.

37. Jappe U, Reinhold D, Bonnekoh B. Arthus reaction to lepirudin, a new recombinant hirudin, and delayed-type hypersensitivity to several heparins and heparinoids, with tolerance to its intravenous administration. Contact Dermatitis 2002;46:29–32.

38. Trautmann A, Bröcker EB, Klein CE. Intravenous challenge with heparins in patients with delayed-type skin reactions after subcutaneous administration of the drug. Contact Dermatitis 1998;39:43–4.

39. Gaigl Z, Klein CE, Großmann R, et al. [Managing allergy to heparin]. Dtsch Arztebl 2006;103:2877–81 [in German].

40. Lindhoff-Last E, Kreutzenbeck HJ, Magnani HN. Treatment of 51 pregnancies with danaparoid because of heparin intolerance. Thromb Haemost 2005;93:63–9.

41. Ludwig RJ, Beier C, Lindhoff-Last E, et al. Tolerance of fondaparinux in a patient allergic to heparins and other glycosaminoglycans. Contact Dermatitis 2003;49:158–9.

42. Ludwig RJ, Schindewolf M, Alban S, et al. Molecular weight determines the frequency of delayed type hypersensitivity reactions to heparin and synthetic oligosaccharides. Thromb Haemost 2005;94:1265–9.

43. Utikal J, Peitsch WK, Booken D, et al. Hypersensitivity to the pentasaccharide fondaparinux in patients with delayed-type heparin allergy. Thromb Haemost 2005;94:895–6.

44. Hirsch K, Ludwig RJ, Lindhoff-Last E, et al. Intolerance of fondaparinux in a patient allergic to heparins. Contact Dermatitis 2004;50:383–4.

45. Hohenstein E, Tsakiris D, Bircher AJ. Delayed-type hypersensitivity to the ultra-low-molecular-weight heparin fondaparinux. Contact Dermatitis 2004;51:149–51.

46. Maetzke J, Hinrichs R, Staib G, et al. Fondaparinux as a novel therapeutic alternative in a patient with heparin allergy. Allergy 2004;59:237–8.

47. Reininger CB, Greinacher A, Graf J, et al. Platelets of patients with peripheral arterial disease are hypersensitive to heparin. Thromb Res 1996;81:641–9.
48. Greinacher A, Michels I, Liebenhoff U, et al. Heparin-associated thrombocytopenia: immune complexes are attached to the platelet membrane by the negative charge of highly sulphated oligosaccharides. Br J Haematol 1993;84:711–6.
49. Greinacher A, Warkentin TE. Recognition, treatment, and prevention of heparin-induced thrombocytopenia: review and update. Thromb Res 2006;118:165–79.
50. Eichler P, Raschke R, Lubenow N, et al. The new ID-heparin/PF4 antibody test for rapid detection of heparin-induced antibodies in comparison with functional and antigenic assays. Br J Haematol 2002;116:887–91.
51. Warkentin TE, Greinacher A. Heparin-induced thrombocytopenia: recognition, treatment, and prevention: the seventh ACCP conference on antithrombotic and thrombolytic therapy. Chest 2004;126:311–37.
52. Shelley WB, Sayen JJ. Heparin necrosis: an anticoagulant-induced cutaneous infarct. J Am Acad Dermatol 1982;7:674–7.
53. Yates P, Jones S. Heparin skin necrosis–an important indicator of potentially fatal heparin hypersensitivity. Clin Exp Dermatol 1993;18:138–41.
54. Balestra B. [Skin necrosis: a paradoxical complication of anticoagulation]. Schweiz Med Wochenschr 1995;125:361–4 [in German].
55. Warkentin TE, Roberts RS, Hirsh J, et al. Heparin-induced skin lesions and other unusual sequelae of the heparin-induced thrombocytopenia syndrome: a nested cohort study. Chest 2005;127:1857–61.
56. Kelly RA, Gelfand JA, Pincus SH. Cutaneous necrosis caused by systemically administered heparin. JAMA 1981;246:1582–3.
57. Alving BM. How I treat heparin-induced thrombocytopenia and thrombosis. Blood 2003;101:31–7.
58. Hirsh J, Heddle N, Kelton JG. Treatment of heparin-induced thrombocytopenia: a critical review. Arch Intern Med 2004;164:361–9.
59. Lubenow N, Kempf R, Eichner A, et al. Heparin-induced thrombocytopenia: temporal pattern of thrombocytopenia in relation to initial use or re-exposure to heparin. Chest 2002;122:37–42.
60. Warkentin TE, Kelton JG. Temporal aspects of heparin-induced thrombocytopenia. N Engl J Med 2001;344:1286–92.
61. Potzsch B, Klovekorn WP, Madlener K. Use of heparin during cardiopulmonary bypass in patients with a history of heparin-induced thrombocytopenia. N Engl J Med 2000;343:515.
62. Selleng S, Lubenow N, Wollert HG, et al. Emergency cardiopulmonary bypass in a bilaterally nephrectomized patient with a history of heparin-induced thrombocytopenia: successful re-exposure to heparin. Ann Thorac Surg 2001;71:1041–2.
63. Harr T, Scherer K, Tsakiris DA, et al. Immediate type hypersensitivity to low molecular weight heparins and tolerance of unfractionated heparin and fondaparinux. Allergy 2006;61:787–8.
64. Bottio T, Pittarello G, Bonato R, et al. Life-threatening anaphylactic shock caused by porcine heparin intravenous infusion during mitral valve repair. J Thorac Cardiovasc Surg 2003;126:1194–5.
65. Bircher AJ, Czendlik CH, Messmer SL, et al. Acute urticaria caused by subcutaneous recombinant hirudin: evidence for an IgG-mediated hypersensitivity reaction. J Allergy Clin Immunol 1996;98:994–6.
66. Greinacher A, Lubenow N, Eichler P. Anaphylactic and anaphylactoid reactions associated with lepirudin in patients with heparin-induced thrombocytopenia. Circulation 2003;108:2062–5.

67. Greinacher A, Eichler P, Albrecht D, et al. Antihirudin antibodies following low-dose subcutaneous treatment with desirudin for thrombosis prophylaxis after hip-replacement surgery: incidence and clinical relevance. Blood 2003;101: 2617–9.

68. Blossom DB, Kallen AJ, Patel PR, et al. Outbreak of adverse reactions associated with contaminated heparin. N Engl J Med 2008;359:2674–84.

69. Chan YC, Valenti D, Mansfield AO, et al. Warfarin induced skin necrosis. Br J Surg 2000;87:266–72.

70. Roche-Nagle G, Robb W, Ireland A, et al. Extensive skin necrosis associated with warfarin sodium therapy. Eur J Vasc Endovasc Surg 2003;25:481–2.

71. Nazarian RM, Van Cott EM, Zembowicz A, et al. Warfarin-induced skin necrosis. J Am Acad Dermatol 2009;61:325–32.

72. Miura Y, Ardenghy M, Ramasastry S, et al. Coumadin necrosis of the skin: report of four patients. Ann Plast Surg 1996;37:332–7.

73. Anderson DR, Brill-Edwards P, Walker I. Warfarin-induced skin necrosis in 2 patients with protein S deficiency: successful reinstatement of warfarin therapy. Haemostasis 1992;22:124–8.

74. Denton MD, Mauiyyedi S, Bazari H. Heparin-induced skin necrosis in a patient with end-stage renal failure and functional protein S deficiency. Am J Nephrol 2001;21:289–93.

75. Jillella AP, Lutcher CL. Reinstituting warfarin in patients who develop warfarin skin necrosis. Am J Hematol 1996;52:117–9.

The Complex Clinical Picture of Presumably Allergic Side Effects to Cytostatic Drugs: Symptoms, Pathomechanism, Reexposure, and Desensitization

Mauro Pagani, MD[a,b,*]

KEYWORDS

- Hypersensitivity • Chemotherapy • Drug allergy • Skin tests
- Oxaliplatin • Cisplatin • Paclitaxel • Desensitization

It is estimated that each year more than 10 million people worldwide are diagnosed with cancer, and its incidence is constantly increasing not only in industrialized countries but also in medium- and low-resource countries. The strain cancer produces on health professionals and the health system is substantial and is growing rapidly.[1] In the last years, researchers and clinicians worldwide have made every possible effort to combat this terrible disease and reduce its impact on patients and their families. Hence, the number of drugs used for the treatment of different types of cancers is constantly increasing and actually exceeds 100 distinct chemical formulations.[2]

The use of most cytotoxic agents is associated with potential hypersensitivity reactions, and the constant increase of their administration has caused an increase in incidence of adverse effects, becoming a relevant problem for clinicians. This article is divided into 2 sections. The first section analyzes general remarks regarding the incidence, clinical features, pathogenetic mechanisms, diagnosis, and prevention of allergic reactions to cytostatic drugs. The second section examines, in detail, the characteristics of chemotherapeutic drugs that provoke hypersensitivity reactions.

[a] Allergology and Oncology Service, Medicine Department, Asola Hospital, Mantova, Italy
[b] Medicine Department, Asola Hospital, Azienda Ospedaliera C. Poma, Mantova, Italy
* Presidio Ospedaliero di Asola, Piazza 80°, Fanteria 1, Asola 46041, Mantova, Italy.
E-mail address: mauro.pagani@aopoma.it

Med Clin N Am 94 (2010) 835–852
doi:10.1016/j.mcna.2010.03.002   **medical.theclinics.com**
0025-7125/10/$ – see front matter © 2010 Elsevier Inc. All rights reserved.

GENERAL REMARKS

Hypersensitivity reactions to chemotherapeutic drugs have been documented for most cancer chemotherapies. These reactions are considered to be uncommon, even if their real incidence is not well known.[3] In fact most reactions are usually mild and are not reported by oncologists, so the problem is probably underestimated. However, hypersensitivity reactions represent a significant problem with certain agents, in particular, platinum compounds, taxanes, L-asparaginase, epipodophyllotoxins, and procarbazine, being less problematic with others.[4] In this regard, it is possible to divide the chemotherapeutic agents into 3 groups, namely, drugs with high, intermediate, or low potential to cause hypersensitivity reactions. The reactions can be caused by the parent compound, their metabolites, or the solvent (eg, Cremophor EL).

The clinical manifestations are variable and unpredictable. Symptoms and signs involve the skin (eg, rash, pruritus, urticaria, angioedema, palmar erythema, facial flushing), respiratory tract (eg, bronchospasm), gastrointestinal tract (eg, abdominal pain, nausea, diarrhea), and cardiocirculatory system (alterations in blood pressure and heart rate). More severe reactions provoke chest pain, angina pectoris, anaphylaxis, and even in rare cases, death.[5] Severe reactions always develop during the infusion of the chemotherapy, whereas mild to moderate reactions can occur either during the treatment or in the 24- to 72-hour period after the end of the chemotherapy administration.[4]

The mechanisms of the hypersensitivity reactions have not been intensively analyzed. In analogy with other drug reactions and based on some skin tests and in vitro analysis, the more severe acute reactions seem to involve drug-specific IgE, as demonstrated for platinum compounds. Most mild reactions are probably caused by other mechanisms, such as direct mast cell or basophil activation and degranulation, or activation of the complement cascade.[6] Moreover, cases of types II, III, or IV reactions have been reported. **Table 1** shows examples of these 4 types of reactions.

The correct identification and diagnosis of hypersensitivity reactions to cytostatic drugs plays a crucial role in the treatment of patients with neoplasm, because unlike other drugs (eg, antibiotics) that may be easily replaced and exchanged in case of adverse reactions, chemotherapeutic drugs are often unique and essential for the treatment of the disease. Therefore, if a hypersensitivity reaction occurs, the physician has to decide between the benefit of continuing the treatment and the risk of a potential fatal anaphylactic reaction during the following administration of chemotherapy. Hence, the correct diagnosis of an allergic side effect to a cytostatic drug is crucial and cannot be postponed.

Table 1
Immunopathogenetic mechanisms of hypersensitivity reactions

Type of HSR	Immunopathogenetic Mechanism	Symptoms	Example
I	IgE mediated	Urticaria, angioedema, bronchospasm, anaphylaxis	L-Asparaginase
II	Cytolytic antibodies (IgG or IgM)	Hemolytic anemia	Oxaliplatin
III	Antigen-antibody immune complex	Vasculitis	Methotrexate
IV	Cell-mediated sensitized T lymphocytes	Contact dermatitis	Anthracyclines

Abbreviation: HSR, hypersensitive reaction.

The diagnosis of hypersensitivity reactions to a drug is based on history; clinical manifestations and, if possible, on skin tests, in vitro tests, and provocation tests.[7] The clinical history is difficult because there are many confounding factors. (1) The patients often take many drugs (eg, to relieve pain) or antiemetics that are also able to provoke hypersensitivity reactions. (2) The cancer, probably via the direct activation of mast cells, may cause some clinical manifestations that mimic hypersensitivity reactions. (3) Some epidemiologic studies have shown that certain cancers are associated with an increased risk of allergies.[8] Therefore, the physician must perform a careful clinical history, analyzing the characteristics and chronology of symptoms and their relationship to the intake of cytotoxic or other drugs.

The clinical history is also important because chemotherapy often provokes non–IgE-mediated reactions and actually even non–immune-mediated reactions.[5] In the presumably immune-mediated reactions, some skin tests (prick and intradermal test) performed to detect drug-specific IgE are useful only for few chemotherapeutic drugs, namely, platinum salts, but not for other drug reactions. Recently, some preliminary observations have shown the presence of specific IgE for carboplatin in the serum of allergic patients (Venemalm L, personal communication, 2010). The patch test, another skin test that helps in the diagnosis of delayed reactions, does not seem to be useful in diagnosis of allergies to cytostatic drugs.[9]

When the diagnosis of a hypersensitivity reaction to a chemotherapeutic drug is made, the physician has to decide whether to discontinue the chemotherapy, or to continue it with another drug or with the same drug responsible for the allergic side effect. A decision is normally made on the basis of factors related to the severity of the reaction, to the circumstances of the patient, to the disease, and to the chemotherapy.

The National Cancer Institute has graded the severity of the reactions in 5 levels (**Table 2**).[10] Generally, grade 1 and 2 reactions allow the continuation of the following doses of chemotherapy without modifications. Grade 3 reactions may require the substitution of the culprit drug. If this is not possible, it is recommended to perform, when there is robust evidence of efficacy, a premedication with steroids and antihistamines and/or reduce the rate of infusion. In case of grade 4 reactions the rechallenge should be avoided and the drug replaced, unless the treatment is curative; in this case the application of a desensitization protocol should be evaluated.

Table 2
Grading of hypersensitivity reactions according to National Cancer Institute criteria

Grade	Hypersensitivity Reactions
1	Transient flushing or rash Drug fever 38°C (100.4°F)
2	Rash Flushing Urticaria Dyspnea Drug fever 38°C (100.4°F)
3	Symptomatic bronchospasm with or without urticaria Parenteral medication or medications indicated Allergy-related edema/angioedema Hypotension
4	Anaphylaxis
5	Death

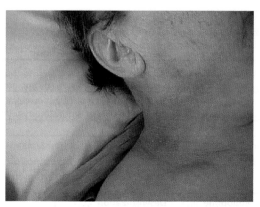

Fig. 1. A 65-year-old woman with generalized urticaria that developed 10 minutes after the sixth course of oxaliplatin was administered for metastatic colorectal cancer. The drug was replaced.

with IgE-mediated reactions; and the positive result of skin tests to oxaliplatin underlines an IgE-mediated mechanism. Indeed, the skin tests are sensitive for the diagnosis of hypersensitivity reactions to oxaliplatin, with a sensitivity ranging from 75% to 100% (**Fig. 2**).[18,28,29] Most reliable results are obtained with an intradermal test, when the reaction has developed during the infusion of oxaliplatin, or within 2 hours after the end of therapy.[9] Patch test, instead, is always negative and is not useful.

Cross-reactivity to other platinum-containing drugs can occur. Leguy-Seguin and colleagues[9] observed positive results of skin tests for oxaliplatin and carboplatin in 3 patients who were allergic to oxaliplatin and were never exposed to carboplatin. On the other hand, 8 patients with allergy tolerated another platinum compound, which showed a negative result in skin test.[9] Similar results were obtained by other investigators.[30] Unfortunately, the efficacy of oxaliplatin is comparable to that of other platinum salts only for the treatment of few cancers, for example, pancreatic or ovarian cancer, whereas it is much higher for other cancers, especially colorectal cancer, where it is not replaceable.

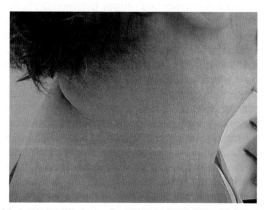

Fig. 2. A 69-year-old woman with generalized urticaria and bronchospasm that appeared 30 minutes after the 10th infusion of oxaliplatin was administered in adjuvant setting for resected colorectal cancer. The therapy was discontinued.

The role of skin tests for the prevention of allergic reaction to oxaliplatin is less evaluated. In an ongoing study the authors have observed positive results of skin tests to oxaliplatin in 3 patients before the allergic reactions appeared in the subsequent administrations of oxaliplatin, although these patients underwent a desensitization procedure (Dr Pagani, personal observation, 2009). Thus, predictive skin testing may become a choice in certain patients.

Premedication schedules performed to prevent hypersensitivity reactions to oxaliplatin have not been reliable, as observed by Brandi and colleagues[13] in 5 of 6 patients with allergy, and confirmed by Thomas and colleagues[31] and Bhargava and Gammon.[32] Therefore, if oxaliplatin is considered fundamental for a patient with a serious allergic reaction, a desensitization protocol is necessary. There are many options for protocols, differing in the rate of infusion or in the concentrations.[20,27,29,33,34] All these protocols were performed on small numbers of patients.

Oxaliplatin can also rarely cause type II hypersensitivity reactions and delayed reactions. Type II reactions such as hemolytic anemia and thrombocytopenia were reported by Garufi and colleagues[35] and Polyzos and colleagues[25]; Santini and colleagues[36] described cases characterized by abdominal cramps, diarrhea, and fever associated with elevation of cytokines, possibly corresponding to a cytokine release syndrome with oxaliplatin acting as a superantigen.

Carboplatin

Carboplatin is a second-generation platinum compound derived by the first synthesized drug of this class, cisplatin. Compared with its parent compound, carboplatin is better tolerated and causes a lower incidence of neurotoxicity, nephrotoxicity, and acute and delayed emesis.[37] Carboplatin is effective in many cancers and plays a major role in ovarian and non–small cell lung cancer.[38] The drug can be administered in monotherapy, and more frequently in combination with other cytostatics, especially taxanes gemcitabine, epipodophyllotoxins, cyclophosphamide, and anthracyclines. Like other platinum compounds, carboplatin can cause hypersensitivity reactions associated with its prolonged use. A review of the literature shows that the incidence of these reactions is less than 1%, 6.5%, 7%, and 19.5% for patients who have undergone less than 5, 6, 7, and 8 cycles of chemotherapy, respectively.[39–41] Because the usual schedules of chemotherapy plan 6 administrations of carboplatin, most allergic reactions will occur when the patient undergoes a retreatment for a relapse of the neoplasm. In particular, Gadducci and colleagues[11] reported that a retreatment interval longer than 2 years seems to be the strongest predictive variable for the development of allergic reactions.

As for oxaliplatin, hypersensitivity reactions to carboplatin vary widely, ranging from mild (grade 1–2) to severe (grade 3–4). About 60% to 70% of carboplatin-induced reactions are mild and appear during and up to 3 days after the end of the treatment. These reactions involve the skin with itching erythema, especially of palms and soles, and facial flushing; normally the symptoms respond to symptomatic therapy with oral antihistamines administered for 3 to 4 days. More severe reactions are less frequent (30%–40% of all reactions), develop about 30 minutes after the beginning of chemotherapy, and involve the skin (eg, facial swelling, diffuse erythroderma), the abdominal tract (eg, abdominal cramps, diarrhea), the respiratory system (eg, dyspnea, bronchospasm, chest pain), and the cardiovascular system (eg, angina pectoris, tachycardia, hypo- or hypertension).[39] The reactions are probably IgE mediated and they develop after several administrations, already cause symptoms during the infusion of carboplatin[40]; especially in more severe cases, skin test results are positive.[42]

administered alone or, more often, in combination with platinum compounds, anthracyclines, or antimetabolites. The adverse effects of docetaxel are similar to paclitaxel, except for fluid retention that seems related to capillary leakage and is dose related.[53]

The solvent in which docetaxel is solubilized is polysorbate 80 and not Cremophor EL, but despite this the incidence of hypersensitivity reactions is high even for this drug (30%). Also for docetaxel, the reactions always occur during the first or second cycle, a few minutes after the start of the infusion. The reactions are usually mild and uniform, and include dyspnea, hypotension, bronchospasm, urticaria, and erythematous rashes. The mechanism of reactions is unknown, but like paclitaxel, are probably not IgE mediated, because they occur during the first 2 administrations.

The premedication decreases the incidence of reactions to 2%, and rarely the therapy has to be discontinued. The protocol is different from that used for paclitaxel and includes oral administration of dexamethasone or its equivalent (16 mg/d) for 3 days, starting 1 day before the chemotherapy.[6] Sharing the same therapeutic indications, docetaxel could potentially substitute paclitaxel in cases of severe hypersensitivity reactions to this drug. Moon and colleagues[54] and Lokich and Anderson[55] obtained good results on 6 patients, but Dizon and colleagues[56] reported a cross-reactivity rate of 90% between the 2 drugs, suggesting that taxane moiety may be responsible for cross-reactivity. Therefore, the substitution of one taxane with the other because of hypersensitivity is actually not recommended.

Other Cytostatic Drugs with High Potential for Hypersensitivity

L-Asparaginase

L-Asparaginase is an enzyme used for the treatment of acute lymphoblastic leukemia. The sources of L-asparaginase used in clinics are bacterial in origin: an *Escherichia coli* derivative or an *Erwinia chrysanthemi* derivative, it is also available in a polyethylene glycol form: PEG-asparaginase. The adverse events related to L-asparaginase include nausea, vomiting, myelotoxicity, hepatic failure, and hypersensitivity reactions, this drug being the one with the highest potential to cause these events.

The incidence of allergic reactions ranges between 6% and 43%, with serious anaphylactic reactions occurring in fewer than 10% of patients treated.[57,58] The overall risk of a reaction per drug dose is 5% to 8% with an increase to 33% after the fourth dose.[12] There are several factors that increase the risk of allergic reactions to L-asparaginase. First, intravenous infusion causes higher and more reactions compared with intramuscular administrations; a time interval of a week or more between the infusions of therapy greatly increases the incidence of reactions compared with daily administration of the drug.[5] Moreover, a previous exposure to L-asparaginase is a risk factor. Muller and colleagues[59] showed that retreatment of patients exposed to the chemotherapy months or years earlier is associated with hypersensitivity reactions in 24% of cases. Other risk factors include doses higher than 6000 IU/m^2/d and single-agent chemotherapy.[58]

The clinical features are those typical of type I reactions: they usually occur within an hour of drug administration and are represented initially by pruritus, dyspnea, urticaria, and hypotension. Life-threatening anaphylaxis may ensue. Evans and colleagues[60] reported that 44% of the patients with reactions had anaphylaxis, indicating that there is great potential for serious problems when a patient is allergic to this drug.

The pathogenetic mechanisms of hypersensitivity to L-asparaginase are not fully explained. Khan and Hill[61] described 5 patients in whom, by means of skin and Prausnitz-Küstner test, they revealed an IgE-mediated hypersensitivity. Fabry and colleagues[62] performed a study on 8 patients with allergy, concluding that anaphylaxis can be explained by complement activation induced by the formation of immunocomplexes of L-asparaginase and specific antibodies of IgM and IgG classes.

Skin tests used to diagnose or prevent hypersensitivity reactions are of no value because they can give false-positive and false-negative results. Test doses are also of no value because they are often false negative.[12]

There are several possibilities in the treatment of patients who have developed hypersensitivity reactions to L-asparaginase and need to continue therapy. Discontinuation of therapy with E coli–derived L-asparaginase and substitution with Erwinia–derived L-asparaginase or PEG-asparaginase is preferred. Beard and colleagues[63] were the first who showed the safety of Erwinia preparations in patients who presented hypersensitivity reactions to E coli–derived L-asparaginase, and their results were confirmed by other investigators.[64] However, cross-reactivity has been reported to occur during the first dose of Erwinia-derived formulation, or the patients may produce specific antibodies to the drug, which could provoke anaphylaxis. Therefore in the cases of hypersensitivity to E coli and Erwinia-derived L-asparaginase, the option is to use PEG-asparaginase, which is less immunogenic than the 2 other forms. When used as a substitute in patients with previous reactions, it is tolerated in more than 70% of cases.[65]

Unfortunately, the availability of Erwinia-derived L-asparaginase and PEG-asparaginase is limited in many parts of the world, so premedication or desensitization protocols are necessary alternatives. Soyer and colleagues[66] performed a premedication with steroids and antihistamines and a desensitization protocol on 16 patients with previous allergic reactions to L-asparaginase. The investigators were able to complete the chemotherapy in almost 70% of the patients. Hence, in countries with shortages of alternative asparaginase preparations, this approach might be a suitable option.

Procarbazine

Procarbazine is an oral chemotherapeutic drug indicated for the treatment of Hodgkin disease, brain neoplasms and, more rarely, for non-Hodgkin lymphomas, melanoma, and lung cancer. The dose-limiting toxicity is myelosuppressive. Other adverse effects include nausea, anorexia, and stomatitis. Hypersensitivity does occur and includes Gell and Coombs type I, III, and IV reactions. The incidence of hypersensitivity reactions ranges between 6% and 18%, and the clinical features involve the skin, with maculopapular rashes most often; but urticaria, fixed drug eruption, and even toxic epidermal necrolysis have been observed.[12] Type III reactions rarely cause pulmonary toxicity. There are 9 cases described in medical literature in which cough, dyspnea with interstitial pneumonitis, restriction on pulmonary function tests, and sometimes eosinophilia develop after the second dose of procarbazine.[67] There is no way to prevent hypersensitivity reactions to procarbazine, because it always appears at rechallenge. Therefore, patients have to discontinue this therapy.[12]

Epipodophyllotoxins

Teniposide

Teniposide is a chemotherapeutic drug used for the treatment of hematologic and neurologic malignancies. Hypersensitivity reactions have long been recognized as one of its toxic effects.

The overall incidence of reactions varies from 6.5% observed by O'Dwyer and colleagues, especially in the treatment of brain cancers, to 41% reported by Kellie on 108 children with leukemia.[6]

Most of the reactions (>90%) are of grade 1 or grade 2 severity, even if cases of anaphylaxis occur. The reactions appear after the first dose but more often after many doses, either within the first few minutes of infusion or hours after administration.[12] The pathogenetic mechanism is not well elucidated. Teniposide is dissolved in Cremophor EL, which is considered by many as being responsible for the reactions. However, Nolte and colleagues[68] showed that teniposide degranulated basophils of 9 patients who were sensitized, whereas Cremophor EL failed to do so.

Etoposide

Etoposide was introduced into clinical practice 30 years ago for the treatment of small cell lung cancer and refractory testicular cancer, and can cause hypersensitivity reactions less commonly than teniposide. It is available for intravenous and oral formulations. The clinical characteristics of reactions are similar to teniposide and are associated only with the intravenous compound, which is dissolved in polysorbate 80. This fact supports the hypothesis that the solvent may be the culprit of reactions.[12]

Premedication with histamine (H1 and H2) blockers and a slow infusion rate may reduce the risk of further hypersensitivity reactions on rechallenge with epipodophyllotoxins.[69] Hudson and colleagues[70] reported a successful rechallenge in 75% of 24 children with hypersensitivity reactions to etoposide. Moreover, they observed 3 cases of reactions in 5 children when etoposide was replaced by teniposide. Therefore this substitution is not recommended.

Drugs with Intermediate Potential to Cause Hypersensitivity Reactions

Anthracyclines (doxorubicin, daunorubicin, epirubicin, idarubicin)

These drugs are antibiotics used for the treatment of several types of cancer, including breast and hematologic neoplasms. The main toxic effects are myelosuppression, cardiotoxicity, and alopecia. The most recent formulation, liposomal doxorubicin, often provokes palmar and plantar erythrodysesthesia, which is occasionally severe and dose limiting.[71]

Anaphylactic-like reactions caused by doxorubicin, epirubicin, and daunorubicin were described by some investigators. The symptoms usually involve the skin, but there are reports of more serious reactions. Doxorubicin and epirubicin can elicit reactions with intravenous or intravesical administration.[12] In this case normally the reactions are local and self-limiting, but Okumura and colleagues[72] described a case of severe generalized erythema after intravesical infusion of epirubicin for a bladder cancer.

The pathogenetic mechanisms have not been widely investigated; however, Szebeni and colleagues[73] showed a direct complement activation by liposomal doxorubicin. No exact data exist on prevention of these hypersensitivity reactions; but a slower infusion rate may protect the patient from reactions, whereas premedication is not effective. Moreover, Castells and colleagues[20] desensitized 5 patients with allergy to liposomal doxorubicin without any problem.

6-Mercaptopurine and azathioprine

6-Mercaptopurine is an analogue antimetabolite, available for oral use, approved for the treatment of acute lymphoblastic leukemia, and is more rarely used for other hematological malignancies. In recent years this drug has also been used to treat inflammatory bowel diseases.[74] In these types of patients mercaptopurine provokes hypersensitivity reactions rather frequently, as reported in a retrospective review of Korelitz and colleagues,[74] in which 16 of 591 patients developed hypersensitivity reactions during treatment with mercaptopurine. In these cases the drug was substituted by its imidazolyl derivative, azathioprine, which caused the same reactions in 5 of 6 patients. However, 4 patients underwent a desensitization protocol that permitted the prosecution of the therapy.

Cross-reactivity between azathioprine and mercaptopurine also was reported by Nagi and colleagues,[75] who observed reactions to mercaptopurine in 1 of 3 of patients who suffered from previous reactions to azathioprine.

Methotrexate

Methotrexate is an antifolate antimetabolite used for a wide spectrum of neoplasms, namely, acute leukemia, lymphomas, sarcoma, breast cancer, and bladder cancer, and also for rheumatic diseases. Low and high doses of methotrexate can precipitate type I reactions that range from grade 1 to 2 to anaphylaxis.[12]

The incidence of allergic reactions is low, but there are several reports that describe severe cases associated with methotrexate.[76,77] Successful desensitization protocols were developed in the last years by Kohli and colleagues[78] and Davis and colleagues[79] Indeed desensitization, as well as premedication, are effective in some patients and are promising procedures for severe cases.

Methotrexate-associated pulmonary toxicity has been well described. Pulmonary infiltrates are the most commonly encountered form; these infiltrates resemble hypersensitivity lung disease and are associated with hilar adenopathy, rashes, and blood eosinophilia, suggesting a type III or type IV reaction.[77] Corticosteroids are normally effective in reversing the pneumonitis, but in rare cases the pulmonary reaction is fatal.

Moreover, methotrexate may induce cutaneous vasculitis and other forms of skin toxicity, such as erythematous rash or Stevens-Johnson syndrome–like exanthema.[80] The pathogenetic mechanism is unknown but could be T-cell mediated.

Drugs with Low Potential to Cause Hypersensitivity Reactions

Cytarabine

This antimetabolite is used for the treatment of acute leukemia and non-Hodgkin lymphomas.

Type I reactions have been described only in case reports and are uncommon. The clinical features usually observed are dyspnea, chest pain, urticaria, and hypotension. The pathogenetic mechanism is unknown, but Blanca and colleagues[81] reported on a positive result in a skin test to cytarabine in a child with allergy, and assumed that specific IgE could play an important role in the development of the reactions.

Immunologic mechanisms were postulated by some investigators to explain the pathogenesis of other symptoms related to cytarabine such as conjunctivitis and palmar-plantar erythema, but they are probably caused by a direct toxicity of this drug without involvement of the specific immune system.[82]

Cyclophosphamide and ifosfamide

Cyclophosphamide is a derivative of nitrogen mustard that is converted to 4-hydroxy cyclophosphamide in the liver. In tissue, it is either converted to inactive metabolites or to the active alkylating agents, phosphoramide mustard and acrolein. Recognized toxic effects of cyclophosphamide include bone marrow suppression; gonadal dysfunction; and pulmonary, cardiac, and urological (hemorrhagic cystitis) toxicity. Cancer of the bladder may be a late consequence. Ifosfamide is a closely related analogue.[5]

Cyclophosphamide is used for the treatment of many types of cancer including breast, ovarian, non-Hodgkin lymphoma, and sarcoma, as well as nonmalignant immunopathological diseases.[2] The incidence of hypersensitivity reactions to cyclophosphamide is less than 1%, as observed in the case study of Popescu and colleagues.[83] The symptoms are typical type I reactions; are variable in severity, ranging from urticaria to anaphylaxis; and usually appear in the first minutes of infusion, even if some cases develop up to 12 hours later. Skin tests were performed for cyclophosphamide and its metabolites, with contrasting results. In the largest study, Popescu and colleagues[83] performed skin tests on 5 patients with delayed-onset hypersensitivity and observed positive reactions to the metabolites but not for cyclophosphamide itself. The investigators concluded that IgE-mediated allergic drug reactions may have a delayed onset, if the allergen is a time-dependent drug metabolite.

Cyclophosphamide is also available in tablets for oral use, which can provoke hypersensitivity reactions. Allergy usually develops 10 to 14 days after the initial dose. The clinical features are less florid than the previously reported reactions to intravenous cyclophosphamide and require a week to resolve.[84,85] The delay in presentation probably reflects the oral dosing regime or a delayed immune mechanism (T cells).

The incidence of hypersensitivity reactions to ifosfamide is less than 1%. The reaction is infused with mesna, widely used for the prevention of cyclophosphamide-related hemorrhagic cystitis. It is possible that the reactions to cyclophosphamide and ifosfamide are partly caused by this antidote.[86] Indeed, mesna has been associated with hypersensitivity-like cutaneous and systemic reactions in adult patients.

SUMMARY

All chemotherapeutic drugs, except nitrosoureas, have caused at least some hypersensitivity reaction. Most frequent are IgE-mediated and probably non–immune-mediated hypersensitivity reactions. The former (eg, caused by platinum-containing drugs) typically appear after 4 to 6 cycles of chemotherapy and may cause anaphylactic reactions. Intradermal skin tests often show positive results for these drugs. Pretreatment with antihistamines and corticosteroids are not effective, whereas desensitization protocols seem to be successful and allow completion of the therapy.

By contrast, milder reactions (urticaria) mostly appear at the first or second exposure. Typical drugs are taxanes. These reactions can be suppressed by pretreatment with antihistamines and corticosteroids. Some of these reactions are caused by the drug itself, others by the solvent (Cremophor EL).

Experience with the drug or drug class, knowledge of cross-reactivity, skin testing, and experience with desensitization or premedication determine the further procedure (see **Table 3**). In most instances this balanced approach allows the continuation of cytostatic therapy with effective drugs.

REFERENCES

1. Boyle P, Levin B. Introduction in: World Cancer Report 2008. IARC Nonserial publication.
2. Freter CE, Perry MC. Systemic therapies. In: Abeloff MD, Armitage JO, Niederhuber JE, et al, editors. Clinical oncology, vol. 1. 4th edition. Churchill-Livingstone; 2008. p. 453, 463.
3. Syrigou E, Syrigos K, Saif MW. Hypersensitivity reactions to oxaliplatin and other antineoplastic agents. Curr Allergy Asthma Rep 2008;8:56–62.
4. Zanotti KM, Markman M. Prevention and management of antineoplastic-induced hypersensitivity reactions. Drug Saf 2001;24:767–79.
5. Shepherd GM. Hypersensitivity reactions to chemotherapeutic drugs. Clin Rev Allergy Immunol 2003;24:253–62.
6. Lee C, Gianos M, Klausermeyer WB. Diagnosis and management of hypersensitivity reactions related to common cancer chemotherapy agents. Ann Allergy Asthma Immunol 2009;102:179–87.

7. Demoly P, Bousquet J. Drug allergy diagnosis work up. Allergy 2002;57(Suppl 72): 37–40.
8. Wang H, Diepgen TL. Is atopy a protective or a risk for cancer? A review of epidemiological studies. Allergy 2005;60:1098–111.
9. Leguy-Seguin V, Jolimoy G, Coudert B, et al. Diagnosis and predictive value of skin testing in platinum salts hypersensitivity. J Allergy Clin Immunol 2007;119:726–30.
10. National Cancer Institute. Common Terminology Criteria for Adverse Events v3.0 (CTCAE). Published date August 9, 2006.
11. Gadducci A, Tana R, Teti G, et al. Analysis of the pattern of hypersensitivity reactions in patients receiving carboplatin retreatment for recurrent ovarian cancer. Int J Gynecol Cancer 2008;18:615–20.
12. Weiss RB. Hypersensitivity reactions. Semin Oncol 1992;19:458–77.
13. Brandi G, Pantaleo MA, Galli C, et al. Hypersensitivity reactions related to oxaliplatin (OHP). Br J Cancer 2003;89:477–81.
14. Maindrault-Goebel F, Andrè T, Turnigard C, et al. Allergic-type reactions to oxaliplatin: retrospective analysis of 42 patients. Eur J Cancer 2005;41:2262–7.
15. Dizon DS, Sabbatini PJ, Aghahanian C. Analysis of patients with epithelial ovarian cancer of fallopian tube carcinoma retreated with cisplatin after the development of a carboplatin allergy. Gynecol Oncol 2002;84:378–82.
16. Polyzos A, Tsavaris N, Kosmos C, et al. Hypersensitivity reactions to oxaliplatin: cross-reactivity to carboplatin and the introduction of a desensitization schedule. Oncology 2001;61:129–33.
17. Markman M, Zanotti K, Peterson G, et al. Expanded experience with an intradermal skin test to predict for the presence or absence of carboplatin hypersensitivity. J Clin Oncol 2003;21:4611–4.
18. Pagani M, Bonadonna P, Senna GE, et al. Standardization of skin test for diagnosis and prevention of hypersensitivity reactions to oxaliplatin. Int Arch Allergy Immunol 2008;145:54–7.
19. Castells MC. Rapid desensitization for hypersensitivity reactions to chemotherapy agents. Curr Opin Allergy Clin Immunol 2006;6:271–7.
20. Castells MC, Tennant NM, Sloane DE, et al. Hypersensitivity reactions to chemotherapy: Outcomes and safety of rapid desensitization in 413 cases. J Allergy Clin Immunol 2008;122:574–80.
21. Andrè T, Boni C, Mounedji-Boudiaf L, et al. Oxaliplatin with high dose leucovorin and 5-fluorouracil 48-hour continuous infusion in pretreated metastatic colorectal cancer. N Engl J Med 2004;350:2343–51.
22. Chollet P, Bensmaine MA, Brienza S, et al. Single agent activity of oxaliplatin in heavily treated advanced epithelial ovarian cancer. Ann Oncol 1996;7:1065–70.
23. Germann N, Brienza S, Rotarsky M, et al. Preliminary results of the activity of oxaliplatin (L-OHP) in refractory/recurrent non-Hodgkin's lymphoma patients. Ann Oncol 1999;10:351–4.
24. Lee MY, Yang MH, Liu IH, et al. Severe anaphylactic reactions in patients receiving oxaliplatin therapy: a rare but potentially fatal complication. Support Care Cancer 2007;15:89–93.
25. Polyzos A, Tsavaris N, Gogas H, et al. Clinical features of hypersensitivity reactions to oxaliplatin: a 10-year experience. Oncology 2009;76:36–41.
26. Gowda A, Goel R, Berdzik J, et al. Hypersensitivity reactions to oxaliplatin: incidence and management. Oncology 2004;18:1671–4.
27. Herrero T, Tomero P, Infante S, et al. Diagnosis and management of hypersensitivity reactions caused by oxaliplatin. J Investig Allergol Clin Immunol 2006;16: 327–30.

28. Garufi C, Cristaudo A, Vanni B, et al. Skin testing and hypersensitivity reactions to oxaliplatin. Ann Oncol 2003;14:497–502.

29. Meyer L, Zuberbier T, Worm M, et al. Hypersensitivity reactions to oxaliplatin: crossreactivity to carboplatin and the introduction of a desensitization schedule. J Clin Oncol 2002;20:1146–7.

30. Elligers KT, Davies M, Sanchis D, et al. Rechallenge with cisplatin in a patient with pancreatic cancer who developed a hypersensitivity reaction to oxaliplatin. Is skin test useful in this setting? J Pancreas 2008;9:197–202.

31. Thomas RR, Quinn MG, Schuler B, et al. Hypersensitivity and idiosyncratic reactions to oxaliplatin. Cancer 2003;97:2301–7.

32. Bhargava P, Gammon D. Hypersensitivity and idiosyncratic reactions to oxaliplatin. Cancer 2004;100:211–2.

33. Mis L, Fernando LH, Hurwitz HI, et al. Successful desensitization to oxaliplatin. Ann Pharmacother 2005;39:966–9.

34. Gammon D, Bharghava P, Mc Cormick MJ. Hypersensitivity reactions to oxaliplatin and the application of a desensitization protocol. Oncologist 2004;9:546–9.

35. Garufi C, Vaglio S, Brienza S, et al. Immunohemolytic anemia following oxaliplatin administration. Ann Oncol 2000;11:497.

36. Santini D, Tonini G, Salerno A, et al. Idiosyncratic reaction after oxaliplatin infusion. Ann Oncol 2001;12:132–3.

37. Bookman MA, Mc Guire WP III, Kilpatrick D, et al. Carboplatin and paclitaxel in ovarian carcinoma. A phase I study of the Gynecologic Oncology Group. J Clin Oncol 1996;14:1895–902.

38. Markman M, Kennedy A, Webster K, et al. Carboplatin plus paclitaxel in the treatment of gynecologic malignancies: the Cleveland Clinic experience. Semin Oncol 1997;24(Suppl 15):26–9.

39. Markman M, Kennedy A, Webster K, et al. Clinical features of hypersensitivity reactions to carboplatin. J Clin Oncol 1999;17:1141–5.

40. Polyzos A, Tsavaris N, Kosmas C, et al. Hypersensitivity reactions to carboplatin administration are common but not always severe: a 10-year experience. Oncology 2001;61:129–33.

41. Sliesoraitis S, Chikhale PJ. Carboplatin hypersensitivity. Int J Gynecol Cancer 2005;15:13–8.

42. Menczer J, Barda G, Glezerman M, et al. Hypersensitivity reactions to carboplatin. Results of skin tests. Eur J Gynaecol Oncol 1999;3:214–6.

43. Basu R, Rajkumar A, Datta NR. Anaphylaxis to cisplatin following nine previous uncomplicated cases. Int J Clin Oncol 2002;7:365–7.

44. Goldberg A, Altaras MM, Mekori YA, et al. Anaphylaxis to cisplatin: diagnosis and value of pretreatment in prevention of recurrent allergic reactions. Ann Allergy 1994;73:271–2.

45. Rowinsky EK, Donehower RC. Paclitaxel (Taxol). N Engl J Med 1995;332:1004–14.

46. Weiss RB, Donehower RC, Wiernik PH, et al. Hypersensitivity reactions from Taxol. J Clin Oncol 1990;8:1263–8.

47. Gradishar WJ, Tjulandin S, Davidson N, et al. Phase III trial of nano-particle albumin-bound paclitaxel compared with polyethylated castor oil-based paclitaxel in women with breast cancer. J Clin Oncol 2005;23:7794–803.

48. Essayan DM, Kagey-Sobotka A, Colarusso PJ, et al. Successful parenteral desensitization to paclitaxel. J Allergy Clin Immunol 1996;97:42–6.

49. Kintzel PE. Prophylaxis for paclitaxel hypersensitivity reactions. Ann Pharmacother 2001;30:367–71.
50. Olson JK, Sood AK, Sorosky JI, et al. Taxol hypersensitivity: rapid retreatment is safe and cost effective. Gynecol Oncol 1998;68:25–8.
51. Markman M, Kennedy A, Webster K, et al. Paclitaxel-associated hypersensitivity reactions: experience of the gynecologic oncology program of the Cleveland Clinic Cancer Center. J Clin Oncol 2000;18:102–5.
52. Feldweg AM, Lee CW, Matulonis UA, et al. Rapid desensitization for hypersensitivity reactions to paclitaxel and docetaxel: a new standard protocol used in 77 successful treatments. Gynecol Oncol 2005;96:824–9.
53. Semb KA, Aamdal S, Oian P. Capillary protein leak syndrome appears to explain fluid retention in cancer patients who receive docetaxel treatment. J Clin Oncol 1998;16:3426–32.
54. Moon C, Verschraegen CF, Bevers M, et al. Use of docetaxel (Taxotere) in patients with paclitaxel (Taxol) hypersensitivity. Anticancer Drugs 2000;11:565–8.
55. Lokich J, Anderson N. Paclitaxel hypersensitivity reactions: a role for docetaxel substitution. Ann Oncol 1998;9:573–4.
56. Dizon DS, Schwartz J, Rojan A, et al. Cross-sensitivity between paclitaxel and docetaxel in a women's cancer program. Gynecol Oncol 2006;100:149–51.
57. Woo MH, Hak LJ, Storm MC, et al. Anti-asparaginase antibodies following *E. coli* asparaginase therapy in pediatric acute lymphoblastic leukemia. Leukemia 1998; 12:1527–33.
58. Narta UK, Kanwar SS, Azmi W. Pharmacological and clinical evaluation of L-asparaginase in the treatment of leukemia. Crit Rev Oncol Hematol 2007;61:208–21.
59. Muller H, Beier R, Loning L, et al. Pharmacokinetics of native *Escherichia coli* asparaginase (Asparaginase medac) and hypersensitivity reactions in ALL-BFM 95 reinduction treatment. Br J Haematol 2001;114:794–9.
60. Evans WE, Tsiatis A, Rivera G, et al. Anaphylactoid reactions to *Escherichia coli* and *Erwinia* asparaginase in children with leukemia and lymphoma. Cancer 1982; 49:1378–83.
61. Khan A, Hill JM. Atopic hypersensitivity to L-asparaginase: resistance to immunosuppression. Int Arch Allergy Appl Immunol 1971;40:463–9.
62. Fabry U, Korholz D, Jurgens H, et al. Anaphylaxis to L-asparaginase during treatment for acute lymphoblastic leukemia in children. Evidence of a complement-mediated mechanism. Pediatr Res 1985;19:400–8.
63. Beard MEJ, Crowther D, Galton DAG, et al. L-asparaginase in treatment of acute leukemia and lymphosarcoma. Br Med J 1970;1:191–5.
64. Ohnuma T, Holland JF, Meyer P. *Erwinia carotovora*, asparaginase patients with prior anaphylaxis to asparaginase from *E. coli*. Cancer 1972;30:376–81.
65. Hak LJ, Relling MV, Cheng C, et al. Asparaginase pharmacodynamics differ by formulation among children with newly diagnosed acute lymphoblastic leukemia. Leukemia 2004;18:1072–7.
66. Soyer OU, Aytac S, Tuncer A, et al. Alternative algorithm for L-asparaginase allergy in children with acute lymphoblastic leukemia. J Allergy Clin Immunol 2009;123:895–8.
67. Mahmood T, Mudad R. Pulmonary toxicity secondary to procarbazine. Am J Clin Oncol 2002;25:187–8.
68. Nolte H, Carstensen H, Hertz H. VM-26 (teniposide)-induced hypersensitivity and degranulation of basophils in children. Am J Pediatr Hematol Oncol 1988;10: 308–12.

69. De Souza P, Friedlander M, Wilde C, et al. Hypersensitivity reactions to etoposide. A report of three cases and review of the literature. Am J Clin Oncol 1994;17: 387–9.
70. Hudson MM, Weinstein HJ, Donaldson SS, et al. Acute hypersensitivity reactions to etoposide in a VEPA regimen for Hodgkin's disease. J Clin Oncol 1993;11: 1080–4.
71. Chan A, Shih V, Tham Chee Kian. Liposomal doxorubicin-associated acute hypersensitivity despite appropriate preventive measures. J Oncol Pharm Pract 2007; 13:105–7.
72. Okumura A, Oishi N, Kaji K, et al. Drug eruption due to intravesical instillation of both epirubicin and mitomycin C. J Dermatol 2009;36:419–22.
73. Szebeni J, Baranyi L, Savay S, et al. Role of complement activation in hypersensitivity reactions to doxil and hynic PEG liposomes: experimental and clinical studies. J Liposome Res 2002;12:165–72.
74. Korelitz BI, Zlatanic J, Goel F, et al. Allergic reactions to mercaptopurine during treatment for inflammatory bowel disease. J Clin Gastroenterol 1999;28:341–4.
75. Nagy F, Molnar T, Szepes Z, et al. Efficacy of 6-mercaptopurine treatment after azathioprine hypersensitivity in inflammatory bowel disease. World J Gastroenterol 2008;14:4342–6.
76. Ozguven AA, Uysal K, Gunes D, et al. Delayed renal excretion of methotrexate after a severe anaphylactic reaction to methotrexate in a child with osteosarcoma. J Pediatr Hematol Oncol 2009;31:289–91.
77. Lateef O, Shakoor N, Balk RA. Methotrexate pulmonary toxicity. Expert Opin Drug Saf 2005;4:723–30.
78. Kohli A, Ferencz TM, Calderon JG. Readministration of high-dose methotrexate in a patient with suspected immediate hypersensitivity and T-cell acute lymphoblastic lymphoma. Allergy Asthma Proc 2004;25:249–52.
79. Davis KA, Williams P, Walker JC. Successful desensitization to high-dose methotrexate after systemic anaphylaxis. Ann Allergy Asthma Immunol 2003;90:87–9.
80. Hani N, Casper C, Groth W, et al. Steven-Johnson syndrome-like exanthema secondary to methotrexate histologically simulating acute graft-versus-host disease. Eur J Dermatol 2000;10:548–50.
81. Blanca M, Torres MJ, Girón M, et al. Successful administration of cytarabine after a previous anaphylactic reaction. Allergy 1997;52:1009–11.
82. Cetkovská P, Pizinger K, Cetkovský P. High-dose cytosine arabinoside-induced cutaneous reactions. J Eur Acad Dermatol Venereol 2002;16:481–5.
83. Popescu NA, Sheehan MG, Kouides PA, et al. Allergic reactions to cyclophosphamide: delayed clinical expression associated with positive immediate skin tests to drug metabolites in five patients. J Allergy Clin Immunol 1996;97:26–33.
84. Rosas-Vargas MA, Casas-Becerra B, Velázquez-Armenta Y, et al. Cyclophosphamide hypersensitivity in a leukemic child. Ther Drug Monit 2005;27:263–4.
85. Stratton J, Warwicker P, Farrington K. Allergic reactions to oral cyclophosphamide therapy in immunologically-mediated renal disease. Nephrol Dial Transplant 2001;16:1724–5.
86. Khaw SL, Downie PA, Waters KD, et al. Adverse hypersensitivity reactions to mesna as adjunctive therapy for cyclophosphamide. Pediatr Blood Cancer 2007;49: 341–3.

NSAID Hypersensitivity (Respiratory, Cutaneous, and Generalized Anaphylactic Symptoms)

Mario Sánchez-Borges, MD[a,b,*]

KEYWORDS

- Angioedema • Aspirin • Asthma
- Nonsteroidal anti-inflammatory drugs • Urticaria

Adverse reactions to drugs have been classified as predictable (related to the pharmacologic actions of the drug) and unpredictable (related to the individual's immunologic response or genetic susceptibility). The term "drug hypersensitivity" refers to the symptoms or signs initiated by an exposure to a drug at a dose normally tolerated by nonhypersensitive persons. "Drug allergy" refers to immunologically mediated drug hypersensitivity reactions, which may be either Immunoglobulin E (IgE)–mediated (immediate) or non–IgE-mediated (delayed). "Nonallergic hypersensitivity reactions" refer to adverse drug reactions that are not mediated by immunologic mechanisms.[1]

Nonsteroidal anti-inflammatory drugs (NSAIDs) are a group of substances of variable chemical composition that antagonize inflammation by interfering with the function of cyclooxygenases (COXs). COXs are enzymes that participate in the conversion of arachidonic acid (AA) into prostaglandins (PGs) and thromboxanes, which are strong mediators of the inflammatory process. This inhibition results in the shunting of AA metabolism toward the 5-lipoxygenase pathway, resulting in the increased release of cysteinyl leukotrienes (**Fig. 1**).

There are 2 isoforms of COXs: constitutive and inducible. COX-1 is the constitutive form present in all cells, whereas the inducible isoenzyme COX-2 is expressed

[a] Department of Allergy and Clinical Immunology, Centro Médico-Docente La Trinidad, Carretera La Trinidad-El Hatillo, Estado Miranda, Venezuela
[b] Department of Allergy and Clinical Immunology, Clínica El Avila, Sexta Transversal Urbanización, Altamira, Piso 8, Consultorio 803, Caracas 1060, Venezuela
* Department of Allergy and Clinical Immunology, Clínica El Avila, Sexta Transversal Urbanización, Altamira, Piso 8, Consultorio 803, Caracas 1060, Venezuela.
E-mail address: sanchezbmario@gmail.com

Med Clin N Am 94 (2010) 853–864
doi:10.1016/j.mcna.2010.03.005
0025-7125/10/$ – see front matter © 2010 Elsevier Inc. All rights reserved.

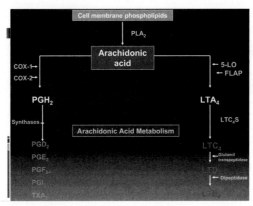

Fig. 1. Metabolic pathways of arachidonic acid. 5-LO, 5-lipoxygenase; FLAP, 5-LO activating protein; LTA$_4$, leukotriene A$_4$; LTC$_4$, leukotriene C$_4$; LTC$_4$S, leukotriene C$_4$ synthase; LTD$_4$, leukotriene D$_4$; LTE$_4$, leukotriene E$_4$; PGD$_2$, prostaglandin D$_2$; PGE$_2$, prostaglandin E$_2$; PGF$_{2\alpha}$, prostaglandin F$_{2\alpha}$; PGH$_2$, prostaglandin H$_2$; PGI$_2$, prostaglandin I$_2$; PLA$_2$, phospholipase A$_2$; TXA$_2$, thromboxane A$_2$.

exclusively in inflammatory cells after stimulation by cytokines, growth factors, bacterial lipopolysaccharide, tumor promoters, and other factors. While acetylsalicylic acid (ASA), also known as aspirin, and the classic NSAIDs inhibit both isoforms of COX, the new, selective COX-2 inhibitors are devoid of COX-1 inhibition and therefore have less ability to decrease gastric PG E$_2$ (PGE$_2$), producing less gastric irritation and ulceration (**Table 1**).

NSAIDs induce allergic and nonallergic hypersensitivity reactions. The second group of reactions is commonly described in medical literature as intolerant, pseudoallergic, or idiosyncratic reactions. In this article, the current knowledge on hypersensitivity reactions to NSAIDs is discussed.

HYPERSENSITIVITY REACTIONS TO NSAIDS

According to the temporal pattern of reactions, hypersensitivity to NSAIDs is classified as acute reactions occurring immediately or hours after exposure to the drug and delayed reactions, which manifest after more than 24 hours of administration of the drug.[2] Acute reactions are far more frequent and are the focus of this article. The

Table 1	
Classification of NSAIDs according to their selectivity for COX isoenzymes	
Selectivity	**Drugs**
Weak COX inhibitors	Acetaminophen, salsalate
Inhibitors of COX-1 or COX-2	Piroxicam, indomethacin, sulindac, tolmetin, ibuprofen, naproxen, fenoprofen, meclofenamate, mefenamic acid, diflunisal, ketoprofen, diclofenac, ketorolac, etodolac, nabumetone, oxaprozin, flurbiprofen
Preferential COX-2 inhibitors	Nimesulide, meloxicam
Selective COX-2 inhibitors	Celecoxib, rofecoxib, valdecoxib, etoricoxib, parecoxib, lumiracoxib

following 2 groups of patients with underlying disease and 2 groups of patients without obvious underlying disease are included:

1. NSAID-exacerbated respiratory disease, presently designated as aspirin-exacerbated respiratory disease (AERD).
2. NSAID-exacerbated cutaneous disease, in particular, urticaria and angioedema in patients with chronic idiopathic urticaria (CIU). In analogy to AERD, it could be called NSAID- or aspirin-exacerbated cutaneous disease (AECD).
3. Multiple NSAID–triggered urticaria, angioedema, and anaphylaxis in patients without other underlying disease.
4. Urticaria, angioedema, and anaphylaxis induced by a single NSAID.

Respiratory Reactions: AERD

Definition
AERD was previously known as ASA triad, asthma triad, Fernand Widal syndrome, Samter syndrome, and aspirin-intolerant asthma. More recently, a denomination of AERD has been proposed to emphasize that the condition evolves independently of administration of aspirin or NSAID, although these drugs will provoke asthmatic attacks in affected individuals.

Prevalence
AERD has been estimated to be prevalent in the range of 4.3% to 11% in adult asthmatics and in about 25% of patients who have asthma and nasal polyposis. One study reported a prevalence between 11% and 20% determined through a questionnaire, 3% through a medical record, and 21% through an oral provocation test.[3] AERD has similar effects on women and men.

Clinical picture
The classic ASA triad consists of chronic rhinosinusitis, nasal polyposis, persistent asthma, and aspirin or NSAID hypersensitivity. The triad of symptoms may develop stepwise over years, and occasionally only 2 of the 3 main symptoms are present. Intake of aspirin or any other NSAID causes, within a few minutes to approximately 120 minutes, symptoms such as a flush reaction in the face and upper thorax, rhinitis, conjunctivitis, feeling of blocked nose, and an often severe exacerbation of asthma with severe breathlessness, which may require emergency treatment. The underlying asthma is generally severe and steroid dependent, and it may be life threatening. The exacerbation due to NSAID intake is clearly dose dependent and probably also dependent on the potency of the COX inhibition of the particular NSAID. The threshold for aspirin doses for asthma exacerbations ranges between 3 and 100 mg and rarely more than 100 to 600 mg. In consequence, such patients may also react to an aspirin dosage given for cardioprotective purposes (100 mg/d).

Pathogenesis
The COX hypothesis proposed by Szczeklik[4] states that inhibition of COX-1, resulting in increased production of leukotrienes and decreased synthesis of PGE_2 (a modulator of mast cell mediator release), is responsible for airway inflammation, rhinosinusitis, and asthma observed in patients with AERD. Multiple observations support this theory, including increased urinary leukotriene (LT) E_4 (LTE_4) levels, and increased expression of the enzyme LT C_4 synthase (LTC_4S) and LT receptors in this patient population.[5,6]

A genetic predisposition for the development of AERD has been proposed, and various genes seem to be involved, including some HLA alleles, single nucleotide polymorphisms in cysteinyl LT receptor 1 (CysLTR1) and CysLTR2 receptors, LTC_4S, thromboxane receptors (TBXA2R), high-affinity receptor for IgE (FcεRIb), T-box transcription factor TBX21, PGE receptor (EP2 type), and tumor necrosis factor α promoter.[7] However, none of these genes are strongly associated with AERD.

Diagnosis

The diagnostic approach for AERD is based on the clinical picture of chronic rhinosinusitis and moderate to severe asthma, with exacerbations occurring when NSAIDs are taken. Aspirin hypersensitivity is confirmed by single-blind oral provocation, which is commonly used in the United States.[8] The test should be performed when asthma is stable (forced expiratory volume in the first second of expiration [FEV_1]>70%, with diurnal variability <10%). In Europe, inhalation or nasal challenges with lysine-aspirin are used.[9] All these tests bear the risk of severe asthma exacerbations, and should be done only by trained specialists with easily available equipment and medication for the treatment of acute asthma attacks if they develop.

In vitro assays measuring sulfidoleukotriene release, such as basophil activation tests and the 15-hydroxyeicosatetraenoic acid generation assay (Aspirin Sensitive Patient Identification Test), are still under study and need further validation at this time.[6]

Multiple protocols for oral ASA provocation are used in different centers,[8–10] and some provocation tests are immediately followed by desensitization.[10] Examples are presented in **Tables 2** and **3**.

Management

Patients with AERD are advised to avoid all COX-1 inhibitors, including aspirin and the classic NSAIDs, to prevent serious asthma exacerbations. For the treatment of pain and inflammation, NSAIDs that do not inhibit (or weakly inhibit) COX-1, such as acetaminophen in doses less than 1000 mg, and COX-2 inhibitors are recommended. It is advisable to challenge these alternatives under supervision to exactly define the tolerated dose, because approximately 10% of patients with AERD also react to acetaminophen, at least in higher doses (>500–800 mg) It is also advisable to strictly instruct the affected patients to use only the controlled alternative drugs, if needed. A list of available and forbidden NSAIDs should be explained and given to the patients, as well as an emergency card (bracelet).

Aspirin desensitization is useful for patients who require continuous therapy, such as those with ischemic heart disease or chronic arthritis.[10] Persistent asthma and rhinosinusitis should be treated with the approaches given by international guidelines such as the Global Initiative for Asthma and European Position Paper on Rhinosinusitis and Nasal Polyps.[11,12]

Table 2
Protocols for oral challenge with aspirin in patients with AERD

Time	Day 1	Day 2	Day 3
7 AM	Placebo	ASA, 30 mg	ASA, 100–150 mg
10 AM	Placebo	ASA, 45–60 mg	ASA, 150–325 mg
1 PM	Placebo	ASA, 60–100 mg	ASA, 325–650 mg

Positive if FEV_1 decreases greater than or equal to 20% and/or a prominent naso-ocular reaction.
Data from Stevenson DD. Aspirin desensitization in patients with AERD. Clin Rev Allergy Immunol 2003;24:159–67. (Stevenson DD, Scripps Clinic and the Scripps Research Institute, La Jolla, CA).

Table 3 Protocols for oral challenge with aspirin in patients with AERD according to EAACI/GA²LEN guidelines	
Day 1	**Day 2**
Placebo	ASA, 27 mg
Placebo	ASA, 44 mg
Placebo	ASA, 117 mg
—	ASA, 312 mg

Doses administered every 1.5 to 2 hours.

Positive if FEV_1 decreases greater than or equal to 20% or symptoms (which are bronchial, in the upper airways, ocular, cutaneous, gastrointestinal) occur.

Abbreviations: EAACI, European Academy of Allergy and Clinical Immunology; GA²LEN, Global Allergy and Asthma European Network.

Data from Nizankowska-Mogilnicka E, Bochenek G, Mastalerz L, et al. EAACI/GA2LEN guideline: aspirin provocation tests for diagnosis of aspirin hypersensitivity. Allergy 2007;62(10):1111–8.

NSAID-Exacerbated Urticaria and Angioedema in Patients with Chronic Urticaria

Prevalence and clinical picture

Reactions to NSAIDs are responsible for 21% to 25% of all adverse reactions to drugs and occur in 0.5% to 1.9% of the general population. Exacerbations of a preexisting urticaria or angioedema after taking aspirin or classic NSAIDs are observed in up to one-third of patients with controlled chronic urticaria and up to two-thirds of patients with active CIU (**Fig. 2**).[13] Analogous to AERD, an NSAID-exacerbated cutaneous disease or AECD could be considered.

Pathogenesis

Mastalerz and colleagues[14] observed that patients with chronic urticaria and aspirin intolerance had increased basal urinary LTE_4 when compared with patients with

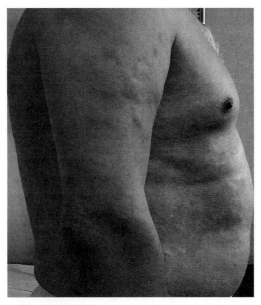

Fig. 2. CIU exacerbated by aspirin.

CIU tolerant to aspirin. Further increases of LTE_4 occurred in the first group but not in ASA-tolerant individuals when patients from both groups were challenged with aspirin. These results suggest that exacerbations of urticaria induced by aspirin in patients with CIU are mediated by inhibition of COX-1.

Asero[15] has recently observed the positive results from autologous serum skin tests and autologous plasma skin tests in more than 90% of patients with chronic urticaria and NSAID intolerance. This observation would suggest a possible association among CIU, autoimmunity, and aspirin hypersensitivity.

Diagnosis

In general, patients have a history of recurrent urticaria without a known precipitating factor, and they may provide, spontaneously or after questioning, information on the aggravation of cutaneous symptoms when exposed to NSAIDs. Some patients may have had only a generalized pruritus with scarce urticarial wheals (eg, after pressure), but NSAID intake may have caused a generalization and aggravation of their urticaria and first manifestation of angioedema. Confirmation by oral challenge may be necessary in some patients (see later discussion on multiple NSAID–triggered urticaria).

Management

Patients with CIU who do not tolerate ASA or NSAIDs should avoid all inhibitors of COX-1. Alternative drugs such as acetaminophen (tolerated by about 89% of these patients) or COX-2 inhibitors may be used after single-blinded oral challenge.[16,17] Compared with patients with AERD, most patients exhibiting cutaneous symptoms caused by multiple NSAIDs need higher doses, for example, of aspirin (approximately 300 mg), to cause an exacerbation of their disease.

The treatment of chronic urticaria is done with nonsedating antihistamines alone or combined with other drugs, as recommended by recent guidelines.[18]

Multiple NSAID–Triggered Urticaria, Angioedema, and Anaphylaxis in Patients Without Other Underlying Disease

Definition and prevalence

In the cases of patients who do not have chronic urticaria and experience urticaria and/or angioedema after treatment with COX-1 inhibitors of various chemical groups, the drugs more frequently involved depend on the prescription pattern predominant in the area. A heteroaryl group of NSAIDs (such as naproxen, diclofenac, ibuprofen) has been more often incriminated.[19,20]

Although no history of underlying disease is obtained, the authors have observed that these reactions occur more often in atopic individuals with rhinitis and/or asthma.[21] ASA and NSAIDs are the 2 major causes of anaphylaxis.[22–24] Cutaneous reactions to COX-2 inhibitors in hospitalized patients are observed in 0.008% of treated subjects,[25] about 50% less frequently than reactions to classic NSAIDs (with a relative risk 0.96 vs 1.77).[26]

Pathogenesis

The mechanisms of multiple NSAID reactions in this patient subpopulation are not known. The observation that urticaria and angioedema are provoked by drugs that share a common pharmacologic mechanism of action would suggest that COX-1 inhibition is involved. On the other hand, it is puzzling that some patients seem to tolerate certain NSAIDs (eg, ibuprofen), but react to others (eg, aspirin, diclofenac, and naproxen).

Clinical picture

Facial angioedema is the most common clinical manifestation (**Fig. 3**).[27] Up to 37% of patients may develop chronic urticaria in the future.[28] Some patients with multiple NSAID hypersensitivity exhibit an increased risk for developing oral mite anaphylaxis (pancake syndrome).[29]

Diagnosis

The medical history discloses the presence of episodes of urticaria or angioedema occurring after exposure to various COX-1 inhibitors of unrelated chemical groups. If necessary, confirmation by means of single-blind oral provocation as depicted in **Table 4** is performed.

Management

Patients are advised to avoid COX-1 inhibitors. Acetaminophen and COX-2 inhibitors are alternative drugs suitable for analgesia and treatment of pain and inflammation in this group of subjects (**Fig. 4**). At present, COX-2 inhibitors are not recommended for chronic use because of the increased risk of cardiovascular accidents, especially in people with a history of coronary or cerebrovascular disease.

Urticaria, Angioedema, and Anaphylaxis Induced by a Single NSAID

Definition and prevalence

Reactions to a single NSAID class are seen more often in patients treated with pyrazolones,[30,31] but they have been reported for many other NSAIDs (mainly diclofenac, and also rarely for others such as acetaminophen, aspirin, ibuprofen, ketorolac, indomethacin, sulindac, zomepirac, fenoprofen, meclofenamate, naproxen, piroxicam, tolmetin, and celecoxib).[32]

These reactions constitute about 30% of all cases of NSAID hypersensitivity, and about 30% of patients have concomitant chronic urticaria. An increased prevalence of atopy has been reported.[21]

Clinical picture

Any of the following clinical manifestations may be observed: urticaria, angioedema, laryngeal edema, systemic anaphylaxis, generalized itching, rhinitis, and bronchospasm.

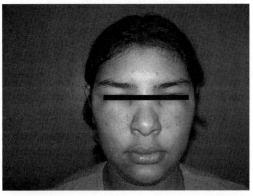

Fig. 3. Facial (periorbital) edema induced by ibuprofen in a 15-year-old female patient with multiple NSAID-triggered angioedema.

Table 4			
Oral provocation with aspirin for patients with urticaria and angioedema			
Day 1	**Day 2**	**Day 3**	**Day 4**
Placebo	ASA, 100 mg	ASA, 325 mg	ASA, 650 mg
Placebo	ASA, 200 mg		

On days 1 and 2, doses given every 2 hours.
   Skin scores recorded every 2 hours.
   In patients with active chronic urticaria, rule of nines (as calculated in cases of patients having burns) may be used.
   In Europe, the recommended consecutive doses of ASA are 71 mg, 117 mg, 312 mg, and 500 mg.[9]

Pathogenesis
In some patients at least, an allergic sensitization mediated by drug-specific IgE to a certain NSAID is likely. Specific IgE can be demonstrated by means of prick or intradermal skin tests or in vitro by immunoassays,[33] which have been well documented for patients with hypersensitivity to pyrazolones and may also play a role in other reactions, although this is less well documented.[34]

Diagnosis
In patients with a history of reaction to a single NSAID and no additional exposure to a second NSAID, skin testing is possible and may reveal a selective sensitization. IgE tests are not commercially available. It may be convenient to confirm the diagnosis by oral challenge, although this should be done cautiously because low concentrations of

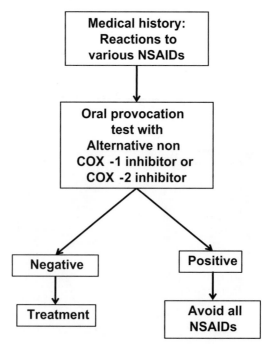

Fig. 4. Algorithm for the management of patients with urticaria and angioedema triggered by multiple NSAIDs.

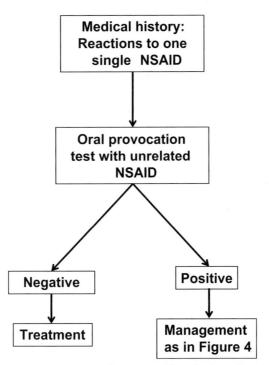

Fig. 5. Algorithm for the management of patients with urticaria and angioedema triggered by a single NSAID.

the drug may already cause symptoms. If the results are positive, another NSAID of a different chemical group should be tested to demonstrate single reactivity (**Fig. 5**). A history of systemic anaphylaxis would be a contraindication to perform the provocation tests with the incriminated substance.

Table 5
Chemical classification of NSAIDs

Group	Drugs
Salicylic acid derivatives	Aspirin, sodium salicylate, choline magnesium trisalicylate, salsalate, diflunisal, salicylsalicylic acid, sulfasalazine, olsalazine
Para-aminophenol derivatives	Acetaminophen
Indole and indene acetic acids	Indomethacin, sulindac, etodolac
Heteroaryl acetic acid	Tolmetin, diclofenac, ketorolac
Arylpropionic acid	Ibuprofen, naproxen, flurbiprofen, ketoprofen, fenoprofen, oxaprozin
Anthranilic acid (fenamates)	Mefenamic acid, meclofenamic acid
Enolic acid	Oxicams (piroxicam, tenoxicam), pyrazoledinediones (phenylbutazone, oxyphentathrazone)
Alkanones	Nabumetone
Pyrazolic derivatives	Antipyrine, aminopyrine, dipyrone

Management

Once the diagnosis of single drug reaction is confirmed, avoidance of the drug and other chemically similar NSAIDs should be advised. These patients can be treated with other non–cross-reacting NSAIDs (**Table 5**).

SUMMARY

Reactions to NSAIDs are a major cause of hypersensitivity to drugs, occupying second place after reactions to antibiotics. The most common acute clinical manifestations involve the respiratory tract (rhinosinusitis and asthma), the skin (urticaria and angioedema), or are generalized (anaphylaxis). The affected patients often already have an underlying respiratory or cutaneous disease, and the intake of various NSAIDs can precipitate more severe symptoms. Early diagnosis and treatment, proper medical advice on drug use, and referral to an allergy specialist when indicated are of paramount importance to prevent unnecessary morbidity and the potential risk of death from these severe reactions.

REFERENCES

1. Johansson S, Bieber T, Dahl R, et al. Revised nomenclature for allergy for global use: report of the Nomenclature Review Committee of the World Allergy Organization, October 2003. J Allergy Clin Immunol 2004;113(5):832–6.
2. Kowalski ML, Makowska JS, Bochenek G, et al. Hypersensitivity to non-steroidal anti-inflammatory drugs (NSAIDs). Classification, diagnosis and management. Review of the EAACI/ENDA and GA2LEN, in preparation.
3. Jenkins C, Costello J, Hodge L. Systematic review of prevalence of aspirin induced asthma and its implications for clinical practice. Br Med J 2004; 328(7437):434–40.
4. Szczeklik A. The cyclooxygenase theory of aspirin-induced asthma. Eur Respir J 1990;3(5):588–93.
5. Picado C. The role of cyclooxygenase in acetylsalicylic acid sensitivity. Allergy Clin Immunol Int 2006;18(4):154–7.
6. Kowalski ML, Makowska JS. Aspirin-exacerbated respiratory disease. An update on diagnosis and management. Allergy Clin Immunol Int 2006;18(4):140–9.
7. Kim SH, Park HS. Genetic markers for differentiating aspirin hypersensitivity. Yonsei Med J 2006;47(1):15–21.
8. Stevenson DD. Aspirin desensitization in patients with AERD. Clin Rev Allergy Immunol 2003;24:159–67.
9. Nizankowska-Mogilnicka E, Bochenek G, Mastalerz L, et al. EAACI/GA2LEN guideline: aspirin provocation tests for diagnosis of aspirin hypersensitivity. Allergy 2007;62(10):1111–8.
10. Hope AP, Woessner KA, Simon RA, et al. Rational approach to aspirin dosing during oral challenges and desensitization of patients with aspirin-exacerbated respiratory disease. J Allergy Clin Immunol 2009;123(2):406–10.
11. Global Initiative for Asthma. Revision: GINA report, global strategy for asthma management and prevention. Global Strategy for Asthma Management and Prevention 2006. Available at: http://www.ginasthma.org/GuidelineItem.asp?intId=1388. Accessed October 29, 2009.
12. Thomas M, Yawn BP, Price D, et al. EPOS Primary Care Guidelines: European position paper on the primary care diagnosis and management of rhinosinusitis and nasal polyps 2007—a summary. Prim Care Respir J 2008;17(2):79–89.

13. Doeglas HM. Reactions to aspirin and food additives in patients with chronic urticaria, including the physical urticarias. Br J Dermatol 1975;93(2):135–44.
14. Mastalerz L, Setkowicz M, Sanak M, et al. Hypersensitivity to aspirin: common
eicosanoid alterations in urticaria and asthma. J Allergy Clin Immunol 2004;
113(4):771–5.
15. Asero R. Predictive value of autologous plasma skin test for multiple nonsteroidal
anti-inflammatory drug intolerance. Int Arch Allergy Immunol 2007;144(3):
226–30.
16. Sánchez-Borges M, Capriles-Hulett A, Caballero-Fonseca F, et al. Tolerability to
new COX-2 inhibitors in NSAID-sensitive patients with cutaneous reactions.
Ann Allergy 2001;87(3):201–4.
17. Asero R. Tolerability of rofecoxib. Allergy 2001;56(9):916–7.
18. Zuberbier T, Asero R, Bindslev-Jensen C, et al. Position paper. EAACI/GA²LEN/
EDF/WAO guideline: management of urticaria. Allergy 2009;64(10):1427–43.
19. Van Puijenbroek EP, Egberts AC, Meyboom RH, et al. Different risks for NSAID-
induced anaphylaxis. Ann Pharmacother 2002;36(1):24–9.
20. Quiralte J, Blanco C, Delgado J, et al. Challenge-based clinical patterns of 223
Spanish patients with nonsteroidal anti-inflammatory-drug-induced reactions.
J Investig Allergol Clin Immunol 2007;17(3):182–8.
21. Sánchez-Borges M, Capriles-Hulett A. Atopy is a risk factor for nonsteroidal anti-
inflammatory drug sensitivity. Ann Allergy Asthma Immunol 2000;84(1):101–6.
22. Kemp SF, Lockey RF, Wolf BL, et al. Anaphylaxis. A review of 266 cases. Arch
Intern Med 1995;155(16):1749–54.
23. Mullins RJ. Anaphylaxis: risk factors for recurrence. Clin Exp Allergy 2003;33(8):
1033–40.
24. Cianferoni A, Novembre E, Mugnaini L, et al. Clinical features of acute anaphylaxis in patients admitted to a university hospital: an 11-year retrospective review
(1985–1996). Ann Allergy Asthma Immunol 2001;87(1):27–32.
25. Layton D, Marshall V, Boshier A, et al. Serious skin reactions and selective COX-2
inhibitors: a case series from prescription-event monitoring in England. Drug Saf
2006;29(8):687–96.
26. Downing A, Jacobsen J, Sorensen HT, et al. Risk of hospitalization for angio-oedema among users of newer COX-2 selective inhibitors and other
nonsteroidal anti-inflammatory drugs. Br J Clin Pharmacol 2006;62(4):
496–501.
27. Quiralte J, Blanco C, Castillo R, et al. Intolerance to nonsteroidal antiinflammatory
drugs: results of controlled drug challenges in 98 patients. J Allergy Clin Immunol
1996;98(3):678–85.
28. Asero R. Intolerance to nonsteroidal anti-inflammatory drugs might precede
by years the onset of chronic urticaria. J Allergy Clin Immunol 2003;111(5):
1095–8.
29. Sánchez-Borges M, Suárez-Chacón R, Capriles-Hulett A, et al. Pancake
syndrome (oral mite anaphylaxis). World Allergy Organiz J 2009;2(5):91–6.
30. van der Klauw MM, Wilson JH, Stricker BH. Drug-associated anaphylaxis: 20
years of reporting in The Netherlands (1974-1994) and review of the literature.
Clin Exp Allergy 1996;26(12):1355–63.
31. Asero R. Oral aspirin challenges in patients with a history of intolerance to
single non-steroidal anti-inflammatory drugs. Clin Exp Allergy 2005;35(6):
713–6.
32. Sánchez-Borges M. Clinical management of nonsteroidal anti-inflammatory drug
hypersensitivity. World Allergy Organiz J 2008;1(2):29–33.

33. Kowalski ML, Bienkiewicz B, Woszczek G, et al. Diagnosis of pyrazolone drug sensitivity: clinical history versus skin testing and in vitro testing. Allergy Asthma Proc 1999;20(6):347–52.
34. Himly M, Jahn-Schmid B, Pitterschatscher K, et al. IgE-mediated immediate-type hypersensitivity to the pyrazolone drug propyphenazone. J Allergy Clin Immunol 2003;111(4):882–8.

Index

Note: Page numbers of article titles are in **boldface** type.

Med Clin N Am 94 (2010) 865–879
doi:10.1016/S0025-7125(10)00085-4
0025-7125/10/$ – see front matter © 2010 Elsevier Inc. All rights reserved.

medical.theclinics.com

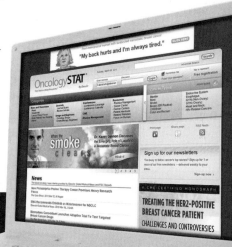

Moving?

Make sure your subscription moves with you!

To notify us of your new address, find your **Clinics Account Number** (located on your mailing label above your name), and contact customer service at:

Email: journalscustomerservice-usa@elsevier.com

800-654-2452 (subscribers in the U.S. & Canada)
314-447-8871 (subscribers outside of the U.S. & Canada)

Fax number: 314-447-8029

Elsevier Health Sciences Division
Subscription Customer Service
3251 Riverport Lane
Maryland Heights, MO 63043

*To ensure uninterrupted delivery of your subscription, please notify us at least 4 weeks in advance of move.